Oral Health in Children

Editors

MAX J. COPPES
SUSAN A. FISHER-OWENS

PEDIATRIC CLINICS
OF NORTH AMERICA

www.pediatric.theclinics.com

Consulting Editor
BONITA F. STANTON

DISCARD

October 2018 • Volume 65 • Number 5

ELSEVIER

1600 John F. Kennedy Boulevard • Suite 1800 • Philadelphia, Pennsylvania, 19103-2899

http://www.theclinics.com

THE PEDIATRIC CLINICS OF NORTH AMERICA Volume 65, Number 5
October 2018 ISSN 0031-3955, ISBN-13: 978-0-323-64223-1

Editor: Kerry Holland
Developmental Editor: Casey Potter

The Pediatric Clinics of North America (ISSN 0031-3955) is published bimonthly by Elsevier Inc., 360 Park Avenue South, New York, NY 10010-1710. Months of issue are February, April, June, August, October, and December. Periodicals postage paid at New York, NY and additional mailing offices. Subscription prices are $216.00 per year (US individuals), $613.00 per year (US institutions), $292.00 per year (Canadian individuals), $816.00 per year (Canadian institutions), $338.00 per year (international individuals), $816.00 per year (international institutions), $100.00 per year (US students and residents), and $165.00 per year (international and Canadian residents and students). To receive students/resident rare, orders must be accompanied by name of affiliated institution, date of term, and the signature of program/residency coordinator on institution letterhead. Orders will be billed at individual rate until proof of status is received. Foreign air speed delivery is included in all *Clinics* subscription prices. All prices are subject to change without notice. **POSTMASTER:** Send address changes to *The Pediatric Clinics of North America*, Elsevier Health Sciences Division, Subscription Customer Service, 3251 Riverport Lane, Maryland Heights, MO 63043. **Customer Service: 1-800-654-2452 (US and Canada). From outside of the US and Canada: 1-314-447-8871. Fax: 1-314-447-8029. For print support, E-mail: JournalsCustomerService-usa@elsevier.com. For online support, E-mail: JournalsOnlineSupport-usa@elsevier.com.**

Reprints. For copies of 100 or more, of articles in this publication, please contact the Commercial Reprints Department, Elsevier Inc., 360 Park Avenue South, New York, NY 10010-1710. Tel.: 212-633-3874; Fax: 212-633-3820; E-mail: reprints@elsevier.com.

The Pediatric Clinics of North America is also published in Spanish by McGraw-Hill Inter-americana Editores S.A., Mexico City, Mexico; in Portuguese by Riechmann and Affonso Editores, Rua Comandante Coelho 1085, CEP 21250, Rio de Janeiro, Brazil; and in Greek by Althayia SA, Athens, Greece.

The Pediatric Clinics of North America is covered in *MEDLINE/PubMed (Index Medicus), Excerpta Medica, Current Contents, Current Contents/Clinical Medicine, Science Citation Index, ASCA, ISI/BIOMED,* and *BIOSIS.*

Printed in the United States of America.

PROGRAM OBJECTIVE
The goal of the *Pediatric Clinics of North America* is to keep practicing physicians and residents up to date with current clinical practice in pediatrics by providing timely articles reviewing the state-of-the-art in patient care.

TARGET AUDIENCE
All practicing pediatricians, physicians and healthcare professionals who provide patient care to pediatric patients.

LEARNING OBJECTIVES
Upon completion of this activity, participants will be able to:
1. Review early childhood caries as well as the management of dental caries in older children
2. Discuss prevention of oral disease and tooth decay
3. Recognize oral health disparities in and special health care needs for children

ACCREDITATION
The Elsevier Office of Continuing Medical Education (EOCME) is accredited by the Accreditation Council for Continuing Medical Education (ACCME) to provide continuing medical education for physicians.

The EOCME designates this enduring material for a maximum of 15 *AMA PRA Category 1 Credit*(s)™. Physicians should claim only the credit commensurate with the extent of their participation in the activity.

All other healthcare professionals requesting continuing education credit for this enduring material will be issued a certificate of participation.

DISCLOSURE OF CONFLICTS OF INTEREST
The EOCME assesses conflict of interest with its instructors, faculty, planners, and other individuals who are in a position to control the content of CME activities. All relevant conflicts of interest that are identified are thoroughly vetted by EOCME for fair balance, scientific objectivity, and patient care recommendations. EOCME is committed to providing its learners with CME activities that promote improvements or quality in healthcare and not a specific proprietary business or a commercial interest.

The planning committee, staff, authors and editors listed below have identified no financial relationships or relationships to products or devices they or their spouse/life partner have with commercial interest related to the content of this CME activity:
Lucas Guimarães Abreu, PhD, MSc, DDS; Jun Aida, PhD; Tahyna Duda Deps Almeida, DDS, MSc; Marcelo Bönecker, PhD; Lauren Boyle; Erica A. Brecher, DMD, MS; Hillary L. Broder, PhD; Paul S. Casamassimo, DDS, MS; Geneviève Castonguay, BSc, PhD; Donald L. Chi, DDS, Phd; Burton L. Edelstein, DDS, MPH; Susan A. Fisher-Owens, MD, MPH, FAAP; Stuart A. Gansky, DrPH; Kimberly Hammersmith, DDS, MPH, FAAP, MS; Alison Kemp; Ashok Kumar, DDS, MS; Charlotte W. Lewis, MD, MPH; Sreenath Madathil, BDS, MSc; Manu Raj Mathur, PhD; Rajkumar Mayakrishnan; Elizabeth Mertz, PhD; Sean Mutchnick, MD; Belinda Nicolau, DDS, MSc, PhD; Bhavna T. Pahel, DDS, MPH, PhD; Howard Pollick, BDS, MPH; Rocio B. Quinonez, DMD, MS, MPH; Anne Rowan-Legg, MD, FRCPC; Wan Kim Seow, BDS, MDSc, PhD, DDSc; Anthony Sheyn, MD; Peter F. Svider, MD; William Murray Thomson, PhD; Renato Venturelli, MSc; Thien Vuong; Richard G. Watt, PhD; John Timothy Wright, DDS, MS; Brian Yuhan, BS.

The planning committee, staff, authors and editors listed below have identified financial relationships or relationships to products or devices they or their spouse/life partner have with commercial interest related to the content of this CME activity:
Max J. Coppes, MD, PhD, MBA, FAAP: is a consultant/advisor for LEO Pharma Inc., Centene Corporation, I-ACT for Children, and WebMD LLC.
Catherine M. Flaitz, DDS, MS: receives research support from GC America, Inc.
Shilpa Sangvai, MD, MPH: owns stock in Procter & Gamble.

UNAPPROVED/OFF-LABEL USE DISCLOSURE
The EOCME requires CME faculty to disclose to the participants:
1. When products or procedures being discussed are off-label, unlabelled, experimental, and/or investigational (not US Food and Drug Administration [FDA] approved); and
2. Any limitations on the information presented, such as data that are preliminary or that represent ongoing research, interim analyses, and/or unsupported opinions. Faculty may discuss information about pharmaceutical agents that is outside of FDA-approved labelling. This information is intended solely for CME

and is not intended to promote off-label use of these medications. If you have any questions, contact the medical affairs department of the manufacturer for the most recent prescribing information.

TO ENROLL

To enroll in the *Pediatric Clinics of North America* Continuing Medical Education program, call customer service at 1-800-654-2452 or sign up online at http://www.theclinics.com/home/cme. The CME program is available to subscribers for an additional annual fee of USD 301.60.

METHOD OF PARTICIPATION

In order to claim credit, participants must complete the following:
1. Complete enrolment as indicated above.
2. Read the activity.
3. Complete the CME Test and Evaluation. Participants must achieve a score of 70% on the test. All CME Tests and Evaluations must be completed online.

CME INQUIRIES/SPECIAL NEEDS

For all CME inquiries or special needs, please contact elsevierCME@elsevier.com.

Contributors

CONSULTING EDITOR

BONITA F. STANTON, MD
Founding Dean, Hackensack Meridian School of Medicine at Seton Hall University, President, Academic Enterprise, Hackensack Meridian Health Robert C. and Laura C. Garrett Endowed Chair for the School of Medicine, Dean Professor of Pediatrics, Nutley, New Jersey, USA

EDITORS

MAX J. COPPES, MD, PhD, MBA, FAAP
Professor and Nell J. Redfield Chair of Pediatrics, University of Nevada Reno, School of Medicine, Physician-in-Chief, Renown Children's Hospital, Reno, Nevada, USA

SUSAN A. FISHER-OWENS, MD, MPH, FAAP
Clinical Professor of Pediatrics, UCSF School of Medicine, Clinical Professor of Preventive and Restorative Dentistry, UCSF School of Dentistry, San Francisco, California, USA

AUTHORS

LUCAS GUIMARÃES ABREU, PhD, MSc, DDS
Professor, Department of Pediatric Dentistry and Orthodontics, School of Dentistry, Universidade Federal de Minas Gerais, Belo Horizonte, Minas Gerais, Brazil

JUN AIDA, PhD
Professor, Department of International Health, Graduate School of Dentistry, Tohoku University, Sendai, Miyagi, Japan

TAHYNA DUDA DEPS ALMEIDA, DDS, MSc
Faculty of Dentistry, McGill University, Montreal, Quebec, Canada; Faculty of Dentistry, Federal University of Minas Gerais, Belo Horizonte, Minas Gerais, Brazil

MARCELO BÖNECKER, PhD
Professor, Chairman, Faculdade de Odontologia, Sao Paulo, Brazil

ERICA A. BRECHER, DMD, MS
Assistant Professor, Department of Pediatric Dentistry, School of Dentistry, Virginia Commonwealth University, Richmond, Virginia, USA

HILLARY L. BRODER, PhD
Professor, Cariology and Comprehensive Care, NYU College of Dentistry, New York University, New York, New York, USA

PAUL S. CASAMASSIMO, DDS, MS
Professor Emeritus, The Ohio State University College of Dentistry, Nationwide Children's Hospital, Columbus, Ohio, USA

GENEVIÈVE CASTONGUAY, BSc, PhD
Faculty of Dentistry, McGill University, Montreal, Quebec, Canada

DONALD L. CHI, DDS, PhD
Associate Professor, Department of Oral Health Sciences, University of Washington, School of Dentistry, Seattle, Washington, USA

BURTON L. EDELSTEIN, DDS, MPH
Chair, Population Oral Health, Columbia University College of Dental Medicine, Professor of Dental Medicine and Health Policy and Management, Columbia University Medical Center, New York, New York, USA; Founding Chair Emeritus and Senior Fellow in Public Policy, Children's Dental Health Project, Washington, DC, USA

SUSAN A. FISHER-OWENS, MD, MPH, FAAP
Clinical Professor of Pediatrics, UCSF School of Medicine, Clinical Professor of Preventive and Restorative Dentistry, UCSF School of Dentistry, San Francisco, California, USA

CATHERINE M. FLAITZ, DDS, MS
Professor, The Ohio State University College of Dentistry, Nationwide Children's Hospital, Columbus, Ohio, USA

STUART A. GANSKY, DrPH
Professor, Lee Hysan Chair of Oral Epidemiology, Division of Oral Epidemiology and Dental Public Health, Director, Center to Address Disparities in Children's Oral Health (Known as CAN DO), Philip R. Lee Institute for Health Policy Studies, University of California, San Francisco, San Francisco, California, USA

KIMBERLY HAMMERSMITH, DDS, MPH, MS
Assistant Clinical Professor, The Ohio State University College of Dentistry, Nationwide Children's Hospital, Columbus, Ohio, USA

ASHOK KUMAR, DDS, MS
Associate Clinical Professor, The Ohio State University College of Dentistry, Nationwide Children's Hospital, Columbus, Ohio, USA

CHARLOTTE W. LEWIS, MD, MPH
Associate Professor, Department of Pediatrics, UW School of Medicine, Attending Physician, Seattle Children's Hospital, Seattle, Washington, USA

SREENATH MADATHIL, BDS, MSc
Faculty of Dentistry, McGill University, Montreal, Quebec, Canada

MANU RAJ MATHUR, PhD
Senior Research Scientist and Associate Professor, Department of Dental Public Health, Public Health Foundation of India, Gurgaon, Haryana, India

ELIZABETH MERTZ, PhD
Associate Professor of Preventive and Restorative Dentistry, UCSF School of Dentistry, Associate Professor of Social and Behavioral Sciences, UCSF School of Nursing, San Francisco, California, USA

SEAN MUTCHNICK, MD
Department of Otolaryngology–Head and Neck Surgery, Wayne State University School of Medicine, Detroit, Michigan, USA

BELINDA NICOLAU, DDS, MSc, PhD
Faculty of Dentistry, McGill University, Montreal, Quebec, Canada

BHAVNA T. PAHEL, DDS, MPH, PhD
Adjunct Assistant Professor, Department of Pediatric Dentistry, UNC School of Dentistry, The University of North Carolina at Chapel Hill, Chapel Hill, North Carolina, USA; Private Practice, Village Family Dental, Greensboro, North Carolina, USA

HOWARD POLLICK, BDS, MPH
Director, Dental Public Health Residency Program, Division of Oral Epidemiology and Dental Public Health, Health Sciences Clinical Professor, Department of Preventive and Restorative Dental Sciences, School of Dentistry, University of California, San Francisco, San Francisco, California, USA

ROCIO B. QUINONEZ, DMD, MS, MPH
Professor, Departments of Pediatric Dentistry and Academic Affairs, School of Dentistry, The University of North Carolina at Chapel Hill, Chapel Hill, North Carolina, USA

ANNE ROWAN-LEGG, MD, FRCPC
Assistant Professor, Department of Pediatrics, University of Ottawa, Consultant Pediatrician, Division of Pediatric Medicine, Children's Hospital of Eastern Ontario, Ottawa, Ontario, Canada

SHILPA SANGVAI, MD, MPH
Assistant Clinical Professor, The Ohio State University College of Medicine, Nationwide Children's Hospital, Columbus, Ohio, USA

WAN KIM SEOW, BDS, MDSc, PhD, DDSc
Emeritus Professor, School of Dentistry, The University of Queensland, Herston, Queensland, Australia

ANTHONY SHEYN, MD
Department of Otolaryngology, The University of Tennessee Health Science Center, Department of Pediatric Otolaryngology, LeBonheur Children's Hospital, St. Jude Children's Research Hospital, Memphis, Tennessee, USA

PETER F. SVIDER, MD
Department of Otolaryngology–Head and Neck Surgery, Wayne State University School of Medicine, Detroit, Michigan, USA

WILLIAM MURRAY THOMSON, PhD
Professor of Dental Epidemiology and Public Health, Faculty of Dentistry, The University of Otago, Dunedin, New Zealand

RENATO VENTURELLI, MSc
Research Associate, Epidemiology and Public Health, University College London, London, United Kingdom

THIEN VUONG
Faculty of Dentistry, McGill University, Montreal, Quebec, Canada

RICHARD G. WATT, PhD
Professor of Dental Public Health, Epidemiology and Public Health, University College London, London, United Kingdom

JOHN TIMOTHY WRIGHT, DDS, MS
James Bawden Distinguished Professor, Department of Pediatric Dentistry, School of
Dentistry, The University of North Carolina at Chapel Hill, Chapel Hill, North Carolina, USA

BRIAN T. YUHAN, BS
Department of Otolaryngology–Head and Neck Surgery, Wayne State University School
of Medicine, Detroit, Michigan, USA

Contents

> Orofacial growth and development is a complex process spanning the life course. This article provides an oral health overview in the context of overall growth and physical and social development from infancy through adolescence. It reviews oral health–specific developmental milestones during childhood (0–12 years) and adolescence (≥13 years). It examines issues particular to each age category or spanning multiple ages (eg, pediatric overweight and obesity, tobacco use, and dental trauma) in relation to oral health and development. In addition, the oral microbiome and its potential role in informing personalized oral health care across the life course is discussed.

> It may be easy to discount oral health in infancy because most infants are not born with teeth and only a few teeth erupt during the first year of life. Infancy, however, is a critical time for formation of habits. Positive habits, such as twice-daily brushing with fluoride toothpaste starting at first teeth eruption, provides topical fluoride, which is important for remineralization of the tooth and helps establish a lifelong healthy practice. Negative habits, such as bottle propping and frequent juice consumption, reinforce behaviors that promote caries and obesity. This article reviews normal dental development and eruption. Congenital anomalies affecting the mouth as well as acquired conditions, primarily dental caries, are reviewed. Oral health preventive modalities, including professionally applied products and home-based strategies, are discussed.

> Although there are recommendations to prevent tooth decay by other means, this nonsystematic review finds that fluoride is the key to prevention and control of tooth decay. There are multiple fluoride modalities with effectiveness and safety of fluoride depending on dose and concentration. Prevention of tooth decay occurs at the individual level by fluoride use at home and with professional application and at the community level through fluoridation of water or salt.

Orthodontics is the dental specialty concerned with the position of teeth
and the relationship between the maxilla and mandible. Much evidence
regarding the characteristics of normal occlusion during childhood/
adolescence, the timely referral of children/adolescents to orthodontic
treatment, and the impact of orthodontic outcomes on individuals' physical, functioning, and psychosocial well-being exists in the literature. This
body of evidence may be helpful for pediatricians and primary care physicians. For those willing to be skilled providers of health care to children/ad-
olescents, knowledge of basic concepts of oral health may contribute to
the communication among physicians, the young individual, and the par-
ents/caregivers.

Oral health is integral to general health. The oral cavity may harbor manifestations of systemic disease and can be the harbinger of early onset. Primary care providers (PCPs) can therefore use the oral cavity to support
working diagnoses. Conversely, systemic diseases and treatments can
affect oral health and require interactions between PCPs and dental providers. Acute oral manifestations of systemic disease may involve teeth
and/or gums. This article reviews oral and systemic disease connections
for some diseases, identifies issues that benefit patients through
medical-dental collaboration, and highlights some nondental oral injuries
that might confront PCPs or emergency medical providers.

Oral lesions in children encompass a wide range of causes, including idio-
pathic entities as well as those related to an underlying systemic illness. In
addition, oral masses include benign entities harboring locally destructive
behavior and even malignancies in rare cases. Thorough patient history
and detailed and efficient physical examination are critical for determining
which lesions can be closely observed versus those that require further
diagnostic workup. Understanding normal oral cavity anatomy is crucial
for performing appropriate evaluation. This article describes the appropriate diagnostic and therapeutic strategies for oral cavity lesions and reviews the broad differential diagnosis of oral cavity masses.

This article provides an overview of periodontal diseases and traumatic
dental injuries (TDIs) in children and adolescents, which are serious public

health problems worldwide. Periodontal diseases, including gingivitis and periodontitis, commonly affect the oral soft tissues and teeth and often co-occur with other chronic diseases. TDIs are prevalent from an early age and carry high treatment costs. Behavioral and environmental factors contribute to both TDIs and periodontal diseases, but the cause varies according to population characteristics and case definition. Both conditions may lead to pain, function impairment, esthetic problems, and psychosocial effects, with major consequences on quality of life.

Oral health disease in young children has not decreased, despite adequate modalities for treatment and prevention. Because many children may not see a dentist before oral disease has begun, disease progression can be expected, affecting short-term and long-term oral health. However, most children are seen by other health professionals frequently in their youngest years, providing a unique opportunity to help weave a safety net of oral health care until they are established in a dental home. This article details ways primary care providers can promote oral health, including ways to integrate ancillary dental professionals into the primary care home.

This article describes child oral–health–related quality of life measures and provides some examples of their use in determining the effect of clinical interventions, such as dental treatment under general anesthesia, orthodontic treatment, and treatment of orofacial clefting.

Over recent years, pediatric oral health has become well established in the United States as an essential component of pediatric health policy as evidenced by the programs authorized and funded by Congress. These actions have improved access and utilization of dental care, engaged primary care pediatrics in oral health, and improved children's oral health outcomes. Nonetheless, there remains a host of authorized but unfunded approaches to addressing children's oral health through coverage, workforce, safety net, prevention, and surveillance. Child health advocates and practitioners need to actively engage as advocates if further improvements are to be attained through policymaking.

PEDIATRIC CLINICS OF NORTH AMERICA

THE CLINICS ARE AVAILABLE ONLINE!
Access your subscription at:
www.theclinics.com

PEDIATRIC CLINICS OF
NORTH AMERICA

Foreword

Teeth: Vital to Our Children's Health

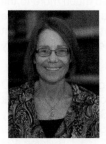

Bonita F. Stanton, MD
Consulting Editor

Not even considered an organ system in its own right (it is part of the digestive system), our primary teeth are now well recognized to be essential contributors to a child's and an adult's health and well-being.

Receiving their just recognition was a long time in coming for our teeth. The first known publication devoted solely to teeth did not appear until the 1500s: *Little Medicinal Book for All Kinds of Diseases and Infirmities of the Teeth* (by Artzney Buchlein, a German). About two centuries later in the 1700s, a French surgeon, Pierre Fauchard, wrote the first known "textbook" about teeth, entitled *The Surgeon Dentist, A Treatise on Teeth*, the first comprehensive guide to dental care ever written.[1]

While the medical profession's understanding of the role of teeth advanced considerably over the ensuing three centuries, confusion regarding the importance of the primary teeth continued to be prevalent. It was not until the last two to four decades that we have come to understand not only the critical role of teeth to health and well-being in general, but also specifically that of the primary teeth. We now know that early childhood caries has significant negative implications for health and well-being not only during childhood but also on into adulthood.[2]

Notwithstanding this now generally accepted awareness of the importance of primary and permanent dentition, oral health remains the largest unmet pediatric health care need in the United States. With nearly half of the children under age 11 having had dental caries, this is arguably the most common chronic childhood disorder in the United States.[3] An abundance of evidence suggests that despite the recommendation from the American Academy of Pediatrics that children visit their dentist every 6 months beginning at age 1 year, this goal is not close to being achieved. Nonetheless, a review of changes in preventative care visitations of children (self-reported by their parents) from 2003 through 2012 found evidence of increasing rates of dental care visits in 45 states. Of concern, and perhaps not surprisingly, children without

Pediatr Clin N Am 65 (2018) xv–xvi
https://doi.org/10.1016/j.pcl.2018.07.002
0031-3955/18/© 2018 Published by Elsevier Inc.

health insurance experienced no reported increase. There were also substantial variations by state.[4]

This regional variation in oral health and health care delivery, both within and between states, has been documented by others. One recent study reported substantial state-to-state level variations in access to dental care and in rates of fair/poor dental care, with two-fold differences between states with the poorest access and care and those with the highest.[5]

Of course, as important as the teeth themselves are, there is so much more to the mouth than "just" the teeth! This issue provides updates on a wide range of the broader topic of oral health and current assessment, and preventative and treatment approaches. Practicing pediatricians and other child care providers will find it very informative and well written.

Bonita F. Stanton, MD
Hackensack Meridian School of Medicine at
Seton Hall University
340 South Orange Street
Building 123
Nutley, NJ 07110, USA

E-mail address:
bonita.stanton@shu.edu

REFERENCES

1. All Around Dental Care. A fun timeline of early dental hisotry. 2018. Available at: https://www.allarounddentalcare.com/blog/a-fun-timeline-of-early-dental-history/. Accessed July 26, 2018.
2. Finucane D. Rational for restoration of carious primary teeth: a review. Eur Arch Paediatr Dent 2012;13(6):281–92.
3. Edelstein BL, Chinn CH. Update on disparities in oral health and access to dental care for America's children. Acad Pediatr 2009;9(6):415–9.
4. Mandal M, Edelstein BL, Ma S, et al. Changes in children's oral health status and receipt of preventive dental visits, United States, 2003-2011/2012. Prev Chronic Dis 2013;10:E204.
5. Fisher-Owens SA, Soobader MJ, Gansky SA, et al. Geography matters: state-level variation in children's oral health care access and oral health status. Public Health 2016;134:54–63.

Preface

Oral Health: A Critical Piece to Develop into a Healthy Adult

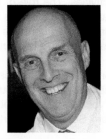   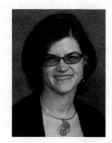

Max J. Coppes, MD, PhD, MBA, FAAP   Susan A. Fisher-Owens, MD, MPH, FAAP
Editors

There are so many aspects that new parents have to consider when raising children. Consequently, there are many issues that pediatricians need to be conversant in when supporting parents in their unique role to take care of their children's needs and assist them in becoming healthy adults. The role of pediatricians of course is not only to manage disease but also increasingly to promote health and preventative care. This role is taken so seriously that the American Academy of Pediatrics, with the support of other organizations, has developed Bright Futures, a "theory-based and evidence-driven" outline of all preventative screens and interventions needed to optimize a healthy development for children up to the age of 21. Rightfully so, this elaborate roadmap includes oral health: with anticipatory guidance starting from before birth, and regular risk assessments and fluoride varnish starting at age 6 months.

This issue of the *Pediatric Clinics of North America* is meant to provide the readership with information that underlies the above-mentioned recommendations and the importance of oral health for the overall well-being of children as they mature into adulthood. Because early childhood caries is five times as common as asthma, much attention throughout is focused on tooth decay or dental caries in its various presentations, the socioeconomic factors attributed to its severity, treatment options, and preventive strategies.

Information is provided on the developmental aspect of oral health, as it is important to be able to distinguish between what one can normally expect to occur and develop in the orally cavity and what is pathologic. The article on infant oral health specifically describes the importance of forming the right habits even before the first teeth become visible.

Attention is also brought to an evolving understanding of the role of the microbiome and more broadly the effects of the interaction between genetic background and environment, in its broadest sense. The environment that we can influence includes the oral

Pediatr Clin N Am 65 (2018) xvii–xix
https://doi.org/10.1016/j.pcl.2018.07.001
0031-3955/18/© 2018 Published by Elsevier Inc.

pediatric.theclinics.com

flora of parents, often taken for granted and "forgotten" as a source of a child's oral health, since most do not realize that dental caries are caused by transmittable bacteria. Other components of the environment that we can control include what children eat and drink, the water they drink, how often they brush their teeth (influenced by how often parents brush their teeth!), and the toothpaste they use, in particular, in communities that lack fluoride in the water.

Our ability to ensure appropriate exposure to fluoride greatly affects the environment in which our teeth and gums perform their daily activities. The role of fluoride in the prevention of tooth decay is mentioned in several articles but also has its own article. In general, discussion about ensuring that children receive fluoride is usually focused on fluoridation of water, but as described here, there are multiple fluoride modalities that can be invoked.

The use of sealants as a means of stopping progression of noncavitated caries lesions in permanent teeth is also described. The use of sealants can and should specifically be considered in older children, teenagers, and young adults, although too often those with greatest need are least likely to receive them. Sealants are particularly apropos for school-based care.

Treatment of malocclusion through orthodontics is discussed, with particular mention of when an orthodontic referral is most appropriate. Special attention is provided to the negative impact on quality of life caused by malocclusion. Ultimately, this can also influence an adult's ability to be hired.

Those with a particularly challenged quality of life are children with special health care needs. Their oral health may be deprioritized given their other health needs, but often their oral health is worsened secondary to medications needed or by their primary disease outright. An article addressing their needs provides guidance on how best to manage the oral health needs of children with special needs.

The peculiar challenges surrounding policymaking for child health and child oral health are discussed. Increasingly in the United States at least, developing policies for oral health issues are fully integrated with developing policies for health in general, promoting a fuller integration between medical and dental care for children.

While many articles focus on the teeth, there is ample evidence that periodontal disease, including gingivitis and periodontitis, are quite common in children and adolescents. Factors that contribute to these diseases include behavioral and socioeconomic ones, which when not properly addressed puts children on a trajectory of chronic oral health challenges.

Special attention is given to measuring oral health–related quality of life in children and adolescents. This is a particularly difficult area to measure since quality of life evolves as children age, often is intimately associated with culture, and may have to measure different aspects depending on the what in the oral cavity is being affected (eg, orofacial clefts vs orthodontic treatments, vs extensive dental caries).

The intimate relationship between the oral cavity as a window into the rest of the body is also described. Many systemic diseases (eg, Crohn disease, gastrointestinal reflux, thrombocytopenia, or immune deficiency) present with symptoms in the oropharynx, and recognizing these as such is of great importance both for the primary care practitioner (PCP) and for the dentist seeing children and teenagers. Similarly, PCPs and urgent care physicians benefit from recognizing atypical symptoms of oral diseases, since children may present to them rather than to a dentist with complaints in the oral cavity.

The oral cavity is of course part of the "head and neck," a body area serviced by ear, nose, and throat (ENT) physicians. One of the contributions focuses on oral lesions often seen by either medical (primary care or ENT) or dental providers. Many lesions are benign, however not all. A description on how best to diagnose and treat oral cavity lesions provides a highly complementary contribution to this overall review of oral health in children.

Given the great burden of oral disease, it is important to understand why pediatric providers should include oral health as a part of their total care. It is reassuring to learn that there are multiple models of how this can be accomplished successfully, and there are other allied health workers who can assist toward achieving the goal of oral health for all children.

As parents and health care providers, we initially teach healthy habits, but to remain effective over time, instruction has to evolve into coaching and encouragement. This is most poignantly illustrated by our ability to instruct and later coach our children habits that promote oral health. We hope that this issue of the *Pediatric Clinics of North America* contributes to a fuller understanding of those priorities that makes us better teachers and better coaches.

Max J. Coppes, MD, PhD, MBA, FAAP
University of Nevada Reno
School of Medicine
Renown Children's Hospital
Reno, NV 89502, USA

Susan A. Fisher-Owens, MD, MPH, FAAP
Department of Pediatrics
UCSF School of Medicine
Zuckerberg San Francisco General Hospital
1001 Potrero Avenue/MS6E37
San Francisco, CA 94110, USA

Department of Preventive and Restorative Dental Sciences
UCSF School of Dentistry
505 Parnassus Avenue
San Francisco, CA 94143, USA

E-mail addresses:
mcoppes@renown.org (M.J. Coppes)
Susan.Fisher-Owens@ucsf.edu (S.A. Fisher-Owens)

A Developmental Approach to Pediatric Oral Health

Bhavna T. Pahel, DDS, MPH, PhD[a,b,]*, Anne Rowan-Legg, MD, FRCPC[c],
Rocio B. Quinonez, DMD, MS, MPH[d]

KEYWORDS

- Oral health • Oral development • Life course • Dentition • Child • Adolescent

KEY POINTS

- Oral health maintenance must be closely linked to oral and craniofacial development.
- Surveillance for many dental developmental milestones can occur at well-visits in pediatric primary care, providing an opportunity for anticipatory oral health guidance.
- Pediatric primary care providers can play an important role in early identification of oral health problems.

INTRODUCTION

Orofacial growth and development is distinct from the rest of the body because it does not cease at the end of epiphyseal growth. Rather, orofacial structures continue to evolve and change over the life course, and can be influenced by factors including genetic background and environment (ie, nutrition, trauma, infection). Using the life course framework, this article moves beyond the biomedical perspective to a more comprehensive approach that acknowledges the multifactorial, dynamic, and cumulative nature of factors affecting orofacial growth and development.[1] As shown in **Fig. 1**, the life course perspective allows for an examination of the cumulative effects of biological, social, and environmental factors from gestation through childhood (and into adulthood) on chronic disease experience and progression.[1] The life course approach has many

Disclosure: None of the authors have any disclosures.
[a] Department of Pediatric Dentistry, UNC School of Dentistry, University of North Carolina at Chapel Hill, 4501B Koury Oral Health Sciences Building, CB# 7450, Chapel Hill, NC 27599-7450, USA; [b] Private Practice: Village Family Dental, 510 Hickory Ridge Drive, Suite 101, Greensboro, NC 27409-9779, USA; [c] Department of Pediatrics, University of Ottawa and Division of Pediatric Medicine, Children's Hospital of Eastern Ontario, 401 Smyth Road, Ottawa, Ontario K1H 8L1, Canada; [d] Departments of Pediatric Dentistry and Academic Affairs, School of Dentistry, The University of North Carolina at Chapel Hill, 1611 Koury Oral Health Sciences Building, CB# 7450, Chapel Hill, NC 27599-7450, USA
* Corresponding author. Department of Pediatric Dentistry, UNC School of Dentistry, University of North Carolina at Chapel Hill, 4501B Koury Oral Health Sciences Building, CB# 7450, Chapel Hill, NC 27599-7450.
E-mail address: bhavna_pahel@unc.edu

Pediatr Clin N Am 65 (2018) 885–907
https://doi.org/10.1016/j.pcl.2018.05.003
0031-3955/18/© 2018 Elsevier Inc. All rights reserved.

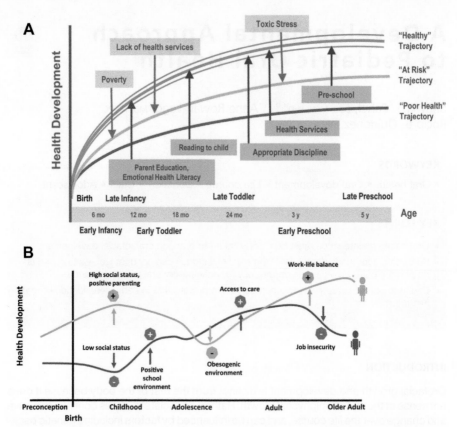

Fig. 1. Parts (*A*) and (*B*) show the effect of various health protective and injurious factors on lifecourse trajectories at different stages of human development. (*From* Halfon N, Larson K, Lu M, et al. Lifecourse health development: past, present and future. Matern Child Health J 2014;18(2):352; with permission.)

lessons to offer on population oral health, considering that the 2 most prevalent oral health conditions (dental caries and periodontal disease) are chronic and cumulative.

This article reviews the role of oral health in overall physical and social development in childhood and adolescence (**Table 1**). It begins with an examination of the effects of maternal oral health on children's oral health, and discusses the importance of establishing oral health maintenance routines in early childhood. It reviews important oral health–specific physical and social developmental milestones during early (0–3 years), middle (3–6 years), and late childhood (6–12 years) and adolescence (≥13 years). These age categories parallel time periods for tooth emergence and maintenance of the primary dentition (0–3 and 3–6 years), followed by the mixed dentition (6–12 years), and finally the permanent dentition (≥13 years). Issues particular to each age group are examined, as well as those spanning multiple age categories, including pediatric overweight and obesity, oral piercings, tobacco use, and dental trauma. It ends with an examination of the oral microbiome and emerging salivary diagnostics as promising research areas that can further the understanding of oral health and development in health and disease as we enter the era of personalized health care.

Although not reviewed in this article, the authors acknowledge that early life experiences and oral health status can have significant influence on oral health throughout the life course. For example, dental disease is a leading cause of school absenteeism,

Table 1
Overview of developmental milestones and related issues in the pediatric population with implications for oral health

| | Prenatal | Early Childhood | | Children | | Adolescents |
		0–2 y	3–5 y	6–12 y		≥ 13 y
Oral/dental development	Lip closure ~6 mo in utero, palate closure ~7–11 wk in utero Formation of primary tooth buds begins at 6 wk in utero, followed closely by tooth buds for permanent teeth	First permanent molars and incisors begin calcification at birth First primary teeth (mandibular central incisors) begin emerging at ~6–8 mo of age	Primary dentition is usually complete by 3 y of age	Permanent teeth emerge anterior to posterior, following their embryologic development, with lower incisors leading as the first primary teeth to exfoliate. Second primary molars are the last primary teeth to exfoliate at ~11-12 y. Lower central incisors and first molars are among the first permanent teeth to emerge		By 13 y, all primary teeth are exfoliated, permanent teeth 12 y molars are emerging Third molars (wisdom teeth) if present emerge at 17–21 y
		Rule of 6: first tooth emerges at ~6 mo, first permanent tooth emerges ~6 y, by 12 y (+6 y) all primary teeth have exfoliated, by ~18 y (+6 y) all permanent teeth present				
Social-emotional Development	—	Early manifestation of temperament Difficult temperament as a risk factor for bottle use at night Parallel play	Developing autonomy. Caregivers still performing oral hygiene	Independence in tasks		Independent decision making Significant peer influence Self-esteem may be related to cosmetic dental issues

(continued on next page)

Table 1
(continued)

	Prenatal	Early Childhood		Children	Adolescents
		0–2 y	3–5 y	6–12 y	≥ 13 y
Speech development	—	25–50-word vocabulary Two-word sentences Knows some body parts	Counts to 10 Tells stories 100% intelligibility Follows 3-step commands	Growing vocabulary	
Fine motor and self-help skills	—	By the end of the stage child is: Using spoon well Drinking from a cup Placing only edibles in mouth	By the end of the stage child is: Toileting alone Copies shapes (drawing) Independent eating and dressing	By the end of the stage child is: Able to perform personal hygiene independently Able to brush teeth independently	
Oral considerations	Maternal nutrition Maternal oral health status and transmission of oral micro-organisms	Teething issues Recommend teeth rings/cold washcloth to chew Avoid topical teething gels containing local anesthetic to prevent toxicity from ingestion Nutrition: Bottle and sippy cup use. Limit milk to 475 mL/d during meals; decrease risk of iron deficiency anemia and dental caries Snacking: see child/adolescent Oral hygiene: brushing with a smear of fluoride toothpaste Gross motor	Nutrition: frequency of snacks and sugar-sweetened beverage consumption (common risk factors with obesity and dental caries) Type of snacks: avoid sticky foods Consideration to vitamin supplements (gummy vitamins)	Exfoliation of primary teeth and eruption of permanent teeth	—

Oral hygiene: brushing with a pea-sized amount of fluoride toothpaste (transition when able to expectorate)
Flossing between teeth that are touching each other
Gross motor developing, transition from caregiver to child oral hygiene

	developing: caregiver performing hygiene Routines: Brush, Book, Bed	~8–10 y Routines: Brush, Book, Bed	
—			Habits: digit sucking, pacifier use, nail biting	Habits: digit sucking, nail biting
—	Trauma: primary tooth trauma (peak age 2–3 y)		Trauma: permanent tooth trauma (peak age 8–9 y) Tongue piercing: tooth and soft tissue trauma
—	—	—	Eating disorders: anorexia nervosa and bulimia nervosa (erosion) Oral sex/HPV, substance/tobacco use/alcohol: oral cancer risk

Abbreviation: HPV, human papillomavirus.

leading to missed opportunities for learning and socializing.[2] Further, socioeconomic status in early childhood as well parents' oral health beliefs are positively associated with individual oral health beliefs during adolescence. Parents' oral health beliefs influence toothbrushing behaviors, dental health care–seeking behaviors, oral health outcomes, and oral health-related quality of life of the offspring in adulthood.[3–5] Thus, early establishment of sound oral health care practices extend those practices into adulthood. In contrast, poor oral health can negatively affect the normal trajectory of childhood development, influencing speech, nutritional status, sleep, socialization, and self-esteem, which are all critical to fostering healthy development.[2,5]

THE PRENATAL PERIOD

Many facial and dental congenital anomalies arise from alterations in the processes occurring during the second phase of organogenesis (4–8 weeks' gestation), a period characterized by morphogenesis and histodifferentiation.[6] Nonsyndromic orofacial clefting (ie, cleft lip and/or cleft palate) is one of the most common congenital anomalies in humans, with an estimated worldwide prevalence of 1.2 per 1000 live births.[7] Facial clefts usually are attributed to failure of neural crest cells to migrate to a certain area, leading to a localized deficiency of mesenchyme. Isolated cleft palate may occur because of the failure of fusion of palatal shelves with each other and the nasal septum. Dental anomalies occur with higher frequency among children with nonsyndromic cleft lip and/or palate, with hypodontia (missing primary and permanent teeth) as a common finding, particularly in the maxillary arch.[8]

Primary and permanent teeth are formed from tissues derived from the ectoderm and mesoderm.[9] A total of 10 tooth germs are formed, each, in the maxilla and the mandible, and represent the 20 future primary teeth (**Fig. 2**). Each developing primary tooth gives rise to the dental lamina for a permanent tooth. Tooth formation begins at approximately 6 weeks of intrauterine life with the formation of the tooth germs from dental lamina, which in turn arises from the basal layer of the oral epithelium. The ectoderm in the tooth germ eventually gives rise to enamel, thus forming the outermost layer of a tooth. The mesoderm gives rise to the dentin and the pulp of the tooth.

MATERNAL ORAL HEALTH

Maternal stress, chronic health conditions, nutrition, medication use, and other exposures can have significant impacts on the developing fetus, with long-lasting developmental and epigenetic effects.[10] Similarly, maternal oral health is related to infant oral health both biologically and behaviorally.[11–13] For example, presence of periodontal disease in pregnant women is associated with preterm delivery, with its attendant complications and low birth weight.[14–16] Research into a possible causal relationship between maternal periodontal disease and adverse pregnancy outcomes needs further elucidation. Regardless, early evidence points to the important role primary care providers can play in providing anticipatory guidance regarding oral health to women before conception and throughout their pregnancies.

Previous research into mother-to-child transmission of cariogenic bacteria emphasized the important role of Streptococcus mutans in dental caries.[17] Emerging evidence suggests increased complexity of the oral microbiome and mechanisms underlying dental disease.[18] For example, the same micro-organisms found in the mother's oral cavity also are reported in the amniotic fluid and the placenta.[19–21] Even the mechanism of delivery seems to affect the microbiota found in the infant. One study reported vaginally delivered infants having more diverse oral microbial taxa compared with those delivered by cesarean section (79 vs 54 species/species clusters, respectively).[22]

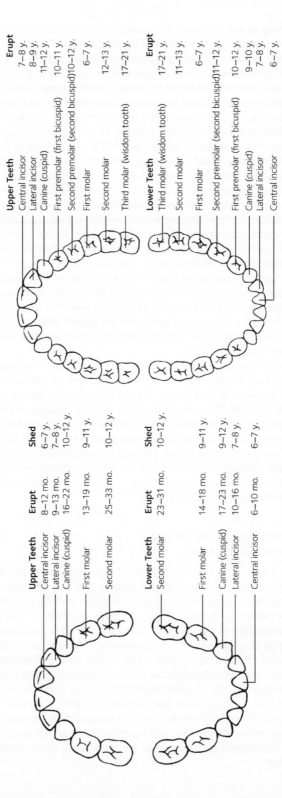

Primary Tooth Development

Upper Teeth	Erupt	Shed
Central incisor	8–12 mo.	6–7 y.
Lateral incisor	9–13 mo.	7–8 y.
Canine (cuspid)	16–22 mo.	10–12 y.
First molar	13–19 mo.	9–11 y.
Second molar	25–33 mo.	10–12 y.

Lower Teeth	Erupt	Shed
Second molar	23–31 mo.	10–12 y.
First molar	14–18 mo.	9–11 y.
Canine (cuspid)	17–23 mo.	9–12 y.
Lateral incisor	10–16 mo.	7–8 y.
Central incisor	6–10 mo.	6–7 y.

Permanent Tooth Development

Upper Teeth	Erupt
Central incisor	7–8 y.
Lateral incisor	8–9 y.
Canine (cuspid)	11–12 y.
First premolar (first bicuspid)	10–11 y.
Second premolar (second bicuspid)	10–12 y.
First molar	6–7 y.
Second molar	12–13 y.
Third molar (wisdom tooth)	17–21 y.

Lower Teeth	Erupt
Third molar (wisdom tooth)	17–21 y.
Second molar	11–13 y.
First molar	6–7 y.
Second premolar (second bicuspid)	11–12 y.
First premolar (first bicuspid)	10–12 y.
Canine (cuspid)	9–10 y.
Lateral incisor	7–8 y.
Central incisor	6–7 y.

Fig. 2. Primary and permanent tooth eruption charts. (*From* American Dental Association (ADA) Eruption Charts. Available at: http://www.mouthhealthy.org/en/az-topics/e/eruption-charts.)

The timing of oral bacterial transmission from mother to child is controversial, with evidence suggesting acquisition before or at birth.[18] Further, conflicting evidence exists regarding transmission from nonmaternal caretakers or between children. Oral bacteria in infants likely remains dormant in crevices of the tongue and tonsils until the nondesquamating surfaces of primary teeth emerge, although direct proof is yet to be ascertained. S mutans and related bacteria more easily colonize newly erupted teeth rather than previously erupted teeth with stable bacterial colonies.

The suboptimal quality and/or quantity of the outermost layer of the tooth (ie, the enamel) can increase dental caries risk.[23] One reason for this finding is that tooth surfaces with developmental defects (eg, enamel hypoplasia) act as retentive niches for bacteria and are colonized more easily and earlier than those without defects. A diet characterized by frequent exposure to fermentable carbohydrates contributes to an increase in cariogenic bacterial counts, including S mutans.

From a social-behavioral perspective, caregivers play a crucial role in helping establish good home oral hygiene and dietary practices. A study among low-income African American preschool children reported that mothers who brushed their own teeth before bedtime on weeknights also were more likely to brush their children's teeth.[24] The investigators also found that mothers with higher oral health knowledge and oral health–specific self-efficacy were likely to have children whose teeth were brushed more frequently. In contrast, parents with low self-efficacy related to brushing, those who did not want to struggle with their preschool children for brushing, and those reporting low social support from family members are less likely to brush their children's teeth twice a day.[25]

Caregivers' dental treatment-related behaviors can influence oral health outcomes in their children. For example, mothers who access dental care regularly have children that are more likely to visit the dentist compared with mothers with an irregular history of past dental visits.[26] In one study, controlling for sociodemographic characteristics, feeding and oral care practices, and maternal oral health, higher maternal salivary bacterial counts (S mutans and Lactobacillus) were associated with doubling of the incidence of early childhood caries (defined as dental caries in a child <72 months old) among their children.[27] In another study, investigators reported that mothers with untreated dental caries are 3 times more likely to have children with higher caries experience (treated and untreated caries).[28]

BIRTH THROUGH 3 YEARS OF AGE
Oral Physical Development

The period from birth through 3 years of age is characterized by dynamic and rapid developmental changes in oral soft tissues and the emergence of teeth beginning around 6 months of age. With respect to oral soft tissues, ankyloglossia is increasingly cited as a reason for breastfeeding problems in infants.[29] The prevalence of ankyloglossia is reported in the range of 0.1% to 12% with a male predilection (1.1:1–3:1) and genetic predisposition.[30] Symptomatic ankyloglossia can be associated with feeding problems and nipple pain in the mother during breastfeeding.[31] The definition and classification of ankyloglossia is not standardized and there is wide variation of opinion regarding its clinical significance and optimal management. A recent Cochrane Review concluded that, based on a limited number of studies with small sample sizes, there is some evidence to suggest that frenotomy for ankyloglossia in infants may reduce nipple pain among breastfeeding mothers, but the effect of frenotomy on breastfeeding outcomes for infants is less clear and needs further investigation.[29]

Regarding oral hard (calcified) tissues, primary teeth begin forming around 7 weeks of intrauterine life and enamel formation on those teeth is complete in the first year of life.[32] In addition, the first permanent molars also exhibit some degree of calcification at birth. Primary teeth begin eruption around 6 months of age and most toddlers have all primary teeth erupted between 24 to 36 months of age. Teeth begin emerging into the oral cavity once three-quarters of their roots are complete and most primary teeth complete their root development by 3 years of age.[32] Mandibular central incisors are usually the first primary teeth to emerge, followed closely by the upper central and lateral incisors and the lower lateral incisors, then the eruption of primary canines, first primary molars, and the second primary molars completes the primary dentition. Spaces observed frequently between primary teeth are desirable because permanent teeth are wider than primary teeth. Lack of spacing in the primary dentition is a harbinger of future crowding.[33]

Social-Emotional Development

Infants develop primitive expressive speech, beginning with vocalization and babbling. Immature jargoning progresses to words over the second year. In parallel, infants learn to bite and chew as the primary dentition emerges and often explore by bringing objects to their mouths. At this stage, the importance of routines with respect to feeding, bathing, sleeping, and toothbrushing for infants' and children's socio-emotional development should be communicated with parents and caregivers. Such routines, if established early in life, are more likely to be carried forward when children enter the more spirited preschool years, when children begin to exert independence; for example, by resisting parental involvement in toothbrushing, leading to parental-child conflict. The Brush, Book, Bed program of the American Academy of Pediatrics (AAP) is a helpful resource about bedtime routines that pediatric providers can use to provide anticipatory guidance to caregivers of children 6 months through 6 years of age.[34]

Oral Health Issues

Primary tooth emergence typically follows the pattern mentioned earlier. However, 1 or more teeth can be present at birth (referred to as natal teeth) or emerge within the first 30 days of life (called neonatal teeth).[35] The prevalence of natal and neonatal teeth is reported at 1:1000 to 1:30,000.[35,36] Natal and neonatal teeth in the anterior region are most frequently early erupting primary teeth. However, presence of these teeth in the posterior region (ie, molars) warrants further evaluation for systemic conditions such as Pfieffer syndrome and histiocytosis X.[37] Although extremely rare, natal and neonatal teeth may be supernumerary or extra teeth that have emerged into the oral cavity before the emergence of the primary dentition.[31] These teeth should be maintained in the arch if at all possible. Significant mobility of natal teeth is a theoretic concern; however, no case of swallowing or aspiration has been reported.[35] These teeth can cause feeding difficulty and repeated contact of the ventral surface of the tongue with the incisal edges of the lower incisors can lead to ulceration of that area of the tongue, referred to as Riga-Fede disease or ulceration.[38] In general, smoothing the incisal edges of the teeth aids in healing of the tongue ulceration, allowing the teeth to be retained.[35,39] Natal and neonatal teeth should be differentiated from 3 developmental lesions often seen as firm, white, round protuberances on an infant's gingiva away from the midline (called Bohn nodules), along the midline of the palate (called Epstein pearls), and on the crest of the alveolar ridge (referred to as a dental lamina cyst).[40] Parents should be reassured that these are transient developmental lesions that involute spontaneously within a few of weeks of their appearance.

Teeth are at risk for dental caries as soon as they emerge into the oral cavity and are exposed to the oral bacteria and fermentable carbohydrates. Early tooth loss caused by advanced dental caries can result in failure to thrive and nutritional deficiencies in young children.[41] Malnutrition and poor weight gain can have long-lasting developmental effects. Thus, parents should be instructed to begin home oral care routines, including brushing with a smear or grain-sized amount of fluoride toothpaste as soon as a tooth is visible in the oral cavity.[42] The amount of fluoride toothpaste can be increased to a pea size once the child is able to expectorate, a skill usually not developed until 3 years of age or later.

With respect to diet-related anticipatory guidance, infants should be weaned off the bottle by 12 months of age; parents should be encouraged not to put their child to bed with a bottle containing milk, formula, or juice.[43] The AAP does not recommend fruit juice before 1 year of age. For children between 1 and 3 years of age, the AAP recommends fruit juice be limited to no more than 120 mL (4 ounces) in a day and only at mealtimes. Mothers should also be advised not to engage in ad-libitum breastfeeding once primary teeth have begun emerging and dietary carbohydrates have been introduced. Children should be encouraged to drink water (preferably fluoridated) between meals.[44] In addition, the early establishment of a dental home as a place to receive comprehensive, coordinated, and culturally sensitive oral health care is widely encouraged as a goal for the first year of an infant's life.[45]

THE PRIMARY DENTITION YEARS (AGES 3–6 YEARS)
Oral Physical Development

Most children should have all 20 of their primary teeth present by 3 years of age. Although rare, there can be congenitally missing (hypodontia) or extra (supernumerary) teeth in the primary dentition. The prevalence of tooth agenesis in the primary dentition is reported to approximate 0.1% to 1.5%, with no sex predilection.[46] The prevalence of supernumerary teeth in the primary dentition is reported at 0.3%.[32]

Once complete, the primary dentition is stable until lower central incisors may be reported as loose or mobile by the child around 5 to 6 years of age. This is followed by their exfoliation and the emergence of the lower permanent central incisors, which are usually the first permanent teeth to emerge. Given the significant variation in exfoliation and emergence of teeth based on race, ethnicity, sex, and body mass index, it is possible for some children to have mobile lower incisors as early as 4 years of age.[47] In such cases, it is important to rule out trauma as a contributing factor to the mobility of 1 or more primary teeth, particularly mandibular incisors. In rare instances, premature primary tooth exfoliation can be attributed to other systemic conditions such as hypophosphatasia.[48] Detailed medical and dental history and a thorough clinical examination are therefore crucial in narrowing the cause of premature exfoliation.

Social Development

Developmentally, 3 years of age marks the beginning of marked social changes, including the emergence of self-identity and social play. The desire to be independent, including eating and trying new skills such as brushing teeth, is strong. Children begin attending school, develop friendships, and are eating at least 1 meal a day independently. Children in this stage may be fearful of a dental visit, particularly if seeing the dentist for the first time or if their parent has dental anxiety, and therefore may depend on the presence of a supportive caregiver.

Oral Health Issues

It is increasingly common for both parents to work outside the home, and single-parent families represent about 20% of all households with children in many countries.[49] This may mean that children are attending preschool or daycare, which can have a significant impact on their diet and routines, for better or worse. As children enter the elementary school years, maintaining a healthy diet can become more challenging because of the competing influences of peers and food choices available at school. Anticipatory guidance should therefore be provided to families regarding healthy snacks and reducing the frequency of highly acidogenic foods that cause the oral cavity pH to decrease to less than 5.5, the critical pH at which enamel begins to lose mineral.

Recent research has established that the frequency of exposure to acidogenic foods plays a larger role in the progression of dental caries than any individual acidogenic exposure.[50] Foods with the following characteristics have been suggested to have low caries risk[32]: (1) high protein content; (2) moderate fat content to encourage clearance of food from the mouth; (3) low in fermentable carbohydrates; (4) good ability to buffer the pH of the oral cavity; (5) high in calcium and phosphorus; (6) maintain the oral cavity's pH at more than 5.5; (7) stimulate salivary flow to encourage clearance of food from the mouth. Therefore, families should be advised to reduce the frequency of consumption of refined carbohydrates such as white bread, chocolate milk, soda, orange juice, raisins, potato chips, and so forth. Instead, they should be encouraged to include fresh fruits and vegetables and high-protein snacks such as cheese and yogurt in their diet. The American Heart Association's dietary recommendations for children and adolescents, endorsed by the AAP and the American Academy of Pediatric Dentistry, is a helpful resource for age group–specific anticipatory guidance.[51]

Oral hygiene routines commenced in the early years should be more established by the time the primary dentition is complete. Once children are 3 years old or able to reliably expectorate, a pea-sized amount of fluoride toothpaste can be used with parental supervision.[42] Of note, as children get closer to 6 years of age and assert their independence, parents may be tempted to completely delegate toothbrushing responsibilities to the child. Given poor toothbrushing skills among children younger than 10 years of age, parental supervision is still recommended.[52]

Child, parental, and environmental factors all influence the likelihood of a behavior such as toothbrushing occurring on a consistent basis.[53] Parental knowledge of appropriate oral health behaviors and beliefs about consequences can contribute to intent. Factors such as child resistance or fatigue can be barriers. Factors such as parental perceived lack of control over the child's behaviors, lack of parenting skills in managing behavior, and lack of capacity to prioritize supervision of toothbrushing or poor skills in maintaining a routine can further complicate performing this desirable practice. Environmental factors, such as competing demands on attention, can be barriers. However, skills to manage behavior and maintain a routine are enablers to successful adoption of good oral health care routines.

Most children with a thumb or finger habit usually stop by about 2 years of age.[54] However, a small percentage of children continue with the habit past their fifth birthday. If there are no associated dental changes such as increased prominence of the upper primary incisors, treatment at this stage is usually not recommended because of compliance concerns. It has been reported that often the habit gets extinguished or reduces in frequency once the child starts school and feels peer pressure to stop the habit.[32] The most important factor in extinguishing the habit is the child's desire to stop. When the child expresses a desire to cease the behavior, the family should be referred to their oral health or primary care provider to explore treatment options to assist with habit elimination.[55] Possible strategies (by themselves or in combination) can include counseling the child about stopping the habit; reminder therapy with a waterproof adhesive bandage on the finger; or a reward for habit elimination, chosen by the child and part of a contract drawn up between the child and parent. If none of these strategies are successful, more advanced adjunctive therapies may be needed. These can include wrapping the child's arm (usually at nighttime, when most habits occur) with a loosely wrapped flexible/elastic bandage that prevents the arm from flexing and the fingers being placed in the mouth. In addition, an intraoral appliance (eg, bluegrass appliance, palatal crib, quad helix) can be fabricated as a physical reminder to discourage children from placing their fingers in their mouths.

Dental trauma is an issue that continues to be important in children 3 to 6 years old. Apart from trauma to the teeth and soft tissues, children often experience trauma to the chin area as a result of falls. When this occurs, mandibular fracture should be ruled out. Signs and symptoms include ecchymosis around the chin, hematoma in the floor of the mouth, numbness in the lower jaw (right, left, or both), and/or an altered bite (occlusion). If facial asymmetry (deviation) is noted on jaw opening and closing, mandibular condylar fracture should be suspected. Although the tongue is often bitten during a fall, it rarely needs medical attention.

THE MIXED DENTITION YEARS (AGES 6–12 YEARS)
Oral Physical Development

Mixed dentition refers to the presence of both primary and permanent teeth in the oral cavity. This period usually begins with the exfoliation of the mandibular primary central incisors, emergence of the mandibular permanent central incisors and first permanent molars around age 6 years, and ends with the exfoliation of the last primary teeth around 12 years of age. The enamel on all permanent teeth except for third molars is complete by 8 years of age.[32] By 12 years of age, most children have all permanent teeth present or actively erupting in their mouths, except for third molars.

Permanent incisors in the maxillary arch are notably larger than their primary predecessors. These teeth therefore exhibit some flaring as they attempt to accommodate in the arch. Such flaring also leads to the presence of spacing between the maxillary anterior teeth; this stage should be considered transitional.[32] Parents often express concerns about whether these spaces will close spontaneously. Parents should be reassured that this spacing is a normal part of growth and development, and most spaces close at the time of emergence of the permanent maxillary canine teeth around 11 to 12 years of age.[32]

Social Development

Health-related routines (oral health, eating, sleeping) should be well established by this stage. Children continue developing friendships and responding to others' emotions and thoughts. Social pressures are strong, and children increasingly try to conform. This tendency can be helpful for extinguishing habits such as thumb-sucking. Children can assume more responsibility in their self-help and hygiene skills, and this can foster confidence and independence. Mental capacity increases and memory of events increases. Therefore, a poor experience with the dentist is likely not easily forgotten at this stage.

Oral Health Issues

Once children are of school age, the potentially strong influence of peers and other role models such as teachers and coaches should not be overlooked. Anticipatory guidance regarding diet, oral hygiene, and trauma prevention should actively engage parents and children. Children involved in contact sports should be advised to use mouth guards. Maxillary permanent incisors are the most often injured permanent teeth in this age group,[56] particularly if the incisors are very flared or prominent.[32] This is also the time when early or phase 1 orthodontic treatment may be considered if it has the potential to alleviate need or amount of time needed for future care (ie, phase 2 orthodontic treatment in the permanent dentition, coinciding with puberty).

Another issue related to children's participation in sports is the increasing consumption of sugared sports drinks, which are often perceived to be healthy by parents. It should be emphasized to parents and children that such drinks are very acidic, contain large amounts of sugars, and may be appropriate for endurance athletes but not necessary for a few hours of physical activity per week.[57]

THE ADOLESCENT YEARS (≥13 YEARS)
Oral Physical Development

By 13 years of age, most individuals have all their primary teeth exfoliated and all permanent teeth, except third molars, have emerged. The third molars typically emerge around 17 to 21 years of age.[32] The roots of most permanent teeth, except third molars, are completely developed by 16 years of age.

Social Development

Adolescence is one of the most dynamic stages of human development. The social and emotional changes of adolescence are accompanied by physical and cognitive changes that present both opportunities and challenges for adolescents, their families, and health professionals. Important social development during adolescence involves a greater self-awareness and a strong desire to be viewed by others in a positive light. This self-awareness can also be the source of great anxiety; for example, about being attractive, loved, and appearing strong. Adolescents with significant oral disease or malocclusion may be embarrassed to smile.

Adolescents often make decisions without parental knowledge. Some of these involve engaging in high-risk behaviors (eg, smoking, alcohol, sexual activity), which can lead to significant morbidity. For example, there is mounting evidence for the role of human papillomavirus (HPV) in oropharyngeal carcinoma, with growing calls for dentists to provide anticipatory guidance on this topic to their patients.[58] Self-esteem, self-efficacy, and confidence are important to foster at this stage.[59] As such, nurturing a sense of self-assurance in adolescents, providing them with knowledge of how to meet life's challenges (and the belief that they can), and reinforcing healthy choices help them develop the social competence and sense of responsibility needed for personal, social, health, and academic achievement.

Oral Health Issues

Numerous issues with implications for oral health seen in adolescence include changing diets and dietary preferences, increasing risk of dental caries, periodontal disease, temporomandibular disorders, and behavioral and sexual practices. Acknowledging the uniqueness and scope of adolescents' oral health issues, the American Academy of Pediatric Dentistry published a comprehensive guideline on adolescent oral health care.[60] The persistent high risk for dental caries observed in adolescence is attributable to high intake of cariogenic foods and sugar-sweetened beverages and suboptimal oral hygiene practices. Of concern, one study attributed 10% to 15% of the total calorie intake among children and adolescents in the United States to sugar-sweetened beverages and 100% fruit juice.[61] Many adolescents are in fixed orthodontic treatment (braces), putting them at higher risk for dental caries and oral soft tissue injuries from dental trauma. The prevalence of gingivitis is higher in adolescence than in prepubertal children. In addition to poor brushing and inadequate flossing, sex hormones are suspected to contribute to this finding, likely through alteration of the subgingival microbiome and/or increase in capillary permeability, leading to increased susceptibility to gingival inflammation.[60]

Temporomandibular disorders can emerge at any time during childhood and adolescent years. However, a higher prevalence of these disorders is noted during adolescence.[62] A recent systematic review noted that about 1 in 6 children and adolescents exhibits signs of temporomandibular joint disorder, ranging from clicking (prevalence = 10%; 95% confidence interval [CI], 11.6–19.9) to locking of the jaw (prevalence = 2.3%; 95% CI, 0.6–5.2).[63] These findings should not be taken lightly, and the family should be encouraged to seek a dentist or orofacial medicine specialist with expertise in the diagnosis and management of temporomandibular disorders.

Sleep bruxism (grinding teeth at night) and daytime clenching is common in children, with most ceasing the habit by adolescence or early adulthood.[64] A mouthguard is usually not recommended because it is not likely to stop the habit and may become a choking hazard if the child breaks a piece of the mouthguard while bruxing. For daytime clenching, children should be encouraged to be more self-aware and cease the habit whenever they notice it occurring. For children who develop symptoms such as frequent headaches and/or soreness in the head and neck musculature, a referral to an orofacial pain specialist should be arranged.

Eating disorders, including anorexia nervosa and bulimia nervosa, may be first noted during adolescence.[65] Eating disorders can have negative effects on the soft tissues of the oral cavity and the developing dentition.[66] Exposure to highly acidic stomach contents can lead to erosive destruction of enamel, the outermost layer of the teeth. This erosive wear is referred to as perimyolysis, and exposes the inner layer, dentin, of the teeth with concomitant dental sensitivity, and increased risk for tooth fractures and dental caries. In addition to a higher prevalence of erosion and dental caries, xerostomia (dry mouth) caused by hyposalivation is often reported because of vomiting (seen in bulimia) or starvation (seen in anorexia).

Developmentally, adolescence is a time when many individuals begin to express their individuality, which can lead to choices with negative effects on individuals' oral health. One example is the practice of piercings in the oral cavity. The tongue is the most common site for a piercing in the mouth, and other sites include the lips, cheeks, and (rarely) the uvula.[67] Oral piercings can lead to difficulty with oral hygiene, increase plaque levels and gingival inflammation, cause gingival recession, increase the risk for dental caries, interfere with speech, and sensitize the person to certain metals leading to a metal allergy/hypersensitivity reaction. Oral piercings are associated with pain, infection, scarring, tooth fractures, and injury to the surrounding soft tissues and should be actively discouraged.[68] For adolescents who chose to have oral piercings, good home oral care and regular visits to the dentist should be encouraged to allow monitoring and timely intervention in case problems develop.

ORAL HEALTH CONSIDERATIONS SPANNING CHILDHOOD AND ADOLESCENCE

Issues such as the effect of trauma on dental development, pediatric overweight and obesity, and tobacco and substance abuse have relevance to oral health and development across the spectrum of childhood and adolescence. For this reason, these issues are discussed separately from the specific age groupings.

TRAUMA AND DENTAL DEVELOPMENT

The prevalence of traumatic dental injuries in primary and permanent teeth ranges from 11% to 47%.[69–75] Oral injuries among children 0 to 6 years old represent 18% of all physical injuries[76] and the prevalence of permanent tooth trauma is approximately 20%.[75] Luxation injuries, particularly intrusion and avulsion, are most commonly reported injuries in the primary dentition.[77] Discoloration of primary teeth occurs in up to 50% of cases following a luxation injury, and the discoloration may or may not fade in intensity over time.[76] Crown fractures are the most common type of injury in the permanent dentition.[77] Children with a skeletal and/or dental malocclusion wherein the maxillary incisors are very prominent (increased incisor protrusion of >2 mm) are particularly prone to experiencing more severe trauma.[78]

When trauma to primary teeth occurs, injury to the permanent successor is an important consideration because of the close proximity of the root apex of the primary tooth to the developing permanent tooth's crown. Intrusion injuries of primary incisors are responsible for most developmental disturbances of permanent teeth, with enamel hypoplasia (defective enamel formation) being the most common side effect.[79] In a longitudinal study of 114 children experiencing 255 primary tooth injuries, 23% of the permanent successors showed enamel hypoplasia, including discoloration and/or enamel defects.[79] The hypoplastic area often appears as a white or brown spot on the permanent incisor when it emerges around 7 to 8 years of age and has a higher probability of occurring if the injury occurred before age 2 years.

Rarely, severe intrusion injuries or avulsion of primary incisors result in malformation or impaction of the permanent successor or cause an alteration in the path of eruption of the permanent tooth. For these reasons, guidelines from the International Association of Dental Traumatology do not recommend replanting avulsed primary teeth to prevent further trauma to the permanent successors.[76] Caregivers of children with a history of traumatic dental injury should be encouraged to have an examination by a dentist. If a primary care provider receives an advice call about an avulsed permanent tooth, they should recommend the caregiver put the tooth back in the socket if they are comfortable doing so, or directly in milk (touching only the crown, and not the root of the tooth) and go to their dentist.

OVERWEIGHT AND OBESITY

The increasing prevalence of pediatric overweight and obesity is of major clinical and public health concern. Apart from the important general health implications, such as increased risk for type II diabetes and cardiovascular disease later in life,[80] there also are important oral health implications of pediatric overweight and obesity. Recent evidence from a nationally representative study in the United States shows that overweight and obesity are positively associated with earlier emergence of first permanent molars, and obesity is associated with earlier emergence of second permanent molars.[47] This dental acceleration is in the time frame of about 6 to 12 months and may have implications for school-based sealant programs that focus on the second and sixth grades to seal newly emerged first and second permanent molars, respectively (please see Howard Pollick's article, "The Role of Fluoride in the Prevention of Tooth Decay," in this issue).

The relationship between pediatric overweight and obesity and dental caries needs further elucidation. A systematic review that included various study types found a significant positive relationship between obesity and dental caries in children from industrialized, but not from newly industrialized, countries (ie, those countries between developed and developing countries, such as Mexico).[81] A more recent systematic review, restricted to longitudinal studies, found inconclusive evidence for the association of preschool-aged and school-aged children's anthropometric measurements with dental caries.[82] Based on these data, pediatric overweight and obesity may not be associated directly with dental caries. However, nutritional choices associated with being overweight/obese,[83] such as frequent consumption of carbonated beverages and 100% fruit juice, are shared risk factors for poor oral health.

Another oral health implication of obesity in children is an increased risk for the occurrence of adverse events during pediatric procedural sedation, a commonly used modality by many pediatric dentists to provide restorative dental care. Scherrer and colleagues[84] reported that obese pediatric patients more frequently needed their airways to be opened by repositioning, required suctioning of excess secretions, and required jaw manipulation (chin lift, jaw thrust). This increase in adverse events is in part attributable to high adipose tissue around the neck and adenotonsillar hypertrophy, also contributing to obstructive sleep apnea, another risk factor for adverse events during sedation.[85] Delayed gastric emptying can also put these children at high risk for aspiration of stomach contents while sedated.

TOBACCO USE

The initiation of tobacco use in the form of cigarettes, cigars, bidis, and chewable tobacco is of great concern in the child and adolescent population. The average age for individuals to begin smoking is 11 to 12 years of age and 90% of tobacco smokers begin smoking at or before 18 years.[86] It is estimated that in the United States, about 20% of high school children (3.5 million individuals) smoke.[87] Among middle school children in the United States, the use of cigarettes, cigars, and bidis decreased between 2004 and 2006; however, smokeless tobacco and pipe use remained the same as in previous years. There was no change in tobacco use among high school children during the same 2-year period, however the use of e-cigarettes is increasing.[87] Recent evidence suggests e-cigarettes are ineffective tools for minimizing use of tobacco products, and do not help users to quit smoking.[88,89]

Among children using tobacco, leukoplakia of the oral mucosa is noted in 50% of users within the first 3 years of initiating use. Anticipatory guidance regarding tobacco use should include facts such as its association with 80% higher risk of oral cancer and 60% higher risk of pancreatic and esophageal cancer. Tobacco use also increases the risk of periodontal problems 4-fold, compromises wound healing in the oral cavity, reduces the user's ability to smell and taste foods, and leads to staining of teeth and restorations.[87] Further, exposure to secondhand tobacco smoke is associated with increased risk for dental caries in the primary dentition[90,91] and enamel hypoplasia in both the primary[92] and permanent dentitions.[93]

SUBSTANCE USE

Substances with a potential for abuse are myriad and include alcohol, medications (benzodiazepines, amphetamines, barbiturates, opioids), marijuana, and cocaine. Data for 2014 from the annual national survey in the United States, *Monitoring the Future*, indicates that the self-reported prevalence of alcohol use in the past 30 days was 9%, 24%, and 37% for grade 8, 10, and 12 students, respectively.[94] Further, in a 2014 National Survey on Drug Use and Health in the United States, approximately 9.4% of adolescents (n = 2.3 million) self-reported to be current users of illicit drugs including marijuana, cocaine, heroin, hallucinogens, and inhalants, and reported abusing prescription medications such as those mentioned earlier.[95] Habitual substance abuse can lead to changes in personality and to cognitive and sensory impairments. There may be evidence of poor oral hygiene and general neglect of oral health, and dangerous drug interactions may occur; for example, with the use of local anesthetic with vasoconstrictors in an individual abusing stimulants (eg, amphetamines).[96] Primary care providers may receive referrals from a dentist's office if such abuse is identified in the dental setting.

CHILDREN WITH SPECIAL HEALTH CARE NEEDS

Poor oral health is common among children with neurodevelopmental conditions (eg, autism, cerebral palsy) and among children with other special health care needs.[97] Access to dental care for this population may be limited by competing medical priorities and costs, distance from a pediatric dental center, and the shortage of pediatric dentists trained in the care of medically complex children. By definition, medically complex children have many chronic and sometimes life-limiting conditions, and oral health care may not be prioritized. Children with autism and behavioral difficulties may be challenging to examine and treat, and, if nonverbal, they may be less likely to express pain related to oral health concerns.[98] In addition, they may have oral sensory aversions that make toothbrushing a difficult task. Medications (eg, asthma medications, anticonvulsants, antidepressants, diuretics) and medical interventions (eg, gastrostomy tube feeding) can alter saliva quality and quantity as a side effect, leading to a higher risk of dental caries. Delays in access to oral care for children with special health care needs can result in the need to postpone medical interventions, such as the administration of chemotherapy, heart surgery, and bone marrow and organ transplants.

FUTURE ORAL HEALTH CONSIDERATIONS IN CLINICAL PRACTICE: THE ORAL MICROBIOME AND SALIVARY DIAGNOSTICS

Personalized health care, with its promise of more efficient, effective, and individualized diagnostics and concomitant therapies, is transforming the health care landscape. It is increasingly being recognized that a better understanding of the development of individuals' microbiomes (and the effects of chronic disease, antibiotic use, nutrition, and so forth) will be helpful to facilitate future diagnostic and therapeutic opportunities in this arena. Current research suggests that acquisition, development, and maturation of the oral microbiome is a dynamic process that begins at, or even before birth. Further, a strong link seems to exist between oral microbial dysbiosis (imbalance between the host and its microbiome) and the development of oral diseases such as periodontal disease and dental caries.[99] Research into the oral microbiome therefore, is one of the most exciting and promising areas in oral health care, with saliva offering a rapid and noninvasive way to realize the needed diagnostic possibilities for developing personalized oral health care.

Genomic studies of dental caries lesions reveal a more complex picture of these disease processes than was previously thought. Emerging evidence suggests a previously unrecognized diversity of the oral microbiome, with more than 700 species currently identified as constituting the complex microbiome of the oral cavity.[100] Earlier studies implicated *S mutans* in the initiation, and *Streptococcus sobrinus* and *Lactobacillus* spp. in the progression, of dental caries. Recent polymerase chain reaction–based analyses suggest a more significant role of other bacterial species, including *Streptococcus sanguinis*, *S sobrinus*, *Streptococcus mitis*, and *Streptococcus intermedius*.[101] Dietary exposures to, for example, highly acidic foods promote the self-selection of acidogenic and aciduric oral microbiota, including, but not limited to *S mutans*. This self-selection in turn promotes progression of dental caries, with a concomitant reduction in the diversity of the oral microbiota to species that can survive in the highly acidic local environment.[101] Studies also have suggested a role for *Candida albicans* in the development of dental caries because of the commonly noted co-occurrence of *Candida* and *S mutans* in early childhood caries.[102,103] Although discussed in various forums, vaccination against organisms causing dental caries remains elusive from a practical standpoint.

Similar to dental caries, great progress is being made in the understanding of periodontal disease initiation and progression. Previous research provided evidence for the central role of *Porphyromonas gingivalis* in initiation of chronic periodontal disease. Further, *Aggregatibacter actinomycetemcomitans* and *Treponema* species are implicated in juvenile aggressive periodontitis observed as early as 6 years of age.[104] However, more recent research suggests additionally complex interactions between minor oral microbial consortia and host immune response in the pathogenesis of periodontal disease.[101] In addition, periodontal pathogens, including *Tannerella forsythia* and *P gingivalis*, are implicated in the pathogenesis of esophageal adenocarcinoma and esophageal squamous cell carcinoma, respectively.[105]

From a developmental perspective, a growing understanding of disease processes can be anticipated using metagenomics approaches that move beyond the isolation and cultivation of individual oral microbial species. For example, salivary diagnostics are already being used for noninvasive testing to identify HPVs related to oral cancers, assess risk for periodontal disease, measure stress levels using salivary cortisol, and identify periodontal pathogens.[106] The possibilities for salivary diagnostics seem endless, with new applications emerging at a rapid pace. These emerging metagenomic innovations, along with the ability to analyze the resulting vast datasets of information should generate new knowledge likely to propel clinicians into the era of precision oral medicine and personalized oral health care.

SUMMARY

This article reviews the unique challenges and opportunities offered by the evolving and dynamic nature of pediatric oral health. It highlights important oral health–related developmental milestones, dental anomalies, and problems affecting oral health that may be observed during children's or adolescents' life courses. Pediatric primary care providers can use this information to identify oral health–related issues and provide anticipatory guidance related to oral health as part of services offered by children's medical homes. Early identification of any oral health problems and coordination of needed care with dental health professionals can assist in maximizing oral health outcomes for children, adolescents, and their families.

REFERENCES

1. Halfon N, Larson K, Lu M, et al. Lifecourse health development: past, present and future. Matern Child Health J 2014;18(2):344–65.
2. Jackson SL, Vann WF Jr, Kotch JB, et al. Impact of poor oral health on children's school attendance and performance. Am J Public Health 2011;101(10):1900–6.
3. Broadbent JM, Zeng J, Foster Page LA, et al. Oral health-related beliefs, behaviors, and outcomes through the life course. J Dent Res 2016;95(7):808–13.
4. Lu HX, Wong MC, Lo EC, et al. Trends in oral health from childhood to early adulthood: a life course approach. Community Dent Oral Epidemiol 2011;39(4):352–60.
5. Heilmann A, Tsakos G, Watt RG. Oral health over the life course. In: Burton-Jeangros C, Cullati S, Sacker A, et al, editors. A life course perspective on health trajectories and transitions. Cham (CH) (Switzerland): Springer; 2015. p. 39–59.
6. Nanci A. Ten Cate's oral histology: development, structure, and function. 6th edition. St Louis (MO): Mosby; 2003.

7. Rahimov F, Jugessur A, Murray JC. Genetics of nonsyndromic orofacial clefts. Cleft Palate Craniofac J 2012;49(1):73–91.
8. Ranta R. A review of tooth formation in children with cleft lip/palate. Am J Orthod Dentofacial Orthop 1986;90(1):11–8.
9. Orban BJ. Orban's oral histology and embryology. St Louis (MO): Mosby; 1991.
10. Rubin LP. Maternal and pediatric health and disease: integrating bio-psychosocial models and epigenetics. Pediatr Res 2016;79(1–2):127–35.
11. Silk H, Douglass AB, Douglass JM, et al. Oral health during pregnancy. Am Fam Physician 2008;77(8):1139–44.
12. Finlayson TL, Gupta A, Ramos-Gomez FJ. Prenatal maternal factors, intergenerational transmission of disease, and child oral health outcomes. Dent Clin North Am 2017;61(3):483–518.
13. Iida H. Oral health interventions during pregnancy. Dent Clin North Am 2017; 61(3):467–81.
14. Offenbacher S, Boggess KA, Murtha AP, et al. Progressive periodontal disease and risk of very preterm delivery. Obstet Gynecol 2006;107(1):29–36.
15. Offenbacher S, Lieff S, Boggess KA, et al. Maternal periodontitis and prematurity. Part I: obstetric outcome of prematurity and growth restriction. Ann Periodontol 2001;6(1):164–74.
16. Goldenberg RL, Culhane JF, Iams JD, et al. Epidemiology and causes of preterm birth. Lancet 2008;371(9606):75–84.
17. da Silva Bastos Vde A, Freitas-Fernandes LB, Fidalgo TK, et al. Mother-to-child transmission of Streptococcus mutans: a systematic review and meta-analysis. J Dent 2015;43(2):181–91.
18. Kilian M, Chapple IL, Hannig M, et al. The oral microbiome - an update for oral healthcare professionals. Br Dent J 2016;221(10):657–66.
19. Vinturache AE, Gyamfi-Bannerman C, Hwang J, et al, Preterm Birth International Collaborative (PREBIC). Maternal microbiome - a pathway to preterm birth. Semin Fetal Neonatal Med 2016;21(2):94–9.
20. Cobb CM, Kelly PJ, Williams KB, et al. The oral microbiome and adverse pregnancy outcomes. Int J Womens Health 2017;9:551–9.
21. Fox C, Eichelberger K. Maternal microbiome and pregnancy outcomes. Fertil Steril 2015;104(6):1358–63.
22. Lif Holgerson P, Harnevik L, Hernell O, et al. Mode of birth delivery affects oral microbiota in infants. J Dent Res 2011;90(10):1183–8.
23. Hong L, Levy SM, Warren JJ, et al. Association between enamel hypoplasia and dental caries in primary second molars: a cohort study. Caries Res 2009;43(5): 345–53.
24. Finlayson TL, Siefert K, Ismail AI, et al. Maternal self-efficacy and 1-5-year-old children's brushing habits. Community Dent Oral Epidemiol 2007;35(4):272–81.
25. Huebner CE, Riedy CA. Behavioral determinants of brushing young children's teeth: implications for anticipatory guidance. Pediatr Dent 2010;32(1):48–55.
26. Goettems ML, Ardenghi TM, Demarco FF, et al. Children's use of dental services: influence of maternal dental anxiety, attendance pattern, and perception of children's quality of life. Community Dent Oral Epidemiol 2012;40(5):451–8.
27. Chaffee BW, Gansky SA, Weintraub JA, et al. Maternal oral bacterial levels predict early childhood caries development. J Dent Res 2014;93(3):238–44.
28. Dye BA, Vargas CM, Lee JJ, et al. Assessing the relationship between children's oral health status and that of their mothers. J Am Dent Assoc 2011;142(2): 173–83.

29. O'Shea JE, Foster JP, O'Donnell CP, et al. Frenotomy for tongue-tie in newborn infants. Cochrane Database Syst Rev 2017;(3):CD011065.

30. Walsh J, Tunkel D. Diagnosis and treatment of ankyloglossia in newborns and infants: a review. JAMA Otolaryngol Head Neck Surg 2017;143(10):1032–9.

31. Krol DM, Keels MA. Oral conditions. Pediatr Rev 2007;28(1):15–22.

32. Pinkham J, Casamassimo P, McTigue D, et al. Pediatric dentistry: infancy through adolescence. St Louis (MO): Elsevier Saunders; 2005.

33. Leighton BC. The early signs of malocclusion. Eur J Orthod 2007;29(Suppl 1): i89–95.

34. American Academy of Pediatrics (AAP). Brush, book, bed: how to structure your child's nighttime routine. Available at: https://www.healthychildren.org/English/healthy-living/oral-health/Pages/Brush-Book-Bed.aspx. Accessed December 9, 2017.

35. Cunha RF, Boer FA, Torriani DD, et al. Natal and neonatal teeth: review of the literature. Pediatr Dent 2001;23(2):158–62.

36. Leung AK, Robson WL. Natal teeth: a review. J Natl Med Assoc 2006;98(2): 226–8.

37. Galassi MS, Santos-Pinto L, Ramalho LT. Natal maxillary primary molars: case report. J Clin Pediatr Dent 2004;29(1):41–4.

38. Padmanabhan MY, Pandey RK, Aparna R, et al. Neonatal sublingual traumatic ulceration - case report & review of the literature. Dent Traumatol 2010;26(6): 490–5.

39. Goho C. Neonatal sublingual traumatic ulceration (Riga-Fede disease): reports of cases. ASDC J Dent Child 1996;63(5):362–4.

40. Cizmeci MN, Kanburoglu MK, Kara S, et al. Bohn's nodules: peculiar neonatal intraoral lesions mistaken for natal teeth. Eur J Pediatr 2014;173(3):403.

41. Clarke M, Locker D, Berall G, et al. Malnourishment in a population of young children with severe early childhood caries. Pediatr Dent 2006;28(3):254–9.

42. American Academy of Pediatric Dentistry. Guideline on fluoride therapy. Pediatr Dent 2013;35(5):E165–8. Updated guideline available at: http://www.aapd.org/media/policies_guidelines/g_fluoridetherapy.pdf. Accessed June 21, 2018.

43. American Academy of Pediatrics Section On Oral Health. Maintaining and improving the oral health of young children. Pediatrics 2014;134(6):1224–9.

44. Heyman MB, Abrams SA, AAP Section on Gastroenterology, Hepatology, and Nutrition, Nutrition, Committee On Nutrition. Fruit juice in infants, children, and adolescents: current recommendations. Pediatrics 2017;139(6):e20170967.

45. Nowak AJ, Casamassimo PS. The dental home: a primary care oral health concept. J Am Dent Assoc 2002;133(1):93–8.

46. Juuri E, Balic A. The biology underlying abnormalities of tooth number in humans. J Dent Res 2017;96(11):1248–56.

47. Pahel BT, Vann WF Jr, Divaris K, et al. A contemporary examination of first and second permanent molar emergence. J Dent Res 2017;96(10):1115–21.

48. Bloch-Zupan A. Hypophosphatasia: diagnosis and clinical signs - a dental surgeon perspective. Int J Paediatr Dent 2016;26(6):426–38.

49. The Organisation for Economic Co-operation and Development (OECD). The demographic and family environment. In. Babies and Bosses - Reconciling work and family life: a synthesis of findings for OECD countries. Paris: OECD Publishing; 2007. Available at: https://doi.org/10.1787/9789264032477-3-en. Accessed June 12, 2018.

50. Dong YM, Pearce EI, Yue L, et al. Plaque pH and associated parameters in relation to caries. Caries Res 1999;33(6):428–36.

51. Gidding SS, Dennison BA, Birch LL, et al. Dietary recommendations for children and adolescents: a guide for practitioners. Pediatrics 2006;117(2):544–59.

52. Pujar P, Subbareddy VV. Evaluation of the tooth brushing skills in children aged 6-12 years. Eur Arch Paediatr Dent 2013;14(4):213–9.

53. Marshman Z, Ahern SM, McEachan RRC, et al. Parents' experiences of toothbrushing with children: a qualitative study. JDR Clin Trans Res 2016;1(2):122–30.

54. Nowak AJ, Warren JJ. Infant oral health and oral habits. Pediatr Clin North Am 2000;47(5):1043–66, vi.

55. Borrie FR, Bearn DR, Innes NP, et al. Interventions for the cessation of non-nutritive sucking habits in children. Cochrane Database Syst Rev 2015;(3):CD008694.

56. Andersson L, Andreasen JO, Day P, et al. Guidelines for the management of traumatic dental injuries: 2. Avulsion of permanent teeth. Pediatr Dent 2016;38(6):369–76.

57. Schneider MB, Benjamin HJ. American Academy of Pediatrics Committee on Nutrition and the Council on Sports Medicine and Fitness. Clinical report–sports drinks and energy drinks for children and adolescents: are they appropriate? 2011. Available at: http://pediatrics.aappublications.org/content/pediatrics/early/2011/05/25/peds.2011-0965.full.pdf. Accessed December 9, 2017.

58. Vazquez-Otero C, Vamos CA, Thompson EL, et al. Assessing dentists' human papillomavirus-related health literacy for oropharyngeal cancer prevention. J Am Dent Assoc 2018;149(1):9–17.

59. Hagan JF, Shaw JS, Duncan PM, editors. Bright Futures: Guidelines for health supervision of infants, children and adolescents. 4th edition. Itasca (IL): American Academy of Pediatrics; 2017.

60. Clinical Affairs Committee American Academy of Pediatric Dentistry. Guideline on adolescent oral health care. Pediatr Dent 2015;37(5):49–56.

61. Wang YC, Bleich SN, Gortmaker SL. Increasing caloric contribution from sugar-sweetened beverages and 100% fruit juices among US children and adolescents, 1988-2004. Pediatrics 2008;121(6):e1604–14.

62. Wahlund K, List T, Dworkin SF. Temporomandibular disorders in children and adolescents: reliability of a questionnaire, clinical examination, and diagnosis. J Orofac Pain 1998;12(1):42–51.

63. da Silva CG, Pacheco-Pereira C, Porporatti AL, et al. Prevalence of clinical signs of intra-articular temporomandibular disorders in children and adolescents: a systematic review and meta-analysis. J Am Dent Assoc 2016;147(1):10–8.e8.

64. Saulue P, Carra MC, Laluque JF, et al. Understanding bruxism in children and adolescents. Int Orthod 2015;13(4):489–506.

65. Milosevic A. Eating disorders and the dentist. Br Dent J 1999;186(3):109–13.

66. Kisely S, Baghaie H, Lalloo R, et al. Association between poor oral health and eating disorders: systematic review and meta-analysis. Br J Psychiatry 2015;207(4):299–305.

67. De Moor RJ, De Witte AM, Delme KI, et al. Dental and oral complications of lip and tongue piercings. Br Dent J 2005;199(8):506–9.

68. Breuner CC, Levine DA, AAP The committee on adolescence. Adolescent and young adult tattooing, piercing, and scarification. Pediatrics 2018;141(2) [pii: e20173630].

69. Cunha RF, Pugliesi DM, de Mello Vieira AE. Oral trauma in Brazilian patients aged 0-3 years. Dent Traumatol 2001;17(5):210–2.

70. Hargreaves JA, Cleaton-Jones PE, Roberts GJ, et al. Trauma to primary teeth of South African pre-school children. Endod Dent Traumatol 1999;15(2):73–6.

71. Bijella MF, Yared FN, Bijella VT, et al. Occurrence of primary incisor traumatism in Brazilian children: a house-by-house survey. ASDC J Dent Child 1990;57(6): 424–7.

72. Yagot KH, Nazhat NY, Kuder SA. Traumatic dental injuries in nursery schoolchildren from Baghdad, Iraq. Community Dent Oral Epidemiol 1988;16(5):292–3.

73. Pugliesi DM, Cunha RF, Delbem AC, et al. Influence of the type of dental trauma on the pulp vitality and the time elapsed until treatment: a study in patients aged 0-3 years. Dent Traumatol 2004;20(3):139–42.

74. do Espirito Santo Jacomo DR, Campos V. Prevalence of sequelae in the permanent anterior teeth after trauma in their predecessors: a longitudinal study of 8 years. Dent Traumatol 2009;25(3):300–4.

75. Andersson L. Epidemiology of traumatic dental injuries. Pediatr Dent 2013; 35(2):102–5.

76. Malmgren B, Andreasen JO, Flores MT, et al. International Association of Dental Traumatology guidelines for the management of traumatic dental injuries: 3. Injuries in the primary dentition. Dent Traumatol 2012;28(3):174–82.

77. DiAngelis AJ, Andreasen JO, Ebeleseder KA, et al. Guidelines for the management of traumatic dental injuries: 1. Fractures and luxations of permanent teeth. Pediatr Dent 2016;38(6):358–68.

78. Siqueira MB, Gomes MC, Oliveira AC, et al. Predisposing factors for traumatic dental injury in primary teeth and seeking of post-trauma care. Braz Dent J 2013;24(6):647–54.

79. von Arx T. Developmental disturbances of permanent teeth following trauma to the primary dentition. Aust Dent J 1993;38(1):1–10.

80. O'Connor EA, Evans CV, Burda BU, et al. Screening for obesity and intervention for weight management in children and adolescents: evidence report and systematic review for the US preventive services task force. JAMA 2017;317(23): 2427–44.

81. Hayden C, Bowler JO, Chambers S, et al. Obesity and dental caries in children: a systematic review and meta-analysis. Community Dent Oral Epidemiol 2013; 41(4):289–308.

82. Li LW, Wong HM, Peng SM, et al. Anthropometric measurements and dental caries in children: a systematic review of longitudinal studies. Adv Nutr 2015; 6(1):52–63.

83. Shefferly A, Scharf RJ, DeBoer MD. Longitudinal evaluation of 100% fruit juice consumption on BMI status in 2-5-year-old children. Pediatr Obes 2016;11(3): 221–7.

84. Scherrer PD, Mallory MD, Cravero JP, et al. The impact of obesity on pediatric procedural sedation-related outcomes: results from the Pediatric Sedation Research Consortium. Paediatr Anaesth 2015;25(7):689–97.

85. Ehsan Z, Ishman SL. Pediatric obstructive sleep apnea. Otolaryngol Clin North Am 2016;49(6):1449–64.

86. US Department of Health and Human Services. Preventing tobacco use among young people: a report of the surgeon general. Atlanta (GA): US Department of Health and Human Services, Centers for Disease Control and Prevention, Office on Smoking and Health; 1994. Available at: http://profiles.nlm.nih.gov/NN/B/C/L/ Q. Accessed December 9, 2017.

87. Clinical Affairs Committee American Academy of Pediatric Dentistry. Policy on tobacco use. Pediatr Dent 2015;38(6):62–6.

88. Grana RA, Popova L, Ling PM. A longitudinal analysis of electronic cigarette use and smoking cessation. JAMA Intern Med 2014;174(5):812–3.
89. Dutra LM, Glantz SA. Electronic cigarettes and conventional cigarette use among U.S. adolescents: a cross-sectional study. JAMA Pediatr 2014;168(7): 610–7.
90. Phillips M, Masterson E, Sabbah W. Association between child caries and maternal health-related behaviours. Community Dent Health 2016;33(2): 133–7.
91. Leroy R, Hoppenbrouwers K, Jara A, et al. Parental smoking behavior and caries experience in preschool children. Community Dent Oral Epidemiol 2008;36(3):249–57.
92. Needleman HL, Allred E, Bellinger D, et al. Antecedents and correlates of hypoplastic enamel defects of primary incisors. Pediatr Dent 1992;14(3):158–66.
93. Ford D, Seow WK, Kazoullis S, et al. A controlled study of risk factors for enamel hypoplasia in the permanent dentition. Pediatr Dent 2009;31(5):382–8.
94. Johnston LD, O'Malley PM, Miech RA, et al. Monitoring the future national survey results on drug use: 1975-2014: overview, key findings on adolescent drug use. Ann Arbor (MI): Institute for Social Research, The University of Michigan; 2015. Available at: http://www.monitoringthefuture.org/pubs/monographs/mtf-overview2014.pdf. Accessed December 9, 2017.
95. Center for Behavioral Health Statistics and Quality. Behavioral health trends in the United States: results from the 2014 National Survey on Drug Use and Health. (HHS publication no. SMA 15–4927, NSDUH series H-50). 2015. Available at: http://www.samhsa.gov/data/. Accessed December 10, 2017.
96. Clinical Affairs Committee American Academy of Pediatric Dentistry. Policy on substance abuse in adolescent patients. Pediatr Dent 2017;39(6): 77–80.
97. Newacheck PW, McManus M, Fox HB, et al. Access to health care for children with special health care needs. Pediatrics 2000;105(4 Pt 1):760–6.
98. Hennequin M, Faulks D, Roux D. Accuracy of estimation of dental treatment need in special care patients. J Dent 2000;28(2):131–6.
99. Zarco MF, Vess TJ, Ginsburg GS. The oral microbiome in health and disease and the potential impact on personalized dental medicine. Oral Dis 2012; 18(2):109–20.
100. Benn A, Heng N, Broadbent JM, et al. Studying the human oral microbiome: challenges and the evolution of solutions. Aust Dent J 2018;63(1): 14–24.
101. Costalonga M, Herzberg MC. The oral microbiome and the immunobiology of periodontal disease and caries. Immunol Lett 2014;162(2 Pt A):22–38.
102. de Carvalho FG, Silva DS, Hebling J, et al. Presence of mutans streptococci and Candida spp. in dental plaque/dentine of carious teeth and early childhood caries. Arch Oral Biol 2006;51(11):1024–8.
103. Yang XQ, Zhang Q, Lu LY, et al. Genotypic distribution of Candida albicans in dental biofilm of Chinese children associated with severe early childhood caries. Arch Oral Biol 2012;57(8):1048–53.
104. Albandar JM, Tinoco EM. Global epidemiology of periodontal diseases in children and young persons. Periodontol 2000 2002;29:153–76.
105. Peters BA, Wu J, Pei Z, et al. Oral microbiome composition reflects prospective risk for esophageal cancers. Cancer Res 2017;77(23):6777–87.
106. Genco RJ. Salivary diagnostic tests. J Am Dent Assoc 2012;143(10 Suppl): 3S–5S.

Infant Oral Health

Erica A. Brecher, DMD, MS[a], Charlotte W. Lewis, MD, MPH[b],*

KEYWORDS

• Infant • Dental caries • Fluoride • Primary dentition • Prevention

KEY POINTS

• Habits established in infancy affect future oral health.
• Fluoride is the cornerstone of preventive oral health.
• Habits that promote oral health in infants also support normal growth and development and help establish a healthy lifestyle.

INTRODUCTION

At first glance, *infant* (defined as children younger than 12 months of age) and *oral health* may not seem like words that belong together. After all, most infants are born without teeth and usually remain toothless for the first half of their infancy. By the time infants turn 1 year old, they probably only have a few teeth. One might ask, Why even worry about oral health in infancy? As it turns out, infancy is a critical time to establish habits, both good and bad, that have the potential to affect an individual's future oral health as well as overall health and well-being into adolescence and beyond. Maintaining healthy baby teeth, also referred to as primary teeth, is critical to facilitate proper growth and development in children. Primary teeth are important for eating, speaking, and growth of the jaws. Dental caries and premature loss of baby teeth can lead to severe problems in the permanent dentition. Primary pediatric care practitioners typically have multiple visits with infants and their parents before they see a dentist and therefore have a crucial role to play in promoting positive oral health practices and habits.

NORMAL DENTAL DEVELOPMENT AND ERUPTION

Teeth start to develop in utero. The primary dentition initiates formation at approximately 6 weeks to 8 weeks of gestation and dentition begins to calcify by the end of the first trimester. Most of the permanent dentition begins to form at approximately 5 months

Disclosures: Neither author has financial or any other conflict of interest related to the material discussed here.
[a] Department of Pediatric Dentistry, Virginia Commonwealth University School of Dentistry, 521 North 11th Street, PO Box 980566, Richmond, VA 23298, USA; [b] Department of Pediatrics, UW School of Medicine, Seattle Children's Hospital, UW Box 354920, Seattle, WA 98195, USA
* Corresponding author.
E-mail address: cwlewis@uw.edu

of gestation, calcifying after birth. Even though the primary teeth begin to form in utero, most infants do not have erupted teeth present at birth. When erupted teeth are present at birth, estimated to occur in the range of approximately 1 in 2000 births,[1] these are known as natal teeth. If teeth erupt within the first month of life, they are referred to as neonatal teeth. Natal and neonatal teeth are usually mandibular (lower) incisors, and more than 90% represent normal dentition, not extra (supernumerary) teeth. Usually no intervention is required. If natal/neonatal teeth interfere with feeding, cause traumatic ulceration of the tongue (Riga-Fede disease), or are so loose that they may pose an aspiration risk, however, a dentist should be consulted. Because they usually comprise the normal dentition, extraction should be avoided if possible.

More commonly, the first tooth erupts at approximately 6 months of age. There is substantial variability between individuals in dental eruption timing. But neither a 4 month old with 2 teeth nor a 9 month old with no teeth should cause concern. The primary teeth erupt sequentially, at a rate of approximately 1 tooth per month, until all 20 primary teeth have erupted by approximately 24 months to 30 months of age (**Table 1**). The first primary teeth to erupt are typically the mandibular (lower) central incisors. The usual sequence of primary tooth eruption is central incisors, lateral incisors, first molars, canines (cuspids), and finally the second molars (**Fig. 1**). Primary tooth approximate eruption timing is presented in **Table 1**.

Eruption of a tooth may occasionally be preceded by an eruption hematoma or eruption cyst. It appears as a bluish swelling overlying the area where the tooth is about to erupt. These are self-limiting, and the hematoma or cyst subsides as the tooth erupts normally. Commonly, primary teeth eruption, referred to as "teething" is associated with symptoms, such as fussiness, drooling, biting, sucking, sleep disturbances, ear-rubbing, facial rash, mild temperature elevation, and decreased appetite for solids.[2] Teething does not cause diarrhea, respiratory infections, or true fever,[2] although teeth eruption and these entities may be present coincidentally. Some children find a cool teething ring to be soothing, and, occasionally, acetaminophen or ibuprofen may be needed to reduce pain from teething. The Food and Drug Administration has issued warnings against the use of benzocaine or viscous lidocaine and homeopathic teething tablets for teething because these have been associated with serious or fatal side effects in young children.[3,4]

Dental Anatomy

The visible portion of a tooth is called the crown. The crowns of primary teeth, except for the primary molars, are smaller than their permanent successors. The crown consists of 3 layers: enamel (a hard, outer protective layer), dentin (made up of tubules to transport nutrients within a tooth), and pulp (nerves and vascular structures critical for the health

Primary Tooth Name	Eruption Timing	
	Upper[a]	Lower[b]
Central incisor	8–12 mo	6–10 mo
Lateral incisor	9–13 mo	10–16 mo
Canine	16–22 mo	17–23 mo
First molar	13–19 mo	14–18 mo
Second molar	25–33 mo	23–31 mo

Table 1
Approximate ages of primary teeth eruption in the upper and lower jaws

[a] Upper: maxillary.
[b] Lower: mandibular.

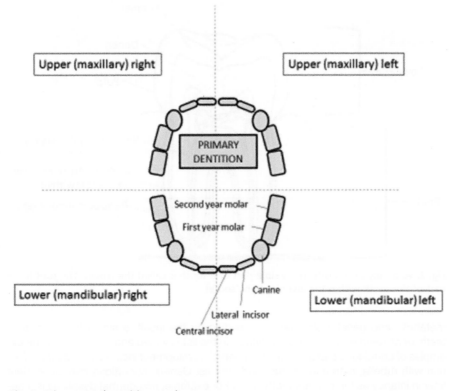

Fig. 1. Primary teeth positions and names.

and viability of the tooth). Primary teeth have thinner layers of enamel and dentin compared with permanent teeth, which make the teeth more susceptible to dental decay. The root is the portion of the teeth within the alveolar bone and is covered with cementum. Teeth are anchored to bone by periodontal ligaments (**Fig. 2**).

PATHOLOGIC CONDITIONS AFFECTING INFANT ORAL HEALTH
Congenital Conditions

Cleft lip and palate
One of the most common congenital anomalies affecting the oral cavity is cleft lip and/ or cleft palate. Oral clefts affect feeding, speech, craniofacial growth and development, and appearance and have important implications for oral health. Children born with clefts may have missing teeth or extra teeth, commonly have malocclusion requiring orthodontic and surgical treatment and are at increased risk for dental caries and periodontal disease.[5] Children born with cleft lip and/or cleft palate should receive specialized care throughout their infancy, childhood, and adolescence from a multidisciplinary cleft or craniofacial team. In addition to surgical and medical specialists, dental professionals on this team may include a pediatric dentist, orthodontist, prosthodontist, and oral surgeon. An overview of various components of cleft care during infancy and childhood is available elsewhere.[5]

Anomalies of dentition
Several congenital factors and prenatal exposures can adversely affect tooth structure and color, including maternal medications, congenital infections, jaundice, and

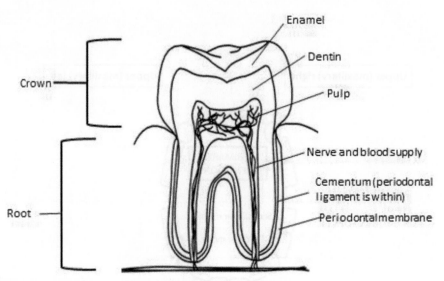

Fig. 2. Anatomy of a tooth. The visible part of a tooth is called the crown. The root is the part of the tooth within the alveolar bone socket.

metabolic and genetic disorders. Depending on the insult, a single tooth, multiple teeth, or all teeth may be affected. Although the list is varied and extensive, some examples of conditions that affect in utero dental development include intrauterine infection with rubella, cytomegalovirus, and syphilis. Genetic conditions may be evident later in infancy as the primary teeth erupt. For example, ectodermal dysplasia is a genetic disorder affecting skin, hair, and teeth. In addition to sweat gland dysfunction and difficulty controlling body temperature, children with ectodermal dysplasia also present with hypodontia (fewer than the normal number of teeth) and malformed (conical) teeth. The jaws of such patients may also be underdeveloped. Other genetic conditions, such as amelogenesis imperfecta and dentinogenesis imperfecta, affect the quality of enamel and dentin, respectively. Although these conditions do not have systemic findings, they can be debilitating in terms of oral findings: painful/sensitive teeth, high caries risk, multiple abscesses and necrotic teeth, and poor esthetics.

Although only primary dentition is present during the first year of life, insults during infancy may adversely affect permanent dentition. For example, a local dental infection in early childhood, such as a periapical abscess involving a primary tooth, can affect the development of the underlying permanent tooth. Especially in children younger than 3 years of age (because this is when the permanent incisor crowns are developing within the jaw), orofacial trauma that causes damage or displacement to the primary teeth can result in malformation or hypomineralization defects in the underlying permanent teeth. In the event of trauma, after evaluation by a physician, patients should be referred to their dentist for further assessment and management.

Acquired Conditions Affecting Infant Oral Health

Dental caries

Prevention of dental caries, the most common chronic disease of childhood, should begin in the prenatal period. During 2011 to 2014, 24% of US children between 2 years and 5 years of age had experienced caries.[6] Dental caries can be a transmissible infectious disease in which cariogenic bacteria are passed from caregiver, usually the mother, to child.[7] The earlier that a child is infected, the higher the risk for early caries onset.[8,9] The maternal caries status is strongly associated with that of their children.[10,11] In high-caries risk groups, babies are colonized with cariogenic bacteria before their first teeth erupt.[11,12] The potential for transmission of cariogenic bacteria from parent to infant emphasizes the importance of oral health for the entire family and of establishing and maintaining healthy habits in infancy. The American Academy of Pediatric Dentistry (AAPD) provides caries risk assessment tools for physicians and can be used as an important education tool for families and caregivers (**Fig. 3**).[13]

Once teeth erupt, cariogenic bacteria and carbohydrate substrate are all that are needed to initiate the caries process. Cariogenic bacteria, including *Streptococcus mutans* and lactobacilli, produce acid as the end product of carbohydrate metabolism. In turn, the acid dissolves the calcium-phosphate mineral of the tooth's enamel in a process called demineralization. Demineralization of a tooth begins with a chalky white spot lesion and eventually causes collapse of the tooth's structure resulting in cavitation (**Fig. 4**). Saliva contains calcium, phosphorus, fluoride, antibodies, and buffering agents that can assist in remineralizing the tooth.

This ongoing demineralization-remineralization dynamic can be pushed in the direction of demineralization if the biofilm pH persistently remains below 5.5. Ongoing acidic conditions occur, for example, with frequent snacking on carbohydrate-rich foods/beverages (**Fig. 5**). When snacking is less frequent, there is more time for the biofilm pH to return to normal, which favors remineralization. Although seemingly simplistic, a complex interplay of behavioral, social, environmental, and genetic variables—some better understood than others—influences the caries process.

Factors	High Risk	Low Risk
Biological		
Mother/primary caregiver has active cavities	Yes	
Parent/caregiver has low socioeconomic status	Yes	
Child has >3 between meal sugar-containing snacks or beverages per day	Yes	
Child is put to bed with a bottle containing natural or added sugar	Yes	
Child has special health care needs	Yes	
Child is a recent immigrant	Yes	
Protective		
Child receives optimally fluoridated drinking water or fluoride supplements		Yes
Child has teeth brushed daily with fluoridated toothpaste		Yes
Child receives topical fluoride from health professional		Yes
Child has dental home/regular dental care		Yes
Clinical Findings		
Child has white spot lesions or enamel defects	Yes	
Child has visible cavities or fillings	Yes	
Child has plaque on teeth	Yes	

Circling those conditions that apply to a specific patient helps the health care worker and parent understand the factors that contribute to or protect from caries. Risk assessment categorization of low or high is based on preponderance of factors for the individual. However, clinical judgment may justify the use of one factor (e.g., frequent exposure to sugar containing snacks or beverages, visible cavities) in determining overall risk.

Overall assessment of the child's dental caries risk: High ☐   Low ☐

Fig. 3. Caries risk assessment tool for physicians and other nondental health care providers. (*From* American Academy of Pediatric Dentistry. Caries-risk assessment and management for children, infants, and adolescents. Reference Manual. Pediatr Dent 2017;39(6):198; with permission.)

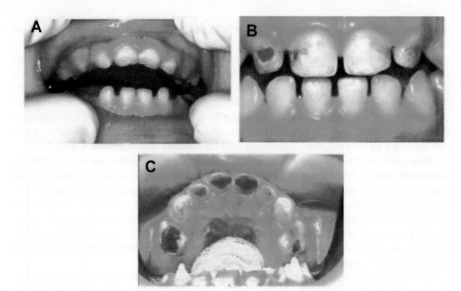

Fig. 4. ECC. Progression from white spot lesions to extensive involvement of the entire dentition. (*A*) white spots represent earliest visible stage of ECC. (*B*) Decay has progressed through enamel in moderate ECC. (*C*) Extensive ECC affecting all of the primary dentition.

Caries in infants and young children are referred to as early childhood caries (ECC). Previously referred to as baby bottle tooth decay or nursing bottle caries, ECC is defined as caries occurring in children younger than 6 years of age. Typically, ECC first affects the maxillary (upper) incisors, initially appearing as chalky white spots along the gingival margin (see **Fig. 4**), and spares the mandibular (lower) incisors.[14] This pattern

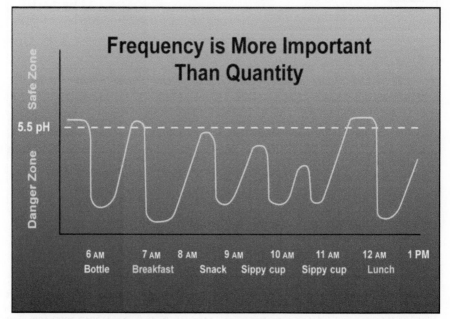

Fig. 5. Dietary practices influence oral pH. (*Courtesy of* RB. Quinonez, DMD, and Dave Krol, MD.)

of caries is hypothesized to result from prolonged and frequent exposure of the teeth to sweetened liquids, such as falling asleep with a bottle of juice or milk in the mouth or prolonged nighttime breastfeeding. ECC may progress quickly to involve most of the remaining primary dentition (see **Fig. 4**B, C). If an infection is left untreated it can progress locally to the developing permanent tooth or can spread systemically, producing serious effects on a child's health.

PREVENTING ORAL DISEASE AND PROMOTING ORAL HEALTH IN INFANCY

Preventing caries and promoting oral health begins with establishing healthy habits in infancy. Modeled after the medical home concept, the dental home should ideally be established by 1 year of age, according to the AAPD guidelines.[15] The dental home is defined as the "ongoing relationship between dentist and patient, inclusive of all aspects of oral health care delivered in a comprehensive, continuously accessible, coordinated, and family-centered way." Early establishment of a dental home facilitates access to preventative and emergency services, improves oral health outcomes, and reduces dental care costs for children.[16,17] Pediatric primary care providers also play an essential role in oral health through provision of anticipatory guidance about oral health at well-child-care visits, oral examination, timely referral to a dental home, and application of fluoride varnish (FV). The role of the pediatric primary care provider in promoting oral health is particularly important during infancy—before children have visited a dentist—and when children have difficulty accessing professional dental care.[18]

There are specific modalities for caries prevention, such as fluoride toothpaste (FTP), but optimal oral health is also the product of healthy eating habits that begin in infancy. Healthy eating habits, such as limiting sugary beverages; avoiding high-fat and processed foods; and emphasizing fresh fruits, vegetables, whole grains, lean meats, and low-fat dairy not only support oral health but also promote overall good health and a healthy weight.

Normal Infant Nutrition and Sucking

An understanding of preventive oral health in infancy requires an overview of normal infant diet as well as nutritive and non-nutritive sucking. Healthy full-term newborns are born fully able to suck and to coordinate sucking, swallowing, and breathing when they feed. The first evidence of sucking and swallowing occurs early in gestation, but a more mature and coordinated suck-swallow-breathe pattern emerges at approximately 34 weeks of gestation. Sucking may be nutritive (to obtain nutrition) or non-nutritive (eg, comfort nursing from sucking on a finger or a pacifier). During infancy, non-nutritive sucking serves many beneficial functions including promoting normal craniofacial growth and function and helping babies to calm and to fall asleep on their own. Pacifier use under the age of 1 has also been found to reduce the incidence of sudden infant death syndrome.[19] When non-nutritive sucking persists beyond infancy, it can lead to malocclusion.

Healthy Dietary Practices to Promote Oral Health

Until 5 months or 6 months of age, infants only need liquid nutrition, ideally, human breast milk suckled from the mother's breast. Breast milk has several immunologic, nutritional, digestive, and other benefits. Exclusive breastfeeding, however, is not always possible for a variety of reasons. Breast milk can be pumped from a mother's breast and fed to a baby from a bottle, but when neither breastfeeding nor bottle-fed expressed breast milk is possible, infant formula can be fed via bottle. In such cases, preparing infant formula from a powder is the most economical option, as long as clean water is available. For the first 12 months of life, infants do not need any other beverages except breast milk or infant formula—no juice, soda, or cow's or goat's milk. The American Academy of Pediatrics recommends that juice should not be introduced prior to age 1 year.[20] Juice has no special nutritional benefits and its consumption contributes to obesity and dental caries. In most circumstances, younger babies do not need to be given extra water to drink and it can be unsafe to give water to infants 6 months and younger because of their immature renal function. In the first 6 months of life, healthy babies born at term typically drink at least 150 mL/kg of breast milk or infant formula in 24 hours, feeding on demand every 2 hours to 4 hours to support a normal average weight gain of 20 g/d to 30 g/d.

Healthy infants have an inherent ability to regulate their intake so that they receive the amount of breast milk or formula needed to grow normally. Even newly born babies show cues when they are ready to eat and indicate that they are done eating by falling asleep or stopping sucking. Nevertheless, babies need a caregiver to assess their cues and to feed them when they are hungry and to stop feeding when they are full. When caregivers force feed or push children to eat when they are not hungry, this sabotages the ability to regulate intake to meet needs.

Overfeeding mostly occurs in the setting of bottle feeding rather than breastfeeding. When babies are held by a parent or caregiver when being fed a bottle, this provides a positive association with feeding and a sense of security and comfort for the infant. Holding the baby when feeding also allows the caregiver to monitor the baby's cues, specifically, when the baby show signs of satiety so the feeding can be stopped. When a bottle is propped or, in older babies, given to them to hold themselves in bed, infants are more likely to overfeed or to fall asleep with milk (or even more unfortunately, sweetened beverages like juice) still flowing, allowing it to pool in the baby's mouth where it becomes substrate for cariogenic bacteria.

Being able to hold up one's head, having adequate truncal support, and an extinguishing tongue thrust are developmental indicators, emerging at approximately 5 months to 6 months of age, that a baby is ready for solid food. There is cultural variation in the specific choice of beikost, but babies are often offered fine purees of fruits or vegetables, cereal, porridge, or smooth soup (nothing chunky) as their first solid food. Breast milk or formula should continue to provide the primary source of calories and nutrients for infants even after they start solids.

As babies develop the ability to pick up small objects and transfer them into their mouths, at approximately 9 months to 12 months of age, they become more interested in feeding themselves and can be offered melt-in-the-mouth solids (very small bite-sized pieces of soft meats, cheeses, crustless bread, and soft fruits and cooked vegetables). Infants have no inherent expectation that their food will be particularly salty or sweet, and there is no reason to feed a baby seasoned, sweetened, or processed food. Likewise, it is unnecessary to add any sweetened liquid or powder to a baby's milk bottle or to dip a baby's pacifier in anything sweet—doing so adds unnecessary calories and increases the risk for dental caries and obesity. Infants should never be given honey or have a pacifier dipped in honey because of the risk of botulism, not to mention caries.[21]

Along with initiating solid foods, the second half of the first year of life is an optimal time to introduce a cup, with the goal of eliminating the bottle by approximately 1 year of age. Many women breastfeed babies past the age of 1 year, but there is no reason for a healthy infant to continue a bottle past this age when developmentally they are ready to drink from a cup. It is harder to remove the bottle from toddlers because they develop an attachment to the bottle that is more about security than it is about nutrition (use a stuffed animal or blanket as a toddler attachment object instead of the bottle). Moreover, babies who bottle feed beyond 2 years of age are more likely to develop obesity.[22]

Despite their popularity, sippy cups are not a necessary intermediary between bottle/breast and cup, although from a practical perspective, a cup with a lid makes inevitable spills less messy. Giving a baby a sippy cup in bed or to graze on throughout the day is no better than when a bottle is used in these ways. Developmentally, older infants are ready for 3 discrete meals and 2 to 3 snack times per day. By 12 months of age, a baby should take liquids from a cup only at meals and snack time and not in between. Constantly snacking and drinking throughout the day is not physiologic (ie, on a given day, humans intermittently feed then fast, feed then fast, and so forth) and predisposes to childhood caries and obesity. Consideration for both the total amount and the frequency of sugar intake is important, however, caries risk is greatest if sugars are consumed more frequently.[23,24] Children with caries have a higher frequency of between-meal juice consumption compared with children who are caries-free.[25] To prevent caries and promote a healthy diet, between-meal beverages should be limited to water only. Children do not need juice in their diets, but if it is given, it should be limited to 4 oz per day for children age 1 year to 3 years, and 4 oz to 6 oz per day for children 4 to 6 years of age.[20] Diluting juice should be discouraged because it may increase the frequency that sweetened beverages are consumed, thereby contributing to caries.

Caries Prevention Modalities

Fluoride is the single most important caries preventive agent available.[26] Although parents may worry about fluoride intake during infancy, when the correct amount for the infant's size is used, fluoride is safe and effective in preventing caries. There are 3 ways in which fluoride can be delivered to infants: through fluoridated drinking water, use of over-the-counter FTP, and professionally applied topical fluoride, such as fluoride varnish.

Fluoride acts to prevent caries by pushing the tooth demineralization-remineralization dynamic in the direction of remineralization. Fluoride interacts with the hydroxyapatite of enamel and is incorporated into the tooth structure in the form of fluorapatite, which is harder and more resistant to acid attack than the original enamel that it replaces. Fluoride works best in remineralizing teeth when it is provided in a topical rather than systemic form (ie, fluoride supplements in liquid and tablet forms). Topical exposure to fluoride occurs through drinking optimally fluoridated water, brushing with FTP, and professional fluoride applications. Even when fluoride is swallowed, ingested fluoride ions are absorbed into the circulation and then released into saliva and crevicular fluid, thereby bathing the teeth in fluoride-rich fluids to promote remineralization.

Community water fluoridation

Community water fluoridation, first implemented in the United States in the mid-twentieth century is a cost-effective, safe and proven population-based caries preventive strategy.[26] Community water fluoridation refers to the addition of fluoride to that naturally present in water to attain an optimal fluoride level to prevent caries. In 2010, 72% of Americans on public water systems received community water fluoridation. The current recommended fluoride concentration in US community water fluoridation is 0.7 ppm (1 ppm = 1 mg/L).

How much fluoridated water an infant drinks is influenced by whether the infant drinks primarily breast milk or formula. Minimal fluoride is present in breast milk, such that exclusively breastfed infants receive less fluoride than infants fed with formula prepared with fluoridated water. The fluoride content of ready-to-use infant formula is negligible, ranging from 0.13 mg/L to 0.3 mg/L. This means that the fluoride content of infant formula made from powder reflects the fluoride in the water used to prepare it. At higher concentration of fluoridated water, concerns have been raised about the risk of fluorosis in babies fed with formula prepared with fluoridated water; however, at the current fluoride level of 0.7 ppm in optimally fluoridated community water, the daily intake of fluoride is within the recommended range of 0.05 mg fluoride/kg/d to 0.07 mg fluoride/kg/d. For example, a 10-kg infant who drinks 28 oz of formula prepared with 0.7 ppm of fluoridated water would consume 0.54 mg of fluoride or 0.054 mg/kg of fluoride.[26]

Fluoride toothpaste

FTP is a valuable delivery system for topical fluoride. In the United States, over-the-counter FTP, including those marketed for children, contains 1100 ppm fluoride (as 0.24% sodium fluoride or 0.76% sodium monofluorophosphate). FTP provides a concentrated topical form of fluoride to the tooth surface for ongoing remineralization. When FTP is used twice daily and not rinsed from the mouth after brushing, strong[26] research evidence indicates a significant reduction in caries incidence.

The American Dental Association and the AAPD recommend that all children have their teeth brushed twice daily for 2 minutes with FTP starting at the first sign of tooth eruption.[27] Children younger than 3 years should have their teeth brushed using a rice-grain size of FTP. At 3 years of age, the amount can be increased to a pea size (**Fig. 6**). Using relatively small quantities of toothpaste when brushing children's teeth means that, even when some toothpaste is swallowed, as is inevitable before children learn to spit it out, the quantity of fluoride ingested is small, safe, and less than what is swallowed when the recommended dose of liquid fluoride supplements are given by mouth.[26] Parents should avoid toothpastes marketed as "infant" or "training" toothpaste because these typically do not contain fluoride.

Professionally applied fluoride products

Applying highly concentrated fluoride products to teeth leaves a fluoride-calcium compound on tooth enamel that releases fluoride whenever biofilm (ie, plaque) pH decreases. Among available options, FV is safe and effective for use of children to reduce caries. Because it adheres to the tooth, there is minimal ingestion and thereby it is safe to use in children of all ages, beginning with the first tooth eruption. Systematic

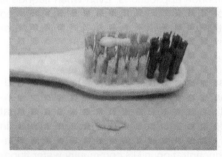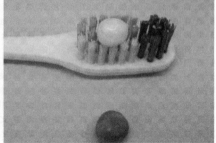

Fig. 6. Appropriate quantity of toothpaste. Children younger than 3 years should have tooth brushed with a rice-sized amount of FTP. Children, 3 years and older, should have their teeth brushed with a pea-sized amount of FTP. (*Courtesy of* Katherine Lewis, PhD, Seattle, WA.)

reviews indicate that regular applications of FV at least 2 times per year reduces caries incidence in primary teeth by 33%.[28] Where access to dental care is difficult, pediatricians and other pediatric health care providers play an important role in delivery of FV by applying it 2 times to 4 times per year to their patients at high risk of caries.[18] Pediatricians and other primary care providers can bill for FV application to low-income children insured by Medicaid.

Fluoride supplementation
Fluoride supplements are systemically ingested fluoride in the form of drops or tablets. Although oral fluoride supplements are still prescribed in the United States for high-caries-risk populations, other countries, including Canada, Australia, New Zealand, and those in the European Union, have abandoned oral fluoride supplements in favor of promoting twice-daily tooth brushing with FTP because FTP is much less expensive, easier to obtain, and more efficacious at caries prevention than oral fluoride supplements.[26] When considering oral fluoride supplementation, all sources of dietary fluoride should be considered, including at home, daycare, and school and in prepared foods and beverages, such as juice, soda, and infant formula. Furthermore, if the fluoride concentration of the home water source is not known, it should be tested to determine the fluoride level (to assess the necessary level of supplementation) and the child's caries risk status should be calculated (see **Fig. 3**). Prior to prescribing fluoride supplements, a physician should consult with the child's dentist to determine if the risks outweigh the benefits.

SUMMARY

Although it might be tempting to believe that oral health in infancy is of little consequence, behaviors and habits initiated in infancy—both positive, such as tooth brushing with FTP, and negative, including drinking sweetened beverages in bed—affect future oral health. Moreover, certain habits that positively influence a baby's oral health, such as limiting juice and snacking, also promote overall health and prevent obesity.

Recommendations
1. Improving mothers' oral health and, in particular, restoring carious lesions during pregnancy reduces risk of cariogenic bacteria transmission and subsequent colonization in infants.
2. Although teeth typically do not erupt their first teeth until approximately 6 months of age, educating parents about infant preventive oral health can begin prenatally and continue at well-baby-care visits.
3. Establishing a dental home by age 1 year helps children and caregivers implement proper preventative practices and reduces the risk of preventable oral disease.
4. Promoting healthy eating habits begins at birth. Young infants need only breast milk or infant formula. Holding a baby while feeding a bottle offer many benefits. Sweetened beverages (eg, juice) should not be introduced before 12 months of age. If given at all, juice should be limited to 4 oz per day for children ages 1 year to 3 years.
5. By 12 months of age, babies are developmentally ready for discrete meals and snacks and to use a cup for drinking beverages. Only water should be consumed between meals and snacks.
6. It is recommended that babies have their teeth brushed twice daily with a rice-grain–sized amount of FTP beginning at first tooth eruption. At age 3, a pea-sized amount of FTP should be used.
7. FV application at least 2 times per year reduces caries.

REFERENCES

1. Leung AKC, Robson WLM. Natal teeth: a review. J Natl Med Assoc 2006;98(2): 226–8.
2. Macknin ML, Piedmonte M, Jacobs J, et al. Symptoms associated with infant teething: a prospective study. Pediatrics 2000;105(4 Pt 1):747–52.
3. Food and Drug Administration. FDA Drug Safety Communication: FDA recommends not using lidocaine to treat teething pain and requires new Boxed Warning. 2014. Available at: https://www.fda.gov/drugs/drugsafety/ucm402240.htm. Accessed December 10, 2017.
4. FDA News Release. FDA confirms elevated levels of belladonna in certain homeopathic teething products. 2017. Available at: https://www.fda.gov/NewsEvents/Newsroom/PressAnnouncements/ucm538684.htm. Accessed December 10, 2017.
5. Lewis CW, Jacob LS, Lehmann CU, Section on Oral Health. The primary care pediatrician and the care of children with cleft lip and/or cleft palate. Pediatrics 2017;139(5) [pii:e20170628].
6. Dye BA, Mitnik GL, Iafolla TJ, et al. Trends in dental caries in children and adolescents according to poverty status in the United States from 1999 through 2004 and from 2011 through 2014. J Am Dent Assoc 2017;148(8):550–65.
7. Caufield PW, Li Y, Dasanayake A. Dental caries: an infectious and transmissible disease. Compend Contin Educ Dent 2005;26(5 Suppl 1):10–6.
8. Law V, Seow WK, Townsend G. Factors influencing oral colonization of mutans streptococci in young children. Aust Dent J 2007;52(2):93–100.
9. Plonka KA, Pukallus ML, Barnett AG, et al. A longitudinal study comparing mutans streptococci and lactobacilli colonisation in dentate children aged 6 to 24 months. Caries Res 2012;46(4):385–93.
10. Reed SG, Cunningham JE, Latham TN, et al. Maternal oral mutans streptococci (MS) status, not breastfeeding, predicts predentate infant oral MS status. Breastfeed Med 2014;9(9):446–9.
11. Plonka KA, Pukallus ML, Barnett AG, et al. Mutans streptococci and lactobacilli colonization in predentate children from the neonatal period to seven months of age. Caries Res 2012;46(3):213–20.
12. Milgrom P, Riedy CA, Weinstein P, et al. Dental caries and its relationship to bacterial infection, hypoplasia, diet, and oral hygiene in 6- to 36-month-old children. Community Dent Oral Epidemiol 2000;28(4):295–306.
13. American Academy on Pediatric Dentistry Council on Clinical Affairs. Policy on use of a caries-risk assessment tool (CAT) for infants, children, and adolescents. Pediatr Dent 2008–2009;30(7 Suppl):29–33.
14. American Academy of Pediatric Dentistry. Policy on Early Childhood Caries (ECC): Classifications, Consequences, and Preventive Strategies. 2016 AAPD Reference Manual. Available at: http://www.aapd.org/policies/. Accessed June 28, 2018.
15. American Academy of Pediatric Dentistry. Definition of Dental Home. 2016 AAPD Reference Manual. Available at: http://www.aapd.org/policies/. Accessed June 28, 2018.
16. Lee JY, Bouwens TJ, Savage MF, et al. Examining the cost-effectiveness of early dental visits. Pediatr Dent 2006;28(2):102–5.
17. Savage MF, Lee JY, Kotch JB, et al. Early preventive dental visits: effects on subsequent utilization and costs. Pediatrics 2004;114(4):e418–23.

18. Dooley D, Moultrie NM, Heckman B, et al. Oral health prevention and toddler well-child care: routine integration in a safety net system. Pediatrics 2016. [Epub ahead of print].
19. Li DK, Willinger M, Petitti DB, et al. Use of a dummy (pacifier) during lseep and risk of sudden infant death syndrome (SIDS): population based case-control study. BMJ 2006;332(7532):18–22.
20. Heyman MB, Abrams SA, Section on Gastroenterology, Hepatology, and Nutrition, Committee on Nutrition. Fruit juice in infants, children, and adolescents: current recommendations. Pediatrics 2017;139(6) [pii:e20170967].
21. Paglia L, Scaglioni S, Torchia V, et al. Familial and dietary risk factors in Early Childhood Caries. Eur J Paediatr Dent 2016;17(2):93–9.
22. Gooze RA, Anderson SE, Whitaker RC. Prolonged bottle use and obesity at 5.5 years of age in US children. J Pediatr 2011;159(3):431–6.
23. Özen B, Van Strijp AJ, Özer L, et al. Evaluation of possible associated factors for early childhood caries and severe early childhood caries: a multicenter cross-sectional survey. J Clin Pediatr Dent 2016;40(2):118–23.
24. Çolak H, Dülgergil ÇT, Dalli M, et al. Early childhood caries update: a review of causes, diagnoses, and treatments. J Nat Sci Biol Med 2013;4(1):29–38.
25. Palmer CA, Kent R Jr, Loo CY, et al. Diet and caries-associated bacteria in severe early childhood caries. J Dent Res 2010;89(11):1224–9.
26. Lewis CW. Fluoride and dental caries prevention in children. Pediatr Rev 2014; 35(1):3–15.
27. American Dental Association Council on Scientific Affairs. Fluoride toothpaste use for young children. J Am Dent Assoc 2014;145(2):190–1.
28. Marinho VC, Higgins JP, Logan S, et al. Fluoride varnishes for preventing dental caries in children and adolescents. Cochrane Database Syst Rev 2002;(3):CD002279.

The Role of Fluoride in the Prevention of Tooth Decay

Howard Pollick, BDS, MPH

KEYWORDS

- Dental caries • Dental decay • Oral health • Fluorides • Primary prevention
- Secondary prevention • Children

KEY POINTS

- Fluoride is the key to prevention of tooth decay.
- There are multiple fluoride modalities.
- Effectiveness and safety of fluoride depend on dose and concentration.
- Individual level fluoride use occurs at home and with professional application.
- Community level prevention occurs through fluoridation of water or salt.

INTRODUCTION
Dental Caries (Tooth Decay) in Children

Early childhood caries (ECC) is defined as the presence of one or more decayed (non-cavitated or cavitated lesions), missing (due to caries), or filled tooth surfaces in any primary tooth in a child younger than 6 years.[1] For children older than 6 years, there is no special category or definition of dental caries (see separate section/chapter on Dental Caries).

Fluoride is the Key to Prevention of Tooth Decay

Fluoride works to reduce the prevalence and severity of dental caries that requires restorative dental care, in preeruptive, posteruptive, systemic, and topical situations.
There are multiple mechanisms by which fluoride works:[2]

- Through reducing demineralization of enamel in the presence of acids produced by cariogenic bacteria in dental plaque breaking down fermentable carbohydrates,
- Through remineralization of early enamel caries, and
- Through inhibition of bacterial activity in dental plaque.

Dental Public Health Residency Program, Division of Oral Epidemiology and Dental Public Health, Department of Preventive and Restorative Dental Sciences, School of Dentistry, University of California San Francisco, 707 Parnassus Avenue, Box 0758, San Francisco, CA 94143-0758, USA
E-mail address: howard.pollick@ucsf.edu

Pediatr Clin N Am 65 (2018) 923–940
https://doi.org/10.1016/j.pcl.2018.05.014
0031-3955/18/© 2018 Elsevier Inc. All rights reserved.

Fluoride accumulates in dental plaque as fluoride ions from saliva, water, toothpaste and rinses, and professionally applied dental products. During daily tooth cleaning, some dental plaque remains, which provides the reservoir of fluoride for the reminer-alization of the tooth surface. High-fluoride modalities, such as fluoride varnish, combine with calcium in dental plaque to form globules of calcium fluoride, which dissociate slowly in the presence of plaque acids (lactic and pyruvic acids produced by bacterial breakdown of fermentable carbohydrates); this occurs because of the presence of a phosphate or protein-rich coating of the globular deposits of calcium fluoride, which releases bioavailable fluoride ions over a longer period of time.[3]

In addition, progression of caries in dentin toward the pulp may be inhibited or slowed by increased fluoride concentration within dentin. Fluoride can be incorpo-rated into the developing tooth if a child swallows fluoride toothpaste or water in com-munities with fluoridated water.[4] There are multiple fluoride modalities, from programs in the community and schools to home-based approaches and professionally applied fluoride in dental offices and other settings.

Community Level Fluoride Programs

The world's population exceeds 7 billion, yet fewer than 1 billion have access to proven community-based water or salt fluoridation programs (and not all those with access take advantage of it). Such programs reduce the prevalence and severity of tooth decay, the most common chronic disease of children, which may be untreated in as much as 95% of the population of some countries.[5]

Water fluoridation

Water fluoridation is practiced in many countries throughout the world. As of 2012, more than 420 million people worldwide have access to either naturally fluoridated wa-ter (about 50 million) or water with adjusted fluoride concentrations at or near optimal (about 370 million).[6] In the United States, more than 211 million people—or about 75% of the population served by public water supplies—have access to fluoridated water.[7] A global systematic Cochrane review has shown that the introduction of community water fluoridation results in a 35% reduction in the mean number of decayed, missing, and filled primary teeth and a 26% reduction in the mean number of decayed, missing, and filled permanent teeth in children. Water fluoridation has also increased the per-centage of children with no decay by 15%, according to the global Cochrane review.[8] Pediatric providers should encourage families to drink tap water where it is fluoridated.

Salt fluoridation

It has been estimated that between 40 million and 280 million people worldwide use salt fluoridation, mainly in European, South American, and Central American coun-tries.[9] Salt fluoridation is sometimes suggested as an option for communities that have a low water fluoride concentration and have no possibility of implementing com-munity water fluoridation. There are no salt fluoridation programs in the United States. The benefits and safety of salt fluoridation are similar to water fluoridation.[10] Although this is effective when no water fluoridation can be achieved, one has to be cautious if both options are available. It is recommended that a national fluoride program use only one of these community-based approaches (water or salt) to minimize the risk for dental fluorosis in young children with developing teeth.[11]

School-Based Fluoride Programs

Fluoridated milk

Although not practiced in the United States, fluoridated milk may be beneficial to schoolchildren, contributing to a substantial reduction in dental caries in primary teeth.[12] Successful milk fluoridation programs have been evaluated in Japan, Scotland, Israel, Hungary, and several other countries, including a study in Louisiana, USA in the 1950s.[13]

Fluoride mouthrinse
Because of the natural swallowing reflex, most children younger than 6 years may not be able to resist swallowing a mouthrinse. For children older than 6 years, regular use of alcohol-free fluoride mouthrinse under supervision has been shown to result in a large reduction in tooth decay in children's permanent teeth.[14] The margin of safety for acute toxicity with school-based 900-ppm fluoride mouthrinse is wide (10 mL contains 9 mg fluoride), which is more than 10 times lower than the probably toxic dose for a 6-year-old child of average weight (20 kg).[6] In communities with low exposure to fluoride in water, school-based fluoride rinsing programs are recommended, but their adoption should be based on the cost of implementation and the caries status of the community.[6]

Home-Based Fluoride

Dietary fluoride supplements
Prescription fluoride supplements (fluoride tablets or drops) have been shown to be effective in reducing caries incidence in permanent teeth, when used as prescribed.[15] However, fluoride tablets and drops have limited application as a public health measure due to poor adherence to the recommended daily schedule,[6] and evidence for ECC prevention with fluoride tablets and drops is insufficient.[16] In the United States, dietary fluoride supplements may be prescribed (with or without vitamins) for children at high risk for caries; the daily dose depends on age and fluoride concentration of the water supply.[17] However, fluoride supplements are not recommended for infants younger than 6 months (or without teeth) or for any children from where the fluoride in the water contains greater than 0.6 mg/L of fluoride (**Table 1**). Where water supplies contain less than 0.3 mg/L fluoride, the following are recommended:

- No fluoride tablets should be prescribed before the age of 6 months;
- Between 6 months and 3 years, prescribe 0.25 mg fluoride per day;
- Between 3 and 6 years 0.50 mg fluoride per day; and
- Between 6 and 16 years 1 mg fluoride per day.

For water supplies with 0.3 to 0.6 mg/L fluoride, the following are recommended:

- Fluoride drops or tablets should not be prescribed before the age of 3 years;
- Between 3 and 6 years, prescribe 0.25 mg of fluoride per day; and
- Between 6 and 16 years 0.5 mg fluoride per day.

Fluoride toothpaste
There is strong evidence that twice-daily use of fluoride toothpaste has a significant caries-reducing effect in young permanent teeth compared with a placebo.[18] Strong evidence suggested a dose–response relationship with enhanced caries protection from toothpastes with 1500 ppm of fluoride compared with formulations with 1000 ppm of fluoride in young permanent teeth following daily use.[19] However, only 1000 to 1100 ppm fluoride toothpaste is currently available in the United States[20] without a prescription. Nevertheless, daily tooth brushing with fluoride toothpaste, even at less than optimal fluoride dosage, from the time of eruption of the first tooth must be regarded as the best clinical practice today, based on moderate quality of evidence.[18] Toothpaste should be applied by the parent, with only a smear for children younger than 3 years and a pea-size amount for those older than 3 years (**Fig. 1**A, B). Toothpaste should be spit out after brushing, without water for rinsing. In addition,

Table 1
Fluoride supplement (tablets and drops) dosage schedule 2010 (Approved by the American Dental Association Council on Scientific Affairs)

Age	Fluoride Ion Level in Drinking Water (ppm)[a]		
	<0.3	0.3–0.6	>0.6
Birth–6 mo	None	None	None
6 mo–3 y	0.25 mg/d[b]	None	None
3–6 y	0.50 mg/d	0.25 mg/d	None
6–16 y	1.0 mg/d	0.50 mg/d	None

Important Considerations When Using Dosage Schedule: (1) If fluoride level is unknown, drinking water should be tested for fluoride content before supplements are prescribed. For testing of fluoride content, contact the local or state health department. (2) All sources of fluoride should be evaluated with a thorough fluoride history. (3) Patient exposure to multiple water sources may complicate proper prescribing. (4) Ingestion of higher than recommended levels of fluoride by children has been associated with an increased risk of mild dental fluorosis in developing, unerupted teeth. (5) To obtain the benefits from fluoride supplements, long-term compliance on a daily basis is required.

[a] 1.0 ppm = 1 mg/L.

[b] 2.2 mg sodium fluoride contains 1 mg fluoride ion.

From American Dental Association. Oral Health Topics. Fluoride: Topical and Systemic Supplements. Available at: http://www.ada.org/en/member-center/oral-health-topics/fluoride-topical-and-systemic-supplements Accessed on May 23, 2018; Copyright © 2018 American Dental Association. All rights reserved. Reprinted with permission.

there are toothpastes on the market that do not have fluoride; pediatric providers should discourage patients from using these.

Prescription strength fluoride toothpaste

There is a strong evidence base for the use of high-fluoride toothpastes (5000 ppm fluoride) in groups at a greater risk of caries.[21] It is recommended to restrict its use in those younger than 6 years to cases where the risk of severe morbidity caused by caries is greater than that of aesthetically objectionable fluorosis. For children younger than 9 years who are at risk for developing dental fluorosis, it is recommended that the toothpaste be rinsed out with water after using high-fluoride toothpaste, whereas when using regular fluoride toothpaste, it is recommended that the toothpaste be spit out after use, rather than rinsed with water.

Fluoride mouthrinse

Mouthrinses for daily home use contain 225 ppm of fluoride, as opposed to the higher 900 ppm of fluoride concentration used in weekly school-based programs. Fluoride

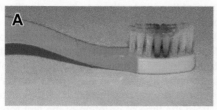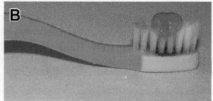

Fig. 1. Toothbrushes with fluoride toothpaste: smear/rice-size amount; pea-size amount. (*A*) Smear amount of toothpaste. (*B*) Pea-sized amount of toothpaste. (*Data from* American Dental Association. Oral health topics. Fluoride: topical and systemic supplements. Available at: http://www.ada.org/en/member-center/oral-health-topics/fluoride-topicaland-systemic-supplements. Accessed May 23, 2018.)

mouthrinses are reserved for children older than 6 years who have outgrown the swallowing reflex and who are at moderate or high caries risk, regardless of fluoride level of the drinking water. It is recommended to rinse for 1 to 2 minutes and spit out the rinse, rather than rinse with water afterward. Benefits of caries prevention from fluoride rinsing were found with and without prior toothbrushing.[22]

Professionally Applied Topical Fluoride

Fluoride gels

Professionally applied high-concentration fluoride gels have been widely used by dental professionals in dental offices to prevent tooth decay in children and adults at high risk for tooth decay, whether in a fluoridated or nonfluoridated area. The application of fluoride gel (12,300 ppm of fluoride as acidulated phosphate fluoride) results in a large reduction in tooth decay in both permanent and primary teeth.[23] Gels are applied to the teeth using gel trays in the dentist's office, which must stay on the patient's teeth for approximately 4 minutes, with adequate suction to reduce swallowing of the gel. Precautions that should be undertaken include the following:[22]

1. Using only the required amount of the fluoride solution or gel to perform the treatment adequately,
2. Positioning the patient in an upright position,
3. Using efficient saliva aspiration or suctioning apparatus, and
4. Requiring the patient to expectorate thoroughly on completion of the fluoride application.

The use of these procedures has been shown to reduce the amount of inadvertently swallowed fluoride to less than 2 mg, which can be expected to be of little consequence. However, the use of these gels has mostly been replaced by the use of fluoride varnish.

Fluoride varnish

Varnishes and gels are equally effective at preventing caries.[24] Increasingly, varnishes are used instead of gels due to the ease of application and low risk from ingestion of large doses, especially for younger children.

Professionally applied 5% sodium fluoride varnish (22,600 ppm of fluoride), in single doses of up to 9 mg fluoride, can remineralize early enamel caries[25] and prevent the need for dental restorations. Varnishes are brushed onto clean, dry teeth, in the dentist's office, the medical office, and increasingly in other sites with children at high caries risk, such as WIC or Head Start. The application takes about 1 minute, and the varnish sets quickly. To keep the varnish on the teeth for several hours, patients are told to eat soft foods and avoid brushing and flossing for the remainder of the day. Fluoride varnish has been shown to be effective in the prevention of caries in both primary and permanent teeth. The interval for frequency of application of fluoride varnish varies depending on the risk of the patient—more frequently for children with higher risk.[26] Although use of fluoride varnish for caries prevention is technically considered an "off-label" use (it is US Food and Drug Administration [FDA] approved for tooth sensitivity), there is a robust evidence base for the efficacy of varnish at preventing caries.[27,28] Varnish can be reapplied every 3 to 6 months, depending on risk, and no cases of fluorosis have been linked to excessive varnish use.

Application of fluoride varnish by primary care providers The FDA has approved fluoride varnish products as medical devices to be used as cavity liners and for the treatment of hypersensitive teeth, but they can be used off-label as caries-preventive agents. Because of its safety, fluoride varnish can be applied without specialized equipment (eg, compressed air or suction) by trained dental and medical personnel (doctor, nurse practitioner, physician assistant, registered nurse, licensed practical nurse, certified medical assistant) to at-risk children and adults in dental and medical offices as well as in a variety of nonmedical clinic venues.[29]

Young children tend to see primary care physicians (PCPs) far more frequently than dentists. In the United States, the American Academy of Pediatrics recommends that a child see PCPs 11 times for a checkup by the age of 2 years. It therefore makes sense to use PCP visits to address oral health in young children. The utilization of PCPs as a first-line provider of preventive dental services in improving children's oral health is an innovative approach that facilitates the integration of the dental and medical communities and oral health inclusion into primary health care. In addition, because medical providers typically have higher rates than dentists of participation in public-funded health care, Medicaid, they can provide preventive oral health services to low-income children as part of well-child care while referring to dentists those who need more complex restorative care.[30]

The potential success of such approach was demonstrated in a program called Into the Mouths of Babes, initiated in North Carolina in 2000. In this program physicians were reimbursed by Medicaid to conduct dental screenings and apply fluoride varnish in children younger than 3 years and counsel parents. This program demonstrated the sustainable long-term success of this initiative.[31] The economic impact of the program demonstrated 32% lower total Medicaid expenditures for hospital episodes.[32]

Combination of fluoride modalities

Topical fluorides (mouthrinses, gels, or varnishes) used in addition to fluoride toothpaste achieve a modest reduction in caries compared with toothpaste used alone.[33] With the exception of fluoride toothpaste, which is the most widely used topically applied fluoride worldwide, topical fluorides are usually recommended for individuals or populations who are considered to be at moderate or high caries risk, after taking into account other exposures to fluoride.[6] Regardless of the type of professionally applied topical fluoride treatments, the results of clinical trials clearly indicate that the benefits of topical fluoride applications are related to the number of treatments and frequency of use.[5]

Preference for fluoride modalities

Fluoride toothpastes, in comparison with mouthrinses or gels, seem to have a similar degree of effectiveness for the prevention of dental caries in children. There is no clear suggestion that fluoride varnish is more effective than mouthrinses and the evidence for the comparative effectiveness of fluoride varnishes and gels and mouthrinses and gels is inconclusive.[34] Therefore, when a child is found to have tooth decay or is deemed to be at high risk for decay, then recommendations to the parents/guardians should be made for them to supervise twice daily use of age-appropriate amounts of fluoride toothpaste for their child, while recommending and obtaining consent to apply fluoride varnish by the health care professional. Note that fluoride mouthrinses for home use are only recommended for children who are able to spit out the rinse and not swallow it.

Frequency of Professionally Applied Fluoride Use

For dental professionals, it is recommended that new patients with active caries, regardless of age, be given an initial series of 4 topical fluoride applications within a period of 2 to 4 weeks. If desired, the initial application can be preceded by a thorough dental prophylaxis (professional cleaning) and the remaining 3 applications of the initial treatment series should be preceded by tooth brushing to remove plaque and oral debris. It should be obvious that this series of treatments can be very conveniently combined with plaque control, dietary counseling, and initial restorative programs that the dental provider has devised for these patients. Following this initial series of treatments, the patient should be given single, topical applications at intervals of 3, 6, or 12 months, depending on the patient's caries status.[35]

Comparing fluoride varnish and dental sealants
Dental sealants, applied by dental professionals, are recommended to seal pits and fissures in the biting surfaces of primary and permanent molars before them showing overt signs of tooth decay. The oral health objectives in Healthy People 2020 include increasing the proportion of children aged 3 to 5 years who have received dental sealants on one or more of their primary molar teeth, as well as increasing the proportion of children aged 6 to 9 years who have received dental sealants on one or more of their permanent first molar teeth and increasing the proportion of adolescents aged 13 to 15 years who have received dental sealants on one or more of their permanent molar teeth.[36] Both dental sealants and fluoride varnish are recommended to provide maximum prevention of tooth decay for those at risk for tooth decay. Fluorides mainly work to prevent decay on the smooth surfaces of teeth, whereas sealants prevent caries on the nonsmooth pit and fissures. Although it should not be a choice between sealants and fluoride varnish, in a community-based oral health program targeted at 6- to 7-year-old children at high caries risk, the application of fluoride varnish as a caries-preventive measure resulted in caries prevention that was not significantly different from that obtained by applying and maintaining dental sealants after 36 months.[37]

Methods to increase compliance with fluoride modalities
A growing number of parents are refusing topical fluoride for their children during preventive dental and medical visits.[38] This refusal is based on readily available erroneous information on the Internet promulgated by antifluoridation rhetoric. Arguments and unproven claims that fluoride causes a multitude of conditions and diseases, such as AIDS, Alzheimer disease, cancer, Down Syndrome, genetic damage, heart disease, lower intelligence, kidney disease, osteoporosis, and bone fracture, have been addressed in authoritative evidence-based information, most notably by the American Dental Association in Fluoridation Facts (2018). It has been proposed that there will be greater compliance with recommended fluoride varnish regimens in families who receive motivational interviewing as compared with families receiving traditional education and counseling.[39]

A focus group study on attitudes to fluoridation[40] made the following conclusions:

- Fluoride advocates should preserve individual choice wherever possible.
- Individual choice takes a back seat, if there is a significant demonstrable benefit and safety to the wider community.
- The scientific evidence indicates that fluoridation offers such benefit and more than adequate safety.

In addition, building trust is essential. The following recommendations were made:

- Experts and advocates need to acknowledge that concerns about fluoride exist and should treat them seriously.
- Simply trying to correct factual misunderstandings without addressing underlying concerns actually increases mistrust.
- The preferred approach should not focus on correcting factual misconceptions or emphasizing positive messages, but on understanding public concerns and building on common ground.

Biomarkers of fluoride exposure

Although fluoride concentrations in plasma, saliva, and urine have some ability to assess fluoride exposure, present data are insufficient to recommend using fluoride concentrations in these body fluids as biomarkers of contemporary fluoride exposure for individuals. Daily fluoride excretion in urine can be considered a useful biomarker of contemporary fluoride exposure for groups of people, and standards for urinary fluoride excretion indicating low, optimal, and high fluoride exposure are available.[6]

Safety of Fluoride

Overall, in the doses listed here, fluoride is very safe. Based on a lowest-observed-adverse-effect level of 0.10 mg/kg/d for moderate enamel fluorosis and an uncertainty factor of 1, a Tolerable Upper Intake Level (UL) of 0.10 mg/kg/d on a daily basis over extended periods of time was established for infants, toddlers, and children through 8 years of age.[41] This should not be interpreted as a limit to prevent acute toxicity, which is much higher in the order of 5 mg/kg or 50 times higher; nor should it be interpreted as a limit for occasional exposure, such as when fluoride varnish is applied. The UL of fluoride is age/weight dependent; for young children the UL varies from 0.7 mg/d to 2.0 mg/d depending on body weight, and because the crowns of permanent teeth have already formed by the age of 9 years, other than the wisdom teeth, for children older than 9 years of age and adults, the daily UL is 10 mg (**Table 2**). Comparisons of fluoride concentration, volume/weight, and total fluoride dose of various topical fluoride products for home use and for professional use can be found in **Tables 3** and **4**.

The most common side effect of chronic high fluoride intake in children younger than 9 years is dental fluorosis. Nonsevere forms of dental fluorosis are not detrimental to health and in fact the milder forms of dental fluorosis have been shown to be associated with increased resistance to dental caries.[42]

Dental Fluorosis

Dental fluorosis is defined as a change in the mineralization of the dental hard tissues caused by long-term ingestion of fluoride during the period of tooth development before eruption into the mouth (first 8 years of life for most permanent teeth excluding third molars). Once the tooth erupts, dental fluorosis refers to a

Table 2
Table of adequate intake and tolerable upper level for fluoride intake by age/weight

Age Group	Reference Weights kg (lbs)[a]	Adequate Intake (mg/d)	Tolerable Upper Intake (mg/d)
Infants 0–6 mo	7 (16)	0.01	0.7
Infants 6–12 mo	9 (20)	0.5	0.9
Children 1–3 y	13 (29)	0.7	1.3
Children 4–8 y	22 (48)	1.0	2.2
Children 9–13 y	40 (88)	2.0	10
Boys 14–18 y	64 (142)	3.0	10
Girls 14–18 y	57 (125)	3.0	10
Men 19 y and older	76 (166)	4.0	10
Women 19 y and older	61 (133)	3.0	10

[a] Value based on data collected during 1988 to 1994 as part of the Third National Health and Nutrition Examination Survey (NHANES III) in the United States.

From American Dental Association. Fluoridation Facts; 2018. p 45: Table 2; Copyright © 2018 American Dental Association. All rights reserved. Reprinted with permission.

Table 3
Professionally applied topical fluoride

Agent	Fluoride Concentration	ppm F (Approx.)	Volume or Weight	Total F Dose	Comments	Time/ Frequency
F Varnish (5% NaF)	2.25%	22,600	0.25 mL	5.65 mg	For <6 y of age	1 min; 3/y
F Varnish (5% NaF)	2.25%	22,600	0.4 mL	9 mg	For >6 y of age	1 min; 3/y
8% SnF_2	1.936%	19,360	5 mL	96.8 mg	Seated, suction, spit	4 min; 2/y
APF Office Gel	1.23%	12,300	5 mL	61.5 mg	Seated, suction, spit	4 min; 2/y
NaF gel/foam (2%)	0.90%	9000	5 mL	45 mg	Seated, suction, spit	4 min; 2/y

range of visually detectable changes in enamel. Dental fluorosis, originally described as mottled enamel, may also be called enamel fluorosis. Changes range from barely visible lacy white markings in milder cases to converged opaque areas, browning, and pitting of the teeth in severe forms. Dental fluorosis cannot develop in teeth after the teeth have formed; once evident, fluorosis does not progress in severity.[43]

Fewer than 1% of individuals in the United States have severe dental fluorosis, a condition recognized as an adverse health effect.[44] The prevalence of severe enamel

Table 4
Home use of topical fluoride

Agent	Fluoride Concentration	ppm F (Approx.)	Volume or Weight	Total F Dose	Comments	Time/ Frequency
Toothpaste (0.22% NaF)	0.10%	1000	1 g	0.1 mg	6 mo to 3 y: smear or rice-size amount	2/d
Toothpaste (0.22% NaF)	0.10%	1000	1 g	0.25 mg	3–6 y: pea-size amount	2/d
Toothpaste (0.22% NaF)	0.10%	1000	1 g	1 mg	Older than 6 y: spit after use	2/d
Prescription toothpaste (1.1% NaF)	0.50%	5000	1 g	5 mg	<9 y: rinse after use	2/d
Home gel (0.4% SnF_2)	0.097%	970	1 g	1 mg	Spit after use	1/d
Mouthrinse (0.05% NaF)	0.025%	225	10 mL	2.25 mg	Spit after use	1/d
Fluoridated water	0.0001%	1	1 L	1 mg	—	Several/d

Adapted from Pollick HF. Topical fluoride therapy. In: Harris NO, Garcia-Godoy F, Nathe CN, editors. Primary Preventive Dentistry (Subscription), 8th Ed., ©2014. Reprinted by permission of Pearson Education, Inc., New York, New York.

fluorosis is very low (near zero) at fluoride concentrations in drinking water below 2 mg/L.[45] (NRC 2006) Nonfluorotic alteration in the appearance of teeth, such as enamel hypoplasia, may be confused with dental fluorosis.[46]

Public health organizations work to keep the dose of fluoride to the minimal necessary while still providing benefit. The recommended fluoride concentration of drinking water was changed in 2015 to a standard 0.7 mg/L across the United States, in part because of higher prevalence of dental fluorosis seen in the NHANES reports.[47] Similarly, the schedule of recommended doses of prescription fluoride supplements was changed in 1994 as a result of evidence of increased dental fluorosis from the earlier recommendation on supplements.[48]

Acute Fluoride Toxicity

Acute fluoride toxicity presents with symptoms of nausea and vomiting, muscle spasms, abdominal pain, possibly leading to coma, convulsions, and cardiac arrhythmias. It can occur with inappropriate and excessive ingestion of fluoride products, such as multiple prescription dietary fluoride supplements at one time, or swallowing excess topical high concentration fluoride applications in a dental office, such as from professionally applied fluoride gels in trays without adequate suction and posttreatment spitting.[45] Immediate action must be taken in such cases.[49]

Chronic fluoride toxicity presents with symptoms and signs of stiffness and pain in the joints and muscles from skeletal fluorosis. This usually results from fluoride exposure over a prolonged period of many years in communities where the water supply (or personal wells) contains a high concentration of fluoride.[50] Most commonly this occurs in areas with naturally fluoridated water. To this effect, the US Environmental Protection Agency has set primary (4 mg/L) and secondary (2 mg/L) maximum contaminant levels for naturally occurring fluoride in drinking water.[51] As a result, community water systems must notify customers, if the secondary maximum contaminant level is exceeded, so that parents and caregivers can see to it that children younger than 9 years do not consume that water on a regular basis, to prevent the development of moderate and severe dental fluorosis.[52] In addition, regulations in the United States stipulate that individual wells must be tested regularly by the owner.[53]

Recommendation on the Use of Infant Formula

There is weak evidence that the fluoride in infant formula reconstituted with fluoridated water could be a cause of enamel fluorosis, as other mechanisms, including swallowing fluoride toothpaste during the tooth developing years, could explain the observed association.[54] When dentists (and other PCPs) advise parents and caregivers of infants who consume powdered or liquid concentrate infant formula as the main source of nutrition, they can suggest the continued use of powdered or liquid concentrate infant formulas reconstituted with optimally fluoridated drinking water while being cognizant of the potential risks of enamel fluorosis development.[55] The Centers for Disease Control states "To lessen this chance, parents may choose to use low-fluoride bottled water some of the time to mix infant formula. These bottled waters are labeled as de-ionized, purified, demineralized, or distilled and are without any fluoride added after purification treatment (FDA requires the label to indicate when fluoride is added)."[56]

Since the USPHS recommendation for optimizing community water supplies to 0.7 ppm of fluoride was instituted, dental fluorosis due to reconstituting infant formula with fluoridated water is expected to be less of an issue.[57]

Silver diamine fluoride

A different fluoride compound is available for secondary prevention and arrest of dentinal caries where a cavity has already been established in a tooth. Silver diamine fluoride (SDF) is effective in arresting dental caries. SDF can arrest caries in the inner dentine of primary and permanent teeth and prevent caries recurrence after treatment. The American Academy of Pediatric Dentistry supports the use of 38% SDF for the arrest of cavitated caries lesions in primary teeth as part of a comprehensive caries management program.[58] SDF is not recommended for primary prevention of caries, although when applied to carious lesions, studies have shown primary prevention in other sites in the mouth.[59] Only specifically trained professionals should apply SDF because of persistent black staining of the carious lesion and soft tissues beyond the cavity, including lips and operator's fingers and clothing. A protocol has been developed for the use of SDF.[60] See **Box 1**[61] for a summary of evidence of effectiveness.

Recommendations for Fluoride Use to Prevent Dental Caries in Children

Despite many similarities, recommendations for the use of topical fluoride vary worldwide by different groups in different countries. The following represent a sample of recommendations for fluoride use to prevent dental caries in children.

American Academy of Pediatrics

For all children (at low or high caries risk)[62]:

Toothpaste: starting at tooth emergence (smear of paste until age 3 y, then pea-size amount)

Fluoride varnish: every 3 to 6 months starting at tooth emergence.

Community water fluoridation.

Dietary fluoride supplements: if drinking water supply is not fluoridated (Note: The American Dental Association does not recommend dietary fluoride supplements for children at low caries risk).

Box 1
American Academy of Pediatric Dentistry: summary of evidence of effectiveness of fluoride

1. There is confirmation from evidence-based reviews that fluoride use for the prevention and control of caries is both safe and highly effective in reducing dental caries prevalence.

2. There is evidence from randomized clinical trials and evidence-based reviews that fluoride dietary supplements are effective in reducing dental caries and should be considered for children at caries risk who drink fluoride-deficient (<0.6 ppm) water.

3. There is evidence from randomized controlled trials and meta-analyses that professionally applied topical fluoride treatments, such as 5% sodium fluoride varnish or 1.23% fluoride gel preparation, are efficacious in reducing caries in children at caries risk.

4. There is evidence from meta-analyses that fluoridated toothpaste is effective in reducing dental caries in children, with the effect increased in children with higher baseline level of caries, higher concentration of fluoride in the toothpaste, greater frequency in use, and supervision. Using no more than a smear or rice-size amount of fluoridated toothpaste for children younger than 3 years may decrease risk of fluorosis. Using no more than a pea-size amount of fluoridated toothpaste is appropriate for children aged 3 to 6 years.

5. There is evidence from randomized clinical trials that 0.2% sodium fluoride mouthrinse and 1.1% sodium fluoride brush-on gels/pastes also are effective in reducing dental caries in children.

From American Academy of Pediatric Dentistry: guidelines on fluoride therapy. 2014. Available at: http://www.aapd.org/media/policies_guidelines/g_fluoridetherapy.pdf. Accessed January 2, 2018.

For children at high caries risk, in addition to recommendations for all children:
Over-the-counter mouthrinse: starting at age 6 years if the child can reliably swish and spit

American Dental Association Council on Scientific Affairs Expert Panel on Topical Fluoride Caries Preventive Agents[63]

For all children: twice daily use of age-appropriate amount of fluoride toothpaste.
For those at risk for caries:
For children younger than 6 years:
- Only 2.26% fluoride varnish at least every 3 to 6 months is recommended
For children older than 6 years:
- Professionally applied 2.26% fluoride varnish at least every 3 to 6 months
  - Or 1.23% fluoride (acidulated phosphate fluoride) gel, at least every 3 to 6 months
- Home use of a prescription-strength, home-use 0.5% fluoride gel or paste twice daily
  - Or 0.09% fluoride mouthrinse daily

Maternal and Child Health Bureau expert panel: topical fluoride for high-risk children

Population-based risk factors[64]:
- Low-income children (eg, enrolled in Head Start, WIC, free/reduced lunch program, Medicaid or SCHIP eligible, or other programs serving low-income children)
- Children with special health care needs
Children younger than 2 years:
Toothpaste:
- Encourage parents and caregivers to take an active role in brushing their children's teeth once the first tooth erupts
- Educate parents and caregivers on proper fluoride toothpaste use
- Brush children's teeth with fluoride toothpaste twice daily
- Use a smear of fluoride toothpaste
- Do not rinse after brushing
Varnish:
- Apply every 3 to 6 months
Children aged 2 to 6 years:
Toothpaste:
- Encourage parents and caregivers to take an active role in brushing their children's teeth
- Educate parents and caregivers on proper fluoride toothpaste use
- Brush children's teeth with fluoride toothpaste, or assist children with tooth brushing, twice a day
- Use no more than a pea-size amount of fluoride toothpaste
- Children should spit out excess toothpaste
- Do not rinse after brushing
Varnish:
- Apply every 3 to 6 months

Academy of Nutrition and Dietetics
It is the position of the Academy of Nutrition and Dietetics to support optimal systemic and topical fluoride as an important public health measure to promote oral health and overall health throughout life.[65]

Box 2
Table of caries risk assessment

Age 6 years and older. Available at: http://www.ada.org/~/media/ADA/Science%20and%20 Research/Files/topic_caries_over6.ashx

Age 6 years and older (For Dental Providers). Available at: http://www.aapd.org/media/policies_ guidelines/g_cariesriskassessment.pdf

Younger than 6 years. Available at: http://www.ada.org/~/media/ADA/Member%20Center/FIles/ topics_caries_under6.pdf?la=en

Younger than 3 years (for physicians and other nondental health care providers). Available at: http://www.aapd.org/media/policies_guidelines/g_cariesriskassessment.pdf

For 0 to 5 years of age (for dental providers). Available at: http://www.aapd.org/media/policies_ guidelines/g_cariesriskassessment.pdf

Recommendations to Reduce Dental Fluorosis

1. Defer the use of fluoride toothpaste until a child is aged between 18 and 36 months unless the child has been assessed as being at increased risk of developing caries (Forum on Fluoridation, 2002; Health Canada, 2010; Australian Research Centre for Population Oral Health, 2012).[4]
2. Use a "smear" of fluoride toothpaste (0.1 mg) for all children younger than 3 years and a pea-size amount (0.25 mg) for those older than 3 years (SIGN 2014; Public Health England, 2014; ADA Council on Scientific Affairs, 2014).
3. Although not available in the United States, some countries recommend the use of low-fluoride toothpaste for young children (EAPD, 2009; Australian Research Centre for Population Oral Health, 2012). The 2012 Australian guidelines recommend the use of low-fluoride toothpaste (500–550 ppm) for children aged 18 months to 5 years.[66]

Other than dental sealants that have been shown to effectively prevent pit and fissure caries (see John Timothy Wright's article, "The Burden and Management of Dental Caries in Older Children," in this issue) (**Box 2**), nonfluoride agents, such as chlorhexidine and xylitol wipes rinse may serve as adjunctive therapeutics for preventing, arresting, or even reversing dental caries, but they are not substitutes for proven fluoride modalities for caries prevention.[67,68]

SUMMARY

Much has been researched and written about fluoride and the prevention of tooth decay (dental caries). There is overwhelming evidence and consensus that fluoride is of paramount importance to prevent tooth decay. In addition to twice daily home use of over-the-counter fluoride toothpaste in the appropriate amounts for different aged children, the most common use is fluoridation of water (or salt), which is effective to reach large number of children simultaneously (population approach). Certain children, mostly those at higher risk for caries, however, need additional fluoride. Numerous modalities are available and each has its advantages and disadvantages. Communication and consultation with dentists will usually develop the best strategy for each individual child. Although any population and/or individual approach to affect health in a positive manner carries risk, fluoridation can result in various levels of dental fluorosis while teeth are developing; it is generally accepted that tooth decay prevention takes precedence. Therefore, as a general recommendation, it is felt that children

Box 3
Further resources

Application of fluoride varnish (link to Youtube video)
  Bertness J, Holt K, editors. Fluoride varnish: a resource guide. 2nd edition. Washington, DC:
  National Maternal and Child Oral Health Resource Center. 2016.
    https://www.mchoralhealth.org/PDFs/ResGuideFlVarnish.pdf
    https://www.youtube.com/watch?v=OzM4UQxP67Q

Application of SDF (link to Youtube video)
  http://www.astdd.org/www/docs/sdf-fact-sheet-09-07-2017.pdf

Abbreviation: SDF, silver diamine fluoride.

should have access to and drink fluoridated water and use recommended amounts of fluoride toothpaste on a twice-daily basis to promote oral health (**Box 3**).

REFERENCES

1. American Academy of Pediatric Dentistry. Policy on Early Childhood Caries (ECC): classifications, consequences, and preventive strategies. 2016. Available at: http://www.aapd.org/media/policies_guidelines/p_eccclassifications.pdf. Accessed January 2, 2018.
2. Recommendations for using fluoride to prevent and control dental caries in the United States. Centers for Disease Control and Prevention. MMWR Recomm Rep 2001;50(RR-14):1–42. Available at: https://www.cdc.gov/mmwr/preview/mmwrhtml/rr5014a1.htm. Accessed May 23, 2018.
3. Pollick HF. Topical fluoride therapy. In: Harris NO, Garcia-Godoy F, Nathe CN, editors. Primary preventive dentistry. 8th edition. Pearson; 2013. p. 248–72 [Chapter 15]. ISBN 13: 9780132845700.
4. O'Mullane DM, Baez RJ, Jones S, et al. Fluoride and oral health. Community Dent Health 2016;33(2):69–99.
5. Beaglehole R, Benzian H, Crail J, et al. The oral health atlas: mapping a neglected global health issue. FDI World Dental Federation. Myriad Editions. 2012. Available at https://issuu.com/myriadeditions/docs/flipbook_oral_health. Accessed January 2, 2018.
6. British Fluoridation Society. One in a million: the facts about water fluoridation. 3rd edition. 2012. Available at: www.bfsweb.org/onemillion/onemillion2012.html. Accessed January 2, 2018.
7. Centers for Disease Control and Prevention. Community water fluoridation. Water fluoridation data & statistics. Available at: https://www.cdc.gov/fluoridation/statistics/index.htm. Accessed January 2, 2018.
8. Iheozor-Ejiofor Z, Worthington HV, Walsh T, et al. Water fluoridation for the prevention of dental caries. Cochrane Database Syst Rev 2015;(6):CD010856.
9. Pollick HF. Salt fluoridation: a review. J Calif Dent Assoc 2013;41(6):395–7, 400-4.
10. Marthaler TM. Salt fluoridation and oral health. Acta Med Acad 2013;42(2):140–55.
11. Horowitz HS. Decision-making for national programs of community fluoride use. Community Dent Oral Epidemiol 2000;28:321–9.
12. Yeung CA, Chong LY, Glenny AM. Fluoridated milk for preventing dental caries. Cochrane Database Syst Rev 2015;(9):CD003876.
13. Bánóczy J, Rugg-Gunn A, Woodward M. Milk fluoridation for the prevention of dental caries. Acta Med Acad 2013;42(2):156–67.

14. Marinho VCC, Chong LY, Worthington HV, et al. Fluoride mouthrinses for preventing dental caries in children and adolescents. Cochrane Database Syst Rev 2016;(7):CD002284.
15. Tubert-Jeannin S, Auclair C, Amsallem E, et al. Fluoride supplements (tablets, drops, lozenges or chewing gums) for preventing dental caries in children. Cochrane Database Syst Rev 2011;(12):CD007592.
16. Twetman S, Dhar V. Evidence of effectiveness of current therapies to prevent and treat early childhood caries. Pediatr Dent 2015;37(3):246–53.
17. Rozier RG, Adair S, Graham F, et al. Evidence-based clinical recommendations on the prescription of dietary fluoride supplements for caries prevention: a report of the American Dental Association Council on Scientific Affairs. J Am Dent Assoc 2010;141(12):1480–9.
18. Twetman S, Axelsson S, Dahlgren H, et al. Caries-preventive effect of fluoride toothpaste: a systematic review. Acta Odontol Scand 2003;61(6):347–55.
19. Walsh T, Worthington HV, Glenny AM, et al. Fluoride toothpastes of different concentrations for preventing dental caries in children and adolescents. Cochrane Database Syst Rev 2010;(1):CD007868.
20. American Dental Association. The ADA/PDR guide to dental therapeutics. 5th edition. Chicago (IL): American Dental Association; 2009.
21. Pretty IA. High fluoride concentration toothpastes for children and adolescents. Caries Res 2016;50(suppl 1):9–14.
22. LeCompte EJ, Doyle TE. Effects of suctioning devices on oral fluoride retention. J Am Dent Assoc 1985;110:357.
23. Marinho VCC, Worthington HV, Walsh T, et al. Fluoride gels for preventing dental caries in children and adolescents. Cochrane Database Syst Rev 2015;(6):CD002280.
24. Seppä L, Leppanen T, Hausen H. Fluoride varnish versus acidulated phosphate fluoride gel: a 3-year clinical trial. Caries Res 1995;29:327–30.
25. Gao SS, Zhang S, Mei ML, et al. Caries remineralisation and arresting effect in children by professionally applied fluoride treatment – a systematic review. BMC Oral Health 2016;16:12.
26. Azarpazhooh A, Main PA. Fluoride varnish in the prevention of dental caries in children and adolescents: a systematic review. J Can Dent Assoc 2008;74:73–9.
27. Beltrán-Aguilar ED, Goldstein JW, Lockwood SA. Fluoride varnishes—a review of their clinical use, cariostatic mechanism, efficacy and safety. J Am Dent Assoc 2000;131(5):589–96.
28. Weintraub J, Ramos-Gomez F, Jue B, et al. Fluoride varnish efficacy in preventing early childhood caries. J Dent Res 2006;85:172–6.
29. American Public Health Association. Policy number: 201010. Fluoride varnish for caries prevention. 2010. Available at: https://www.apha.org/policies-and-advocacy/public-health-policy-statements/policy-database/2014/07/09/07/51/fluoride-varnish-for-caries-prevention. Accessed January 2, 2018.
30. Tellez M, Wolff MS. The public health reach of high fluoride vehicles: examples of innovative approaches. Caries Res 2016;50(Suppl 1):61–7.
31. Rozier RG, Stearns SC, Pahel BT, et al. How a North Carolina program boosted preventive oral health services for low-income children. Health Aff 2010;29(12):2278–85.
32. Stearns SC, Rozier RG, Kranz AM, et al. Cost-effectiveness of preventive oral health care in medical offices for young Medicaid enrollees. Arch Pediatr Adolesc Med 2012;166(10):945–51.
33. Marinho VCC, Higgins JPT, Sheiham A, et al. Combinations of topical fluoride (toothpastes, mouthrinses, gels, varnishes) versus single topical fluoride for

preventing dental caries in children and adolescents. Cochrane Database Syst Rev 2004;(1):CD002781.

34. Marinho VCC, Higgins JPT, Sheiham A, et al. One topical fluoride (toothpastes, or mouthrinses, or gels, or varnishes) versus another for preventing dental caries in children and adolescents. Cochrane Database Syst Rev 2004;(1):CD002780.

35. American Dental Association Council on Scientific Affairs. Professionally applied topical fluoride, evidence-based clinical recommendations. J Am Dent Assoc 2006;137(8):1151–9.

36. Available at: https://www.healthypeople.gov/2020/topics-objectives/topic/oral-health/objectives. Accessed June 22, 2018.

37. Chestnutt IG, Playle R, Hutchings S, et al. Fissure seal or fluoride varnish? A randomized trial of relative effectiveness. J Dent Res 2017;96(7):754–61.

38. Chi DL. Parent refusal of topical fluoride for their children: clinical strategies and future research priorities to improve evidence-based pediatric dental practice. Dent Clin North Am 2017;61(3):607–17.

39. Weinstein P, Harrison R, Benton T. Motivating mothers to prevent caries: confirming the beneficial effect of counseling. J Am Dent Assoc 2006;137(6):789–93.

40. Viewpoint Learning, Inc, Rosell S, Furth I. Effectiveness of population-based interventions to promote oral health: understanding public judgment on science-intensive issues: San Diego dialogues on community water fluoridation. Berkeley (CA): Dental Health Foundation and School of Public Health, University of California; 2007. Available at: http://www.viewpointlearning.com/wp-content/uploads/2011/04/Undetstanding_Public_Judgment_on_Science-Intensive_Issues_San_Diego.pdf. Accessed January 2, 2018.

41. Institute of Medicine (US) Standing Committee on the Scientific Evaluation of Dietary Reference Intakes. Dietary reference intakes for calcium, phosphorus, magnesium, vitamin D, and fluoride. Washington, DC: National Academies Press (US); 1997. Available at: https://www.ncbi.nlm.nih.gov/books/NBK109832/#ch8.s34. Accessed May 23, 2018.

42. Iida H, Kumar JV. The association between enamel fluorosis and dental caries in U.S. schoolchildren. J Am Dent Assoc 2009;140(7):855–62.

43. Beltrán-Aguilar ED, Barker L, Dye BA. Prevalence and severity of dental fluorosis in the United States, 1999-2004. NCHS Data Brief 2010;(53):1–8.

44. National Research Council, Committee on Fluoride in Drinking Water, Board on Environmental Studies and Toxicology. Fluoride in drinking water: a scientific review of EPA's standards. Washington, DC: National Academies Press; 2006.

45. Whitford GM. Acute toxicity of ingested fluoride. Monogr Oral Sci 2011;22:66–80.

46. Sabokseir A, Golkari A, Sheiham A. Distinguishing between enamel fluorosis and other enamel defects in permanent teeth of children. Arany P, ed. PeerJ 2016;4:e1745. Available at: https://peerj.com/articles/1745/. Accessed January 2, 2018.

47. U.S. Department of Health and Human Services Federal Panel on Community Water Fluoridation. U.S. public health service recommendation for fluoride concentration in drinking water for the prevention of dental caries. Public Health Rep 2015;130(4):318–31.

48. Recommendations for using fluoride to prevent and control dental caries in the United States. Centers for disease control and prevention. MMWR Recomm Rep 2001;50(RR-14):1–42. Available at: https://www.cdc.gov/mmwr/preview/mmwrhtml/rr5014a1.htm#tab1. Accessed January 2, 2018.

49. Bayless JM, Tinanoff N. Diagnosis and treatment of acute fluoride toxicity. J Am Dent Assoc 1985;110:209–11. Available at: https://www.ncbi.nlm.nih.gov/pubmed/3856600. Accessed May 23, 2018.

50. World Health Organization. Water-related diseases. Fluorosis. Available at: http://www.who.int/water_sanitation_health/diseases-risks/diseases/fluorosis/en/. Accessed January 2, 2018.
51. US Environmental Protection Agency. Fact sheet. Fluoride. Available at: https://safewater.zendesk.com/hc/en-us/sections/202346337. Accessed January 2, 2018.
52. US Environmental Protection Agency. Questions and answers on fluoride. Available at: https://www.epa.gov/sites/production/files/2015-10/documents/2011_fluoride_questionsanswers.pdf. Accessed January 2, 2018.
53. Association of State and Territorial Dental Directors. Natural fluoride in drinking water fact sheet. 2016. Available at: http://www.astdd.org/docs/natural-fluoride-fact-sheet-9-14-2016.pdf Accessed January 2, 2018.
54. Hujoel PP, Zina LG, Moimaz SA, et al. Infant formula and enamel fluorosis: a systematic review. J Am Dent Assoc 2009;140:841–54.
55. Berg J, Gerweck C, Hujoel P, et al. Evidence-based clinical recommendations regarding fluoride intake from reconstituted infant formula and enamel fluorosis. J Am Dent Assoc 2011;142:79–87.
56. Available at: www.cdc.gov/fluoridation/faqs/infant-formula.html. Accessed on March 8, 2018.
57. American Academy of Pediatric Dentistry. Policy on use of fluorides. 2014. Available at: http://www.aapd.org/media/policies_guidelines/p_fluorideuse.pdf. Accessed January 2, 2018.
58. Crystal YO, Marghalani AA, Ureles SD, et al. Use of silver diamine fluoride for dental caries management in children and adolescents, including those with special health care needs. Pediatr Dent 2017;39(5):E135–45. Available at: http://www.aapd.org/media/Policies_Guidelines/G_SDF.pdf. Accessed January 2, 2018.
59. Contreras V, Toro MJ, Elías-Boneta AR, et al. Effectiveness of silver diamine fluoride in caries prevention and arrest: a systematic literature review. Gen Dent 2017;65(3):22–9.
60. Horst JA, Ellenikiotis H, Milgrom PL. UCSF protocol for caries arrest using silver diamine fluoride: rationale, indications and consent. J Calif Dent Assoc 2016; 44(1):16–28. Available at: https://www.ncbi.nlm.nih.gov/pmc/articles/PMC4778976/. Accessed January 2, 2018.
61. American Academy of Pediatric Dentistry: guidelines on fluoride therapy. 2014. Available at: http://www.aapd.org/media/policies_guidelines/g_fluoridetherapy.pdf. Accessed January 2, 2018.
62. Clark MB, Slayton RL, Section on Oral Health. Fluoride use in caries prevention in the primary care setting. Pediatrics 2014;134:626. Available at: http://pediatrics.aappublications.org/content/134/3/626. Accessed March 16, 2018.
63. Weyant RJ, Tracy SL, Anselmo TT, et al. Topical fluoride for caries prevention-executive summary of the updated clinical recommendations and supporting systematic review. J Am Dent Assoc 2013;144(11):1279–91.
64. Topical fluoride recommendations development of decision support matrix recommendations from MCHB expert panel. 2007. Available at: https://www.mchoralhealth.org/PDFs/TopicalFluorideRpt.pdf Accessed January 2, 2018.
65. Position of the Academy of Nutrition and Dietetics. The impact of fluoride on health. J Acad Nutr Diet 2012;112:1443–53 [Erratum: J Acad Nutr Diet. 2013;113(4):598].
66. Australian Research Center for Population Oral Health. Fluoride consensus workshop 2012. Fluoride review guidelines. Available at: https://www.adelaide.edu.au/arcpoh/dperu/fluoride/ARCPOH_FluorideOct2014.pdf. Accessed March 16, 2018.
67. American Dental Association Council on Scientific Affairs Expert Panel on Nonfluoride Caries-Preventive Agents. Nonfluoride caries-preventive agents:

executive summary of evidence-based clinical recommendations. J Am Dent Assoc 2011;142(9):1065–71.

68. Wang Y, Li J, Sun W, et al. Effect of non-fluoride agents on the prevention of dental caries in primary dentition: a systematic review. PLoS One 2017;12(8): e0182221.

Early Childhood Caries

Wan Kim Seow, BDS, MDSc, PhD, DDSc

KEYWORDS

- Early childhood caries • *Streptococcus mutans* • Prevention • Preschool children
- Primary dentition

KEY POINTS

- Early childhood caries (ECC) is highly prevalent in poor and socially disadvantaged communities.
- The main risk factors for ECC are oral colonization with cariogenic bacteria, frequent consumption of sugar, lack of tooth brushing, and enamel hypoplasia.
- Contributory factors for ECC include environmental and psychological stresses that adversely influence caregiver preventive oral care behaviors.
- Strategies for ECC prevention include reducing mutans streptococci transmission from caregivers to infants, restricting dietary sugars, tooth brushing, topical fluoride applications, and early dental visits.

INTRODUCTION

Early childhood caries (ECC) refers to caries found in the primary ("milk") teeth of children younger than 6 years of age.[1] Despite significant advances in preventive dentistry, ECC continues to affect large numbers of children globally.[2] ECC is one of the most common chronic childhood diseases, and the largest prevalence is found in poor, socially disadvantaged, and minority groups.[3–15] This article aims to provide an overview of ECC based on current understanding of its cause, prevention, and management.

WORLDWIDE PREVALENCE OF EARLY CHILDHOOD CARIES

Although representative data are sparse, general reports from several countries show that the prevalence of ECC in 2- to 3-year-old children is approximately 12% to 27%.[4–8] In 4- to 6-year-old children, the prevalence generally ranges from 27% to 48%,[8–11] with more than 76% reported from the Middle East.[12] Indigenous communities in Australia, United States, and Canada have high ECC prevalence rates of 60% to more than 90%.[13–15]

School of Dentistry, The University of Queensland, 288 Herston Road, Herston, Queensland 4006, Australia
E-mail address: k.seow@uq.edu.au

Pediatr Clin N Am 65 (2018) 941–954
https://doi.org/10.1016/j.pcl.2018.05.004
0031-3955/18/© 2018 Elsevier Inc. All rights reserved.

pediatric.theclinics.com

CLINICAL PRESENTATIONS

ECC usually starts on the maxillary primary incisors (**Fig. 1**), followed sequentially on first molars, canines, and second molars in accordance with the eruption pattern of the teeth. Clinically, the first visible signs of caries may be subsurface lesions appearing as white-yellow linear ("white-spot") lesions adjacent to the gingival (gum) margins (**Fig. 2**). These white-spot lesions usually cavitate within a short period of time because of the relative thinness of primary enamel. A severe form of ECC that is associated with enamel hypoplasia is termed "hypoplasia-associated severe-ECC" (HAS-ECC) (**Fig. 3**).[16] HAS-ECC is commonly seen in very young children living in poverty and needs to be recognized as a separate, high-risk, clinical entity because it usually warrants a different, targeted approach.

COMPLICATIONS OF EARLY CHILDHOOD CARIES

Caries in young children causes mouth pain and dental abscesses, eating difficulties, and reduced weight and body mass index for age compared with healthy children.[17] ECC is associated with poor quality of life,[18] including multiple emergency room visits,[19] sleep disturbances,[20] missed school days, and lower academic performance.[21] Also, early extractions of primary teeth due to ECC may lead to malocclusions. Finally, children with ECC have a higher risk for future caries.[22]

CAUSE OF EARLY CHILDHOOD CARIES

The cause of ECC is multifactorial and complex. The traditionally taught Keyes' etiologic caries triad of bacteria, sugar, and tooth surface is greatly affected by sociocultural and environmental factors that modify oral care behaviors, sugar intake, and access to dental services.[23] The cariogenic bacteria (*Streptococcus mutans*, *Streptococcus sobrinus*, and lactobacilli) reside in the dental biofilm and produce acids by fermenting dietary sugars.[24] When the pH drops below a critical level, the tooth surface starts to demineralize (ie, loss of calcium and phosphate mineral).[25] The mineral loss may be reversed by salivary factors (high salivary flow results in clearance, buffering, and increased calcium supply), and remineralization is facilitated by the presence of fluoride. The processes leading to caries involve dynamic cycles of demineralization and remineralization of the tooth surface.[25] Over time, when the demineralization effects are greater than remineralization, the outcome is a carious lesion.

Although the pathogenesis of ECC is similar to other types of dental caries, ECC is usually widespread and rampant, most likely due to the immaturity of the newly

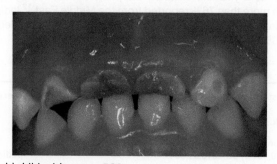

Fig. 1. A 2-year-old child with severe ECC.

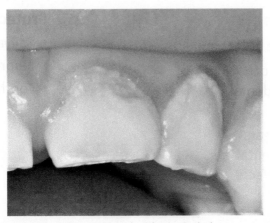

Fig. 2. Primary incisors with caries associated with gingival plaque retention.

erupted primary tooth surfaces, large numbers of cariogenic bacteria, and the highly acidic conditions unbalanced by protective measures.[26]

Fig. 4 depicts the direct risk and protective factors in the development of ECC from a healthy state of the primary incisors (top image) to early cavities associated with "white-spot" lesions (middle image) when the risk factors overwhelm the protective factors. The early lesions usually progress quickly to extensive cavities (bottom image).

Microbial Factors

The most common microorganisms associated with ECC is a group of highly acidogenic and aciduric bacteria known as mutans streptococci (MS), which include the species *S mutans* and *S sobrinus*.[27] Recent studies using molecular techniques have confirmed the predominance of *S mutans* in the dental plaque of children with ECC.[28,29] Longitudinal investigations show that children with very high levels of MS are 6 times more likely to experience additional cavities over time than those without MS at first visit.[30] In addition, children who are colonized with MS at an early age are at higher risk for ECC than children who are colonized at older ages.[6]

The virulence of MS is associated with their ability to generate large amounts of acid and high acid tolerance.[31] The low pH results in demineralization, and the acid

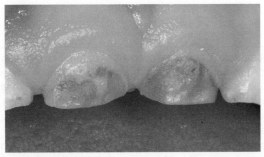

Fig. 3. Advanced ECC with appearance suggestive of preexisting developmental enamel defects in the affected incisors.

Risk factors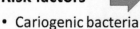

- Cariogenic bacteria
- Retention of microbial dental plaque
- Dietary sugars
- Developmental enamel defects

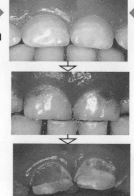

Protective factors

- Saliva
- Fluoride
- Tooth brushing

Fig. 4. The risk and protective factors involved in the development of ECC.

environment created by MS promotes a shift of the microbial species in the dental biofilm toward the aciduric and acidogenic groups, such as lactobacilli.[32] In addition, MS uses sucrose to produce large quantities of extracellular polysaccharides that enable strong cellular adhesion to the tooth surface and greatly increase the pathogenicity of the dental biofilm by limiting acid diffusion.[33]

Other oral acidogenic and aciduric microorganisms in the dental biofilm are also likely to play a role in ECC.[34] To date, *Scardovia wiggsiae*, *Bifidobacterium*, and *Lactobacilli*, species have been identified in the dental plaque of children with ECC, and several investigators have suggested that these microbes contribute to the development of ECC.[35–37] Finally, the presence of *Candida albicans* may increase the cariogenicity of *S mutans* by enhancing biofilm formation and acid production.[38,39]

Children usually acquire MS from their mothers,[40] although transmission from other family members, caregivers, and children may also occur.[41–43] High oral counts of MS in mothers are associated with unrestored caries, poor periodontal health, and inadequate oral hygiene.[44] These maternal oral conditions increase in their children the risk for MS colonization and ECC.[45]

Oral colonization with MS occurs before tooth emergence in at least 20% of children, most likely facilitated by frequent sugar consumption and exposure to MS-rich saliva of family/caregivers.[44,46] However, the colonization rate increases greatly when the first primary teeth emerge, and by the time the primary dentition is fully erupted at approximately 30 months of age, more than 80% of children have acquired MS.[47–49]

Dietary Factors

Sugars play a critical role in the development of caries.[50] Clinical investigations have established that children with ECC more frequently consume between-meal juice and sweetened solid foods than caries-free controls.[6,51] If one combines sugar intake with decreased salivary flow, the effects are cumulative: when children fall asleep with a nursing bottle filled with sweet fluids, the risk for ECC is greatly increased, because salivary flow is reduced during sleep.

Although milk contains lactose, which is a fermentable sugar, the high concentration of calcium and phosphorus will help to prevent dissolution of enamel.[52] In the clinical reports suggesting that ECC is associated with prolonged at-will breast-feeding,[53,54] factors other than breast milk, for example, developmental enamel defects and poor oral hygiene, are likely to have contributed to the caries risk.

A recent systematic review reports that breast-feeding in infancy is protective for ECC.[55] However, the review and other epidemiologic evidence also suggest that breast-feeding longer than 12 months and at night may be associated with increased risk for ECC.[56,57] These results may be explained by the fact that although breast milk has low intrinsic cariogenicity, the effects of breast-feeding beyond 12 months are likely to be strongly modulated by other risk factors, such as oral colonization with cariogenic bacteria, ingestion of dietary sugars, presence of developmental enamel defects, and inadequate oral hygiene.[54,55,58–61] Therefore, clinicians should emphasize the importance of daily tooth brushing, restricting sugars, and regular dental visits for all children in addition to the usual American Academy of Pediatrics (AAP) recommendations regarding breast-feeding.[62]

Tooth Factors

The loss of tooth surface integrity resulting from developmental disruptions of the enamel is now recognized as a major risk factor for ECC.[16,26,63] Developmental defects of enamel (DDE) may be expressed as enamel hypoplasia whereby the enamel is deficient in quantity, and clinically observed as pits, grooves, or large areas of missing or dysplastic enamel.[64] The defects present as rough surfaces that are readily colonized by MS.[65] DDE can also be expressed as hypomineralized enamel, where the mineral content is reduced and less resistant to carious attack than normal enamel.[64] **Fig. 5** shows a primary central incisor with a caries lesion associated with DDE. The location of the caries in **Fig. 5** contrasts with the more common ECC lesions that are associated with plaque retention at the gingival margins (see **Fig. 2**). However, as shown in **Fig. 3**, in many advanced cases of HAS-ECC, the diagnosis of preexisting DDE is difficult because of the extensive destruction by caries.

DDE in the primary dentition is found in approximately 22% to 49% of healthy children and more than 60% of preterm children.[65–67] The major causes of DDE are congenital medical conditions, birth prematurity, childhood metabolic and infectious illnesses, and the intake of certain medications, for example,

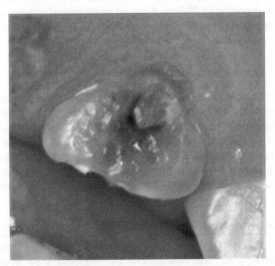

Fig. 5. A primary central incisor with caries associated with enamel hypoplasia.

cytotoxic drugs.[64] The high ECC prevalence observed in children with congenital or acquired conditions may be explained by the fact that many of these conditions disrupt enamel formation,[68] which in turn predisposes the affected enamel to ECC.

Contributory Risk Factors

Environmental factors as well as caregiver psychosocial stresses have been shown to contribute to the development of ECC. Over a decade ago, Fisher-Owens and co-workers[69] proposed a comprehensive model to approach oral health in general. This model includes a broad range of genetic, social, and environmental risk factors that should be taken into consideration when approaching pediatric oral health. Some of the risk factors act through the caregivers, who have a pivotal role for preventing ECC because they provide the oral care for their children.[23]

Previous reports have demonstrated that caregiver health literacy and health beliefs are associated with sociocultural status and may act as barriers to obtaining dental care for their children.[70] Other studies found that caregiver chronic stress is associated with child caries experience,[71] suggesting that chronic stress may have adverse effects on caregivers' ability to adopt preventive behaviors for their children's oral health.

Chronic stress is associated with depression and anxiety.[72] Depression and anxiety in mothers, in turn, are associated with risk for ECC in their children.[73,74] Other investigations also suggest that caregivers from disadvantaged communities have lower self-efficacy and sense of coherence, and that these traits are associated with less preventive oral care and greater presence of caries in their children.[75-77] In addition, mothers with limited absolute financial means or relative social capital are more likely to forgo preventive dental visits and have children with greater unmet dental needs than more advantaged families.[78]

Psychosocial barriers to good oral health, including ECC prevention, may be addressed using intervention methods that involve personal interaction between caregiver and health workers,[79] for example, communication through telephone, social media, or home visits. The positive effects of home visits on ECC prevention were shown in Brazil and the United Kingdom over a decade ago,[80,81] and more recently in Australia,[82] where the cost-effective success of a telephone-based support approach was demonstrated.[83] Parent-based motivational interviewing can enhance the personal interaction of health workers with the caregiver to improve oral health behaviors for ECC prevention.[84]

PREVENTION OF EARLY CHILDHOOD CARIES

There are many possible strategies for prevention of ECC: first, preventing or delaying MS colonization in children by reducing MS transmission from caregivers and improving oral hygiene in both caregivers and children; second, reducing the cariogenicity of the diet by restricting sugars; and third, increasing the caries resistance of newly erupted teeth by applying topical fluoride. These strategies may be included in establishing a dental home for preventing ECC. A caries risk assessment (CRA) is also recommended at the first visit to help develop an appropriate plan for prevention.[85]

Preventing or Delaying Mutans Streptococci Colonization in Infants

Improving maternal oral health can reduce transmission of MS to their children.[86] Mothers can lower their oral MS counts by reducing their sugar consumption, restoring carious lesions, tooth brushing and flossing and using fluoride rinses and xylitol.[87,88] Receiving antenatal oral health education can improve maternal preventive oral care which can lead to less ECC in their children[89]

Oral Hygiene for Infants

Longitudinal trials have established that regular tooth brushing with fluoridated toothpaste is associated with less MS colonization and less ECC.[6,49,90] Tooth brushing disrupts the dental biofilm and reduces bacterial numbers, while the fluoride in toothpaste helps to remineralize carious lesions. To prevent ECC, caregivers should be advised to commence tooth brushing with a soft brush and fluoridated toothpaste as soon as the first teeth erupt.

Restricting Dietary Sugars

To prevent ECC, caregivers should be instructed to restrict the frequency of sweet snacks and drinks. The author suggests that caregivers be advised to follow the AAP recommendations for fruit juice, that is, fruit juice should not be given to children younger than 1 year of age and be limited to 120 mL for 1 to 3 year olds and 120 to 180 mL for 4 to 6 year olds.[91] The dangers of frequent sipping of sweetened drinks and fruit juices from a bottle or a sippy cup, particularly at sleep time should be also emphasized. Furthermore, physicians need to consider the ECC risk posed by sugar-containing syrups when prescribing oral medicines that are consumed frequently for certain chronic medical conditions.[92] At the minimum, families should be reminded to brush the child's teeth after taking the sugar-containing medications.

Increasing Caries Resistance of Tooth Surfaces

Fluoride helps to remineralize the demineralized tooth surfaces caused by caries. It increases the resistance of the tooth and is a mainstay for caries prevention.[93] Fluoride may be delivered in the community drinking water, or as oral supplements, topical varnishes, gels, and rinses. Drinking community fluoridated water provides approximately 35% reduction in caries experience in the primary dentition.[94] Systematic reviews confirm that fluoridated toothpaste is efficacious for controlling caries in children younger than 6 year old.[95,96] Fluoride varnish is a popular topical fluoride agent for ECC prevention. A systematic review of trials involving the primary dentition reports that fluoride varnish use may result in approximately 37% reduction in caries.[97]

Silver diamine fluoride (SDF) has antibacterial and mineralizing properties because of its silver and fluoride content. These properties suggest that it has potential for managing ECC.[98] The main disadvantage of SDF is cosmetic: it stains the carious lesions black. This black stain may be unacceptable to some children and parents.[99] In general, SDF is particularly effective for children who are unable to tolerate extensive restorative treatment, for example, children with certain disabilities and those who lack access to restorative care under general anesthesia. The American Academy of Pediatric Dentistry (AAPD) has recently given conditional recommendation for SDF to be used for arresting cavitated caries lesions in primary teeth.[100]

ESTABLISHING A DENTAL HOME FOR EARLY CHILDHOOD CARIES PREVENTION

An important strategy for ECC prevention is establishing a dental home for all children by 1 year of age.[101,102] A dental home is defined as the continuing relationship between a dentist and the child that encompasses all aspects of oral health care.[103] The dental home focuses on children's access to regular, individualized preventive care, including fluoride varnish applications. A dental home also facilitates anticipatory guidance on regular tooth brushing, the use of fluoridated toothpaste, and limiting snacks and drinks.[104]

Children whose preventive dental care started at a younger age have fewer dental procedures and less treatment costs compared with children who start later.[105] However, establishing a dental home for financially deprived, impoverished, and socially disadvantaged children remains difficult because of psychosocial, economic, and environmental barriers.[23] Most children already have frequent contact with their medical providers, that is, pediatricians, family physicians, and child health nurses, so these interactions can provide opportunities to maximize oral health.[86] With some minimal training, most primary-care medical providers can perform oral health screening, ECC risk assessment, fluoride varnish applications, and timely referral to pediatric dentists for urgent and long-term dental care.

CARIES RISK ASSESSMENT

The AAPD recommends that caries risk assessment (CRA) should be done as part of a child's first dental examination to facilitate an individualized plan of prevention.[85] Current CRA tools generally assess the biological and social ECC risk factors, including low socioeconomic status, recent immigrant status, special health care needs, presence of active caries in the mother/primary caregiver, consumption of more than 3 daily between-meal sugary snacks or beverages, and going to bed with a bottle containing sugar.[85] Included also are factors protective for caries, that is, presence of a dental home, drinking fluoridated water or receiving fluoride supplements, twice daily tooth brushing with fluoridated paste, and receiving topical fluoride.[85] Clinical caries risk indicators, including presence of at least one decayed/missing/filled surface, carious white-spot lesions or enamel defects, elevated MS levels, and visible dental plaque, are also part of the CRA.[85] The child's overall caries risk is determined based on the relative number of risk and protective factors. In addition to assessing caries risk, CRA tools can also be used for discussing preventive and management strategies with parents. A free version is available from the AAP for use in the primary care office (https://www.aap.org/en-us/Documents/oralhealth_RiskAssessmentTool.pdf).

CONVENTIONAL AND NEWER MANAGEMENT APPROACHES FOR EARLY CHILDHOOD CARIES

Dental treatment of caries in the primary dentition historically involves restorations, pulp treatment, and extraction of nonrestorable teeth.[106] Because of young children's inability to tolerate extensive treatment in the dental chair, many affected children require treatment under general anesthesia, which is costly and associated with health risks.[107,108] Conventional restorative and surgical management deal with the result of ECC, but do not prevent further caries. Consequently, relapse rates after standard treatments are high (22%–79%).[109]

A newer approach to treatment of ECC uses a chronic disease management method, which emphasizes preventive procedures applied through parental involvement and postponement of advanced restorations.[110] Other strategies include the institution of preventive programs with active monitoring of ECC lesions,[85] and use of interim therapeutic restorations.[111] These methods are reported to be cost-effective and may be suitable as caries control strategies for children who have to wait long periods to access general anesthesia, or who have no access to restorative care.[112]

SUMMARY

Despite recent advances in preventive dentistry, ECC continues to affect large numbers of young children, particularly those from poor, indigenous, and minority communities. The control of ECC is difficult, most likely due to the complex behavioral problems that stem from social, economic, and other environmental factors operating at the individual, family, and community levels. Preventive strategies should focus on early dental examination, establishing a dental home by one year of age, tooth brushing, restricting sugars and topical fluoride applications.

REFERENCES

1. American Academy of Pediatric Dentistry. Policy on early childhood caries (ECC): classifications, consequences, and preventive strategies. Pediatr Dent 2017;39(6):59–61.
2. Dye BA, Hsu KL, Afful J. Prevalence and measurement of dental caries in young children. Pediatr Dent 2015;37(3):200–16.
3. Heilmann A, Tsakos G, Watt RG. Oral health over the life course. In: Burton-Jeangros C, Cullati S, Sacker A, et al, editors. A life course perspective on health trajectories and transitions. Cham (Switzerland): Springer; 2015. p. 39–59.
4. Zhou Y, Lin HC, Lo ECM, et al. Risk indicators for early childhood caries in 2-year-old children in southern China. Aust Dent J 2011;56(1):33.
5. Dye BA, Thornton-Evans G, Li X, et al. Dental caries and sealant prevalence in children and adolescents in the United States, 2011-2012. NCHS Data Brief 2015;(191):1–8.
6. Plonka KA, Pukallus ML, Barnett AG, et al. A longitudinal case-control study of caries development from birth to 36 months. Caries Res 2013;47(2):117–27.
7. Nobile CG, Fortunato L, Bianco A, et al. Pattern and severity of early childhood caries in Southern Italy: a preschool-based cross-sectional study. BMC Public Health 2014;14:206.
8. Public Health England. National Dental Epidemiology Programme for England: oral health survey of five-year-old children in 2012–a report of prevalence and severity of dental decay. London: Crown Publications; 2013. Available at: http://www.nwph.net/dentalhealth/Oral%20Health%205yr%20old%20children%202012%20final%20report%20gateway%20approved.pdfLondon.
9. Do LG, Spencer AJ. Oral health of Australian children. The national child oral health study 2012-2014. Adelaide (Australia): University of Adelaide Press; 2016.
10. Duangthip D, Gao SS, Lo EC, et al. Early childhood caries among 5- to 6-year-old children in Southeast Asia. Int Dent J 2017;67(2):98–106.
11. Poon BT, Holley PC, Louie AM, et al. Dental caries disparities in early childhood: a study of kindergarten children in British Columbia. Can J Public Health 2015; 106(5):e308–14.
12. Azizi Z. The prevalence of dental caries in primary dentition in 4- to 5-year-old preschool children in northern Palestine. Int J Dent 2014;2014:839419.
13. Indian Health Service. The 1999 oral health survey of American Indian and Alaska Native dental patients: findings, regional differences and national comparisons. Rockville (MD): Indian Health Service, Division of Dental Services; 2002.

14. Australian Institute of Health and Welfare, Dental Statistics and Research Unit, Jamieson LM, et al. Oral health of Aboriginal and Torres Strait Islander children. Canberra (Australia): Australian Institute of Health and Welfare; 2007.

15. Schroth RJ, Smith PJ, Whalen JC, et al. Prevalence of caries among preschool-aged children in a northern Manitoba community. J Can Dent Assoc 2005;71(1):27.

16. Caufield PW, Li Y, Bromage TG. Hypoplasia-associated severe early childhood caries – A proposed definition. J Dent Res 2012;91(6):544–50.

17. Khanh LN, Ivey SL, Sokal-Gutierrez K, et al. Early childhood caries, mouth pain, and nutritional threats in Vietnam. Am J Public Health 2015;105(12):2510–7.

18. Fernandes IB, Pereira TS, Souza DS, et al. Severity of dental caries and quality of life for toddlers and their families. Pediatr Dent 2017;39(2):118–23.

19. Ladrillo TE, Hobdell MH, Caviness AC. Increasing prevalence of emergency department visits for pediatric dental care, 1997-2001. J Am Dent Assoc 2006;137(3):379–85.

20. Vieira-Andrade RG, Gomes GB, de Almeida Pinto-Sarmento TC, et al. Oral conditions and trouble sleeping among preschool children. J Publ Health 2016; 24(5):395–400.

21. Arrow P, Klobas E. Child oral health-related quality of life and early childhood caries: a non-inferiority randomized control trial. Aust Dent J 2016;61(2):227–35.

22. Li Y, Wang W. Predicting caries in permanent teeth from caries in primary teeth: an eight-year cohort study. J Dent Res 2002;81(8):561–6.

23. Seow WK. Environmental, maternal, and child factors which contribute to early childhood caries: a unifying conceptual model. Int J Paediatr Dent 2012;22(3): 157–68.

24. Fejerskov O, Nyvad B, Kidd E. Dental caries: the disease and its clinical management. 3rd edition. Hoboken (NJ): Wiley-Blackwell; 2015.

25. Featherstone JDB. Dental caries: a dynamic disease process. Aust Dent J 2008; 53(3):286–91.

26. Seow WK. Biological mechanisms of early childhood caries. Community Dent Oral Epidemiol 1998;26(S1):8–27.

27. van Houte J, Gibbs G, Butera C. Oral flora of children with "nursing bottle caries". J Dent Res 1982;61(2):382–5.

28. Agnello M, Marques J, Cen L, et al. Microbiome associated with severe caries in Canadian First Nations children. J Dent Res 2017;96(12):1378–85.

29. Ma C, Chen F, Zhang Y, et al. Comparison of oral microbial profiles between children with severe early childhood caries and caries-free children using the human oral microbe identification microarray. PLoS One 2015;10(3):e0122075.

30. Edelstein BL, Ureles SD, Smaldone A. Very high salivary Streptococcus mutans predicts caries progression in young children. Pediatr Dent 2016;38(4):325–30.

31. Loesche WJ. Role of Streptococcus mutans in human dental decay. Microbiol Rev 1986;50(4):353–80.

32. Marsh PD. Dental plaque as a biofilm and a microbial community – implications for health and disease. BMC Oral Health 2006;6(Suppl 1):S14.

33. Leme AFP, Koo H, Bellato CM, et al. The role of sucrose in cariogenic dental biofilm formation—new insight. J Dent Res 2006;85(10):878–87.

34. Takahashi N, Nyvad B. The role of bacteria in the caries process: ecological perspectives. J Dent Res 2011;90(3):294–303.

35. Tanner AC, Kent RL Jr, Holgerson PL, et al. Microbiota of severe early childhood caries before and after therapy. J Dent Res 2011;90(11):1298–305.

36. Kanasi E, Dewhirst FE, Chalmers NI, et al. Clonal analysis of the microbiota of severe early childhood caries. Caries Res 2010;44(5):485–97.

37. de Carvalho FG, Silva DS, Hebling J, et al. Presence of mutans streptococci and Candida spp. in dental plaque/dentine of carious teeth and early childhood caries. Arch Oral Biol 2006;51(11):1024–8.

38. Raja M, Hannan A, Ali K. Association of oral candidal carriage with dental caries in children. Caries Res 2010;44(3):272–6.

39. Falsetta ML, Klein MI, Colonne PM, et al. Symbiotic relationship between Streptococcus mutans and Candida albicans synergizes virulence of plaque biofilms in vivo. Infect Immun 2014;82(5):1968–81.

40. Berkowitz RJ, Turner J, Green P. Maternal salivary levels of Streptococcus mutans and primary oral infection of infants. Arch Oral Biol 1981;26(2):147–9.

41. Mattos-Graner RO, Li Y, Caufield PW, et al. Genotypic diversity of mutans streptococci in Brazilian nursery children suggests horizontal transmission. J Clin Microbiol 2001;39(6):2313–6.

42. Childers NK, Momeni SS, Whiddon J, et al. Association between early childhood caries and colonization with Streptococcus mutans genotypes from mothers. Pediatr Dent 2017;39(2):130–5.

43. Li Y, Caufield PW. The fidelity of initial acquisition of mutans streptococci by infants from their mothers. J Dent Res 1995;74(2):681–5.

44. Wan AK, Seow WK, Purdie DM, et al. Oral colonization of Streptococcus mutans in six-month-old predentate infants. J Dent Res 2001;80(12):2060–5.

45. Chaffee BW, Gansky SA, Weintraub JA, et al. Maternal oral bacterial levels predict early childhood caries development. J Dent Res 2014;93(3):238–44.

46. Plonka KA, Pukallus ML, Barnett AG, et al. Mutans streptococci and lactobacilli colonization in predentate children from the neonatal period to seven months of age. Caries Res 2012;46(3):213–20.

47. Caufield PW, Cutter GR, Dasanayake AP. Initial acquisition of mutans streptococci by infants: evidence for a discrete window of infectivity. J Dent Res 1993;72(1):37–45.

48. Plonka KA, Pukallus ML, Barnett AG, et al. A longitudinal study comparing mutans streptococci and lactobacilli colonisation in dentate children aged 6 to 24 months. Caries Res 2012;46(4):385–93.

49. Wan AK, Seow WK, Purdie DM, et al. A longitudinal study of Streptococcus mutans colonization in infants after tooth eruption. J Dent Res 2003;82(7):504–8.

50. Sheiham A, James WP. Diet and dental caries: the pivotal role of free sugars reemphasized. J Dent Res 2015;94(10):1341–7.

51. Palmer CA, Kent R Jr, Loo CY, et al. Diet and caries-associated bacteria in severe early childhood caries. J Dent Res 2010;89(11):1224–9.

52. Bowen W, Lawrence R. Comparison of the cariogenicity of cola, honey, cow milk, human milk, and sucrose. Pediatrics 2005;116(4):921–6.

53. Dilley GJ, Dilley DH, Machen JB. Prolonged nursing habit: a profile of patients and their families. ASDC J Dent Child 1980;47(2):102–8.

54. Weerheijm KL, Uyttendaele-Speybrouck BFM, Euwe HC, et al. Prolonged demand breast-feeding and nursing caries. Caries Res 1998;32(1):46–50.

55. Tham R, Bowatte G, Dharmage SC, et al. Breastfeeding and the risk of dental caries: a systematic review and meta-analysis. Acta Paediatr 2015;104(467):62–84.

56. Chaffee BW, Featherstone JD, Gansky SA, et al. Caries risk assessment item importance: risk designation and caries status in children under age 6. JDR Clin Trans Res 2016;1(2):131–42.

57. Valaitis R, Hesch R, Passarelli C, et al. A systematic review of the relationship between breastfeeding and early childhood caries. Can J Public Health 2000; 91(6):411–7.

58. Avila WM, Pordeus IA, Paiva SM, et al. Breast and bottle feeding as risk factors for dental caries: a systematic review and meta-analysis. PLoS One 2015; 10(11):e0142922.

59. Nirunsittirat A, Pitiphat W, McKinney CM, et al. Breastfeeding duration and childhood caries: a cohort study. Caries Res 2016;50(5):498–507.

60. Bernabé E, MacRitchie H, Longbottom C, et al. Birth weight, breastfeeding, maternal smoking and caries trajectories. J Dent Res 2017;96(2):171–8.

61. Neves PA, Ribeiro CC, Tenuta LM, et al. Breastfeeding, dental biofilm acidogenicity, and early childhood caries. Caries Res 2016;50(3):319–24.

62. Meek JY, Hatcher AJ. The breastfeeding-friendly pediatric office practice. American Academy of Pediatrics: section on breastfeeding 2017. Available at: http://pediatrics.aappublications.org/content/139/5/e20170647. Accessed June 18, 2018.

63. Seow WK, Leishman SJ, Palmer JE, et al. A longitudinal observational study of developmental defects of enamel from birth to 6 years of age. JDR Clin Trans Res 2016;1(3):285–91.

64. Seow WK. Enamel hypoplasia in the primary dentition: a review. ASDC J Dent Child 1991;58:441–52.

65. Li Y, Navia JM, Bian JH. Prevalence and distribution of developmental enamel defects in primary dentition of Chinese children 3–5 years old. Community Dent Oral Epidemiol 1995;23(2):72–9.

66. Seow WK, Humphrys C, Tudehope DI. Increased prevalence of developmental dental defects in low-birth-weight children: a controlled study. Pediatr Dent 1987;9:221–5.

67. Slayton RL, Warren JJ, Kanellis MJ, et al. Prevalence of enamel hypoplasia and isolated opacities in the primary dentition. Pediatr Dent 2001;23:32–6.

68. Seow WK. Etiology of developmental enamel defects in the primary dentition. Clinical Dentistry Reviewed 2017;1(1):1–8.

69. Fisher-Owens SA, Gansky SA, Platt LJ, et al. Influences on children's oral health: a conceptual model. Pediatrics 2007;120(3):e510–20.

70. Finnegan DA, Rainchuso L, Jenkins S, et al. Immigrant caregivers of young children: oral health beliefs, attitudes, and early childhood caries knowledge. J Community Health 2016;41(2):250–7.

71. Masterson EE, Sabbah W. Maternal allostatic load, caretaking behaviors, and child dental caries experience: a cross-sectional evaluation of linked mother-child data from the Third National Health and Nutrition Examination Survey. Am J Public Health 2015;105(11):2306–11.

72. Bergdahl J, Bergdahl M. Perceived stress in adults: prevalence and association of depression, anxiety and medication in a Swedish population. Stress Health 2002;18(5):235–41.

73. Crowe M, O'Sullivan A, McGrath C, et al. Early childhood dental problems: classification tree analyses of 2 waves of an infant cohort study. JDR Clin Trans Res 2016;1(3):275–84.

74. Seow WK, Clifford H, Battistutta D, et al. Case-control study of early childhood caries in Australia. Caries Res 2009;43(1):25–35.

75. Finlayson TL, Siefert K, Ismail AI, et al. Reliability and validity of brief measures of oral health-related knowledge, fatalism, and self-efficacy in mothers of African American children. Pediatr Dent 2005;27(5):422–8.

76. Reisine S, Litt M. Social and psychological theories and their use for dental practice. Int Dent J 1993;43(3 Suppl 1):279–87.
77. Bonanato K, Paiva SM, Pordeus IA, et al. Relationship between mothers' sense of coherence and oral health status of preschool children. Caries Res 2009; 43(2):103–9.
78. Iida H, Rozier RG. Mother-perceived social capital and children's oral health and use of dental care in the United States. Am J Public Health 2013;103(3):480–7.
79. McLeish J, Redshaw M. Mothers' accounts of the impact on emotional wellbeing of organised peer support in pregnancy and early parenthood: a qualitative study. BMC Pregnancy Childbirth 2017;17:28.
80. Feldens CA, Vitolo MR, Drachler Mde L. A randomized trial of the effectiveness of home visits in preventing early childhood caries. Community Dent Oral Epidemiol 2007;35(3):215–23.
81. Kowash MB, Toumba KJ, Curzon ME. Cost-effectiveness of a long-term dental health education program for the prevention of early childhood caries. Eur Arch Paediatr Dent 2006;7(3):130–5.
82. Plonka KA, Pukallus ML, Barnett A, et al. A controlled, longitudinal study of home visits compared to telephone contacts to prevent early childhood caries. Int J Paediatr Dent 2013;23(1):23–31.
83. Koh R, Pukallus M, Kularatna S, et al. Relative cost-effectiveness of home visits and telephone contacts in preventing early childhood caries. Community Dent Oral Epidemiol 2015;43(6):560–8.
84. Borrelli B, Tooley EM, Scott-Sheldon LAJ. Motivational interviewing for parent-child health interventions: a systematic review and meta-analysis. Pediatr Dent 2015;37:254–65.
85. American Academy of Pediatric Dentistry. Caries-risk assessment and management for infants, children, and adolescents. Pediatr Dent 2017;39(6):197–204.
86. American Academy of Pediatric Dentistry. Perinatal and infant oral health care. Pediatr Dent 2017;39(6):208–12.
87. Isokangas P, Soderling E, Pienihakkinen K, et al. Occurrence of dental decay in children after maternal consumption of xylitol chewing gum, a follow-up from 0 to 5 years of age. J Dent Res 2000;79(11):1885–9.
88. Köhler B, Andréen I. Influence of caries-preventive measures in mothers on cariogenic bacteria and caries experience in their children. Arch Oral Biol 1994; 39(10):907–11.
89. Plutzer K, Spencer AJ. Efficacy of an oral health promotion intervention in the prevention of early childhood caries. Community Dent Oral Epidemiol 2008; 36(4):335–46.
90. Seow WK, Cheng E, Wan V. Effects of oral health education and tooth-brushing on mutans streptococci infection in young children. Pediatr Dent 2003;25(3):223–8.
91. American Academy of Pediatric Dentistry. Policy on dietary recommendations for infants, children, and adolescents. Pediatr Dent 2017;39(6):64–6.
92. Mackie IC. Children's dental health and medicines that contain sugar. BMJ 1995;311(6998):141–2.
93. ten Cate JM. Current concepts on the theories of the mechanism of action of fluoride. Acta Odontol Scand 1999;57(6):325–9.
94. Iheozor-Ejiofor Z, Worthington HV, Walsh T, et al. Water fluoridation for the prevention of dental caries. Cochrane Database Syst Rev 2015;(6):CD010856.
95. Walsh T, Worthington HV, Glenny AM, et al. Fluoride toothpastes of different concentrations for preventing dental caries in children and adolescents. Cochrane Database Syst Rev 2010;(1):CD007868.

96. Wright JT, Hanson N, Ristic H, et al. Fluoride toothpaste efficacy and safety in children younger than 6 years: a systematic review. J Am Dent Assoc 2014; 145(2):182–9.

97. Marinho VCC, Worthington HV, Walsh T, et al. Fluoride varnishes for preventing dental caries in children and adolescents. Cochrane Database Syst Rev 2013;(7):CD002279.

98. Rosenblatt A, Stamford TC, Niederman R. Silver diamine fluoride: a caries "silver-fluoride bullet". J Dent Res 2009;88(2):116–25.

99. Gao SS, Zhao IS, Hiraishi N, et al. Clinical trials of silver diamine fluoride in arresting caries among children: a systematic review. JDR Clin Trans Res 2016;1(3):201–10.

100. American Academy of Pediatric Dentistry. Policy on the use of silver diamine fluoride for pediatric dental patients. Pediatr Dent 2017;39(6):51–3.

101. American Academy of Pediatric Dentistry. Review council policy on oral health care programs for infants, children, and adolescents. Pediatr Dent 2017;39(6): 27–8.

102. Clark MB, Slayton RL. Fluoride use in caries prevention in the primary care setting. Pediatrics 2014;134(3):626–33.

103. American Academy of Pediatric Dentistry. Definition of dental home. Pediatr Dent 2017;39(6):12.

104. American Academy of Pediatric Dentistry. Periodicity of examination, preventive dental services, anticipatory guidance/counseling, and oral treatment for infants, children, and adolescents. Pediatr Dent 2017;39(6):188–96.

105. Nowak AJ, Casamassimo PS, Scott J, et al. Do early dental visits reduce treatment and treatment costs for children? Pediatr Dent 2014;36(7):489–93.

106. American Academy of Pediatric Dentistry. Guideline on restorative dentistry. Pediatr Dent 2016;38(6):250.

107. Sinner B, Becke K, Engelhard K. General anaesthetics and the developing brain: an overview. Anaesthesia 2014;69(9):1009–22.

108. U.S. Food and Drug Administration FDA Drug Safety Communication: FDA review results in new warnings about using general anesthetics and sedation drugs in young children and pregnant women. 2016. Available at: https://www.fda.gov/Drugs/DrugSafety/ucm 532356.htm. Accessed November 20, 2017.

109. Twetman S, Dhar V. Evidence of effectiveness of current therapies to prevent and treat early childhood caries. Pediatr Dent 2015;37(3):246–53.

110. Edelstein BL, Ng MW. Chronic disease management dtrategies of early childhood caries: support from the medical and dental literature. Pediatr Dent 2015;37(3):281–7.

111. American Academy of Pediatric Dentistry. Policy on interim therapeutic restorations (ITR). Pediatr Dent 2017;39(6):57–8.

112. Tonmukayakul U, Arrow P. Cost-effectiveness analysis of the atraumatic restorative treatment-based approach to managing early childhood caries. Community Dent Oral Epidemiol 2017;45(1):92–100.

The Burden and Management of Dental Caries in Older Children

John Timothy Wright, DDS, MS

KEYWORDS

- Pit • Fissure • Occlusal • Caries • Prevalence • Sealant • Cost • Adolescent

KEY POINTS

- Dental caries affects most children.
- Pit and fissure surfaces represent a disproportionate amount of disease compared with the total number of surfaces at risk.
- Pit and fissure sealants are effective in preventing pit and fissure caries.
- Pit and fissure sealants are effective stopping the progression of noncavitated caries lesions.

INTRODUCTION

Dental caries is a complex and multifactorial chronic disease that is endemic in populations around the world. Dental caries continues to be highly prevalent in the United States, beginning for many people in early childhood and continuing throughout their life.[1] Although dental caries is infrequently associated with mortality, it does cause significant morbidity, including pain, suffering, loss of work and school time, loss of income, and the spending of billions of health care dollars.[2] The genetic and environmental determinants associated with disease risk and resistance exert dynamic influences on this disease process. Genetic studies suggest that the heritable influence on pit and fissure caries development varies from about 20% to 50%, indicating that an individual's genetic determinants play an important role in their risk/resistance.[3] The environment is a modifier of caries risk that influences tooth development (eg, fluoride exposure, risk of enamel defects), oral hygiene, topical fluoride exposure, carbohydrate exposure, microbiome exposure, and many other potential dental caries modifiers. Tooth formation is highly regulated at the molecular level and the

Disclosure Statement: The author has no commercial or financial conflicts of interest from any funding source.
Department of Pediatric Dentistry, School of Dentistry, The University of North Carolina, Brauer Hall #7450, Chapel Hill, NC 27599, USA
E-mail address: tim_wright@unc.edu

shape; size, mineralization, and even pit and fissure morphology are strongly determined by the individual's genetic makeup or genome.

It is not surprising that the dental caries experience faced by the 6- to 18-year-old is indeed different in many ways from the disease afflicting the infant/toddler or elderly person. Children younger than 6 years mostly have primary teeth, which are structurally and compositionally different than the permanent dentition, have dynamic diet and feeding issues, and depend on caregivers for their oral health care. As children get older new teeth begin to erupt that are genetically coded for at conception but are then exposed to different environmental influences throughout their development that modified their risk and resistance to dental caries. Emergence of the first permanent molars and subsequent permanent teeth results in having new at-risk dental surfaces (because of increased total number of teeth transitioning from 20 primary to 32 permanent teeth) and provides an opportunity for applying targeted preventive strategies. Alignment and spacing of the early permanent dentition, dietary changes, and exposure to orthodontic appliances are just a few of the factors affecting caries risk in older children. This article focuses on how dental caries continues to affect the 6- to 18-year-old and how different treatment modalities, such as pit and fissure sealants, can be useful for reducing the risk of developing caries lesions.

CARIES PREVALENCE AND RISK FACTORS

The prevalence of dental caries increases with age so that by the time most individuals are young adults they will have experienced dental caries. In 2011 to 2012, 21% of US children aged 6 to 11 years experienced dental caries in permanent teeth.[4] Dental caries is not distributed evenly across populations; in the United States, 27% of hispanic children aged 6 to 11 years are affected compared with 19% of non-Hispanic white children.[4] Children of lower socioeconomic status (SES) have an increased prevalence of caries compared with children of higher SES.[5,6] The prevalence of having experienced dental caries increases to 59% of US adolescents aged 12 to 19 years, with 15% having untreated caries lesions.[4] The severity of caries varies with age and SES but nearly 7% of US 6- to 8-year-olds already are classified as having severe caries (ie, 3 or more decayed surfaces).[5]

The human dentition varies in its anatomy with the anterior teeth having smooth surfaces, whereas the posterior teeth have smooth surfaces between the teeth and more tortuous anatomy on the biting surfaces. Although the smooth surfaces of teeth can develop caries lesions, it is the biting surfaces of the molar teeth that have the greatest risk for having caries. The biting or chewing surfaces of teeth are typically decorated with incompletely coalesced areas of enamel that are seen clinically as pits, fissures, and grooves. These pit and fissure areas of teeth represent stagnation sites for both biofilm and cariogenic substrates. The pit and fissure surfaces account for a disproportionate amount of the caries experience and result in restorations in permanent tooth surfaces in 12- to 19-year-olds.[5] The occlusal or biting surfaces of teeth, which typically have significant pit and fissure anatomy, account for just 12.5% of the at-risk tooth surfaces in the permanent dentition; however, they account for most of the caries. Similar caries prevalence and progression in children aged 6 to 18 years are reported around the world.[6,7] The first permanent molars are the most caries-prone permanent teeth followed by the second permanent molars.[8,9] Although the premolars have occlusal surfaces with pits and fissures, they have a much lower caries prevalence compared with the molars.

Children with caries in the primary dentition are more likely to have caries in the permanent dentition.[6,10] This is most likely best explained because these children have demonstrated, through the development of caries in early life (ie, in the primary dentition), that they have the requisites necessary for developing dental caries. It is thus not surprising that these children continue to experience dental caries in the permanent dentition. Moreover, even when their primary teeth fall out, the mouth is still populated by a biofilm that can cause caries and often continues to have environmental factors (eg, diet, fluoride exposure) conducive to developing caries lesions.

There are a variety of risk factors, some of which are unique for the development of pit and fissure caries. These include pit and fissure biofilm, the morphology of the fissures (more or less deep/pitted), enamel mineralization, and stage of tooth eruption.[10–13] The visual presence of heavy plaque or biofilm on a partially erupted fissure surface has been associated with increased caries risk.[14] The timing of tooth eruption also is a risk factor with women tending to erupt their molars before men, thereby putting female molars at risk for developing caries earlier when compared with male molars. Studies evaluating the biofilm in pits and fissures show there is a unique biofilm architecture and speciation depending on the ecological niche.[15] The presence of roughened and opaque enamel underneath a layer of plaque is associated with the presence of active caries on pit and fissure surfaces.[14]

Permanent molars often have pronounced pit and fissure anatomy that includes small tortuous defects that extend from the tooth surface to the dentin enamel junction. In addition to involving the occlusal surface, the buccal or facial surface of mandibular permanent molars and the lingual surface of maxillary molars are commonly involved (**Fig. 1**).[16] Pits and fissures are not readily cleansable by brushing due to their anatomy (frequently smaller in diameter than a toothbrush's bristle) and they receive less preventive benefit from fluorides compared with the smooth surfaces of the teeth. Pit and fissure caries is thought to be more aggressive than the ability of fluoride to effectively promote remineralization in these stagnation sites and prevent caries progression.

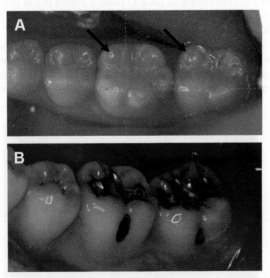

Fig. 1. The first and second permanent molars (*arrows*) often have pits and fissures on the occlusal, buccal, and lingual surfaces (*A*) that frequently become carious and require restoration (*B*) that historically would have been amalgam but today would most often be tooth-colored materials.

In addition to the anatomic pit and fissures contributing to the high prevalence of caries in molar teeth, there can be other developmental malformations caused by genetic changes or environmental stressors that alter mineralization of the enamel.[13,17] First permanent molars frequently have developmental defects such as those seen in molar incisor hypomineralization (MIH). This condition occurs more commonly in children who experience a variety of childhood illnesses (eg, respiratory infections) with a prevalence that ranges from 2% to 40% in populations around the world.[18] Affected teeth have diminished mineral in the enamel that can be localized to a small area or involve the entire crown. The severity is highly variable with severely affected teeth having large areas involved and having such reduced enamel mineralization that it cannot withstand the rigors of the oral cavity resulting in the enamel breaking away from the dentin as the tooth erupts (**Fig. 2**). Once the enamel breaks away from the tooth surface, there is an increased susceptibility to develop caries lesions. Teeth affected with MIH can be associated with hypersensitivity to chemical and thermal stimuli due to the compromised insulating capacity of the poorly mineralized or lost enamel. Teeth with MIH are reported to have an increased prevalence of caries lesions.[19] Treatment of MIH ranges from applying dental sealants to extraction depending on multiple factors, including the severity of the condition.[20]

STRATEGIES FOR MANAGING PIT AND FISSURE CARIES

Implementing strategies to comprehensively manage dental caries in children aged 6 to 18 years must address specific "pit and fissure" management strategies. This is not to be at the exclusion of managing smooth surface caries through fluorides, mechanical plaque control, and other methods, but the focus of this article is on managing the preponderance of caries that involves pits and fissures. Risk assessment includes amongst others evaluation of previous history of pit and fissure caries, tooth anatomy, presence of plaque, stage of tooth eruption, and enamel etching signifying early caries activity. Because the prevalence of pit and fissure caries in the first and second permanent molars is so high in the group of 6- to 18–year-olds, most children of this age should be considered for sealants.

During active tooth eruption, fluorides can be applied to the pit and fissure surfaces to help prevent early caries development. Clinical trials suggest there may be a slightly greater caries protection from fluoride varnish on pits and fissures compared with acidulated fluorophosphate gels when applied topically to the teeth.[21] The results of

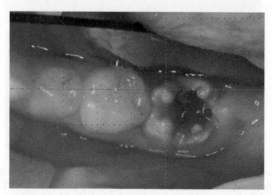

Fig. 2. MIH. This condition varies in its clinical presentation but can result in loss of enamel across the tooth surface as seen in this severely affected mandibular first permanent molar.

primary prevention on pit and fissure surfaces using silver diamine fluorides are variable with some trials showing no benefit, whereas others demonstrating a significant reduction in occlusal caries development in permanent molars.[22] A recent large clinical trial showed no significant difference in pit and fissure caries prevention between pit and fissure sealants versus fluoride varnish,[23] whereas a systematic review indicated that resin sealants are superior to fluoride varnish in preventing pit and fissure caries in first permanent molars.[24] However, this latter conclusion is based on few trials and a low level of evidence. Consequently, additional research is warranted to address whether one is better than the other in preventing pit and fissure caries.

PIT AND FISSURE SEALANTS

Pit and fissure sealants were introduced in the 1960s and have undergone a marked evolution (**Table 1**). There is a variety of materials that are currently marketed and in clinical use as pit and fissure sealants with new materials being marketed each year. Most of the past clinical trials have evaluated resin-based sealants (using resins based on bisphenol-A glycidyl dimethacrylate) and the acid etch technique.[25,26] These early clinical trials showed that sealants were effective at preventing caries, that sealant retention of the resin was necessary for sustained caries prevention, and that sealant loss was not associated with an increased risk for caries development compared with never having had a sealant placed.[27] Polymer chemistry continued to advance and ultraviolet light–cured materials were replaced by autopolymerizing resins.[28,29] Visible light–cured materials were introduced and retain much of the market share to date.[30]

There have been multiple systematic reviews evaluating the effectiveness of sealants in preventing pit and fissure caries and their ability to stop progression of noncavitated caries lesions.[31,32] These reviews, including the evaluation of dozens of randomized controlled clinical trials, have resulted in guidelines for the application of sealants that were jointly developed and adopted by the American Dental Association and the American Academy of Pediatric Dentistry.[31] Multiple meta analyses suggest that sealants can result in upwards of a 70% reduction in pit and fissure caries.[33] Most clinical trials, including some that followed patients for a prolonged period of time, have been completed with resin-based sealants; however, there is insufficient data at this time to indicate that one sealant material is superior to another.[33] The data indicate better retention of resin sealants but similar caries prevention rates in

Table 1
History of pit and fissure sealants

Generation	Material	Mode of Adhesion
1960s	Cyanoacrylate	Self-adhesive
1970s	Bisphenol-A glycidyl dimethacrylate Ultraviolet light cure	Acid etch
1970s	Bisphenol-A glycidyl dimethacrylate Self-cure and visible light cure	Acid etch
1974	Glass ionomer	Self-adhesive
1990s	Resin-modified glass ionomer	Self-adhesive/acid conditioner
2010s	Self-etch resin system	Self-etching
2010s	Moisture-tolerant resin	Acid etch
2010s	Bioactive resins	Acid etch

studies of 48 months duration.[34] Sealants are considered safe. In fact, no adverse outcomes have been reported in any of the clinical studies. Based on urinary bisphenol A excretion measurements, it does not look like the presence of bisphenol A in some resin sealants poses a health hazard.[35] The recommendation, therefore, is not to change practice at this time but follow this matter with additional studies.

Selection of sealant material should be at least partially determined based on the ability to adequately prepare and isolate the tooth surface. Resin materials are traditionally hydrophobic and will have increased bonding failure rates when placed on moist or contaminated surfaces. Moisture contamination of newly erupted molars in young patients can be challenging, especially in areas adjacent to the tissue such as the buccal surfaces of mandibular molars and the occlusal distal-lingual pit/fissure of maxillary molars. The use of bonding agents have been proposed to increase sealant retention, and clinical studies suggest they can significantly improve sealant retention in sites difficult to isolate and maintain moisture control.[36]

When it is considered critical to place a sealant on a newly erupted tooth due to rapid caries development, poorly mineralized enamel (eg, MIH), or other reasons, the clinician should consider using a glass ionomer or resin-modified glass ionomer, because these materials are hydrophillic and thus not as sensitive to moisture contamination as a resin sealant. When moisture contamination is less than ideal, the use of a hydrophilic resin sealant could also be considered. However, these materials do not yet have long-term retention data available (only 12-month studies reported).[37] Resin sealants that are filled for better wear properties, that have fluoride release, or that incorporate amorphous calcium phosphate to add in remineralization have been developed but clinical evidence indicates they all perform similar to traditional resin sealants.[33] Glass ionomer and resin-modified glass ionomer sealants release fluoride and some investigators feel that this could be important in their effectiveness in preventing pit and fissure caries even when most of the sealant material has been lost.[34] Additional long-term clinical studies are needed to clarify whether fluoride release from sealants is of benefit.

Sealant prevalence in permanent teeth in 2011 to 2012 was 31% in 6- to 8–year-olds. The prevalence of having at least one sealed permanent tooth increased to nearly 50% in children aged 9 to 11 years.[4] Based on the National Health and Nutrition Examination Survey data, the Centers for Disease Control and Prevention (CDC) reported that sealant use increased over the past decade. Still less than 40% of low SES children benefit from having sealants.[38] In the low-income child population the decayed/missing/filled rate for first permanent molars was almost 3 times greater than that in higher-income children. The CDC estimated that nearly 6.5 million low-income American children could benefit from sealants.[38] School-based sealant programs have been implemented in many areas of the United States and around the world to increase the utilization of sealants.[39]

BARRIERS TO SEALANT USE

There are numerous and diverse barriers that continue to reduce the adoption of sealants as a noninvasive approach to managing pit and fissure caries. These include failure to diagnose pit and fissure caries, dental education, an emphasis on the surgical management of caries, clinician experience, reimbursement levels, and parental knowledge.[40] Practice-based studies show that clinician experience is a strong determinant of clinical practice.[41] A recent study showed that clinicians making decisions regarding suspicious occlusal caries lesions were more likely to monitor (40%) and recommend oral hygiene instructions (21%) than to place sealants (3%). Surgical intervention was implemented in 39% of suspicious occlusal carious lesions, and of those so treated 61% had dental caries.[42] Because almost a third of these patients did in fact not have dental caries, evidence-based preventative management, including the use of sealants, should have been considered an appropriate alternative. Improved diagnostics directed at discerning whether a tooth had dentinal caries or not, and whether the caries is active or not, would likely increase the use of nonsurgical interventions for pit and fissure caries management. An increased emphasis on sealant use and the role of nonsurgical caries management in dental curricula could improve sealant use as well. Dental education remains largely focused on developing skills and knowledge around a surgical paradigm for caries management. Significant shifts in philosophies in dental education and clinical practice, as well as changes in the current reimbursement schemes, are needed to change the current emphasis on surgical-based approaches for caries management.

SUMMARY

Managing dental caries in the children aged 6 to 18 years involves assessing the child's potential for developing caries lesions and considering the different approaches for addressing how best to help maintain/establish a dentition with no active caries. Given the fact that in this age group diet frequently changes as they transition through school and spend less time at home, and in fact, in the United States at least, sugar-sweetened beverages become a standard part of their diet, caries prevention is of great importance. Caries remains highly prevalent in children aged 6 to 18 years with much of the disease manifesting as pit and fissure caries. Identifying children with increased risk for caries and selectively applying nonsurgical caries management therapeutics, such as pit and fissure sealants, are critical steps in the management of caries as a chronic disease. Sealants have been shown to be effective in reducing caries in this age group and their use is supported by current practice guidelines.

REFERENCES

1. Rozier RG, White BA, Slade GD. Trends in oral diseases in the U.S. population. J Dent Educ 2017;81(8):eS97–109.
2. Jackson SL, Vann WF Jr, Kotch JB, et al. Impact of poor oral health on children's school attendance and performance. Am J Public Health 2011;101(10):1900–6.
3. Shaffer JR, Wang X, Desensi RS, et al. Genetic susceptibility to dental caries on pit and fissure and smooth surfaces. Caries Res 2012;46(1):38–46.
4. Dye BA, Thornton-Evans G, Li X, et al. Dental caries and sealant prevalence in children and adolescents in the United States, 2011-2012. NCHS Data Brief 2015;(191):1–8.
5. Dye BA, Mitnik GL, Iafolla TJ, et al. Trends in dental caries in children and adolescents according to poverty status in the United States from 1999 through 2004 and from 2011 through 2014. J Am Dent Assoc 2017;148(8):550–65.e7.
6. Hall-Scullin E, Whitehead H, Milsom K, et al. Longitudinal study of caries development from childhood to adolescence. J Dent Res 2017;96(7):762–7.
7. Kassebaum NJ, Smith AGC, Bernabe E, et al. Global, regional, and national prevalence, incidence, and disability-adjusted life years for oral conditions for 195 countries, 1990-2015: a systematic analysis for the global burden of diseases, injuries, and risk factors. J Dent Res 2017;96(4):380–7.
8. King NM, Shaw L, Murray JJ. Caries susceptibility of permanent first and second molars in children aged 5-15 years. Community Dent Oral Epidemiol 1980;8(3):151–8.

9. Norrisgaard PE, Qvist V, Ekstrand K. Prevalence, risk surfaces and inter-municipality variations in caries experience in Danish children and adolescents in 2012. Acta Odontol Scand 2016;74(4):291–7.

10. Li Y, Wang W. Predicting caries in permanent teeth from caries in primary teeth: an eight-year cohort study. J Dent Res 2002;81(8):561–6.

11. Ditmyer MM, Dounis G, Howard KM, et al. Validation of a multifactorial risk factor model used for predicting future caries risk with Nevada adolescents. BMC Oral Health 2011;11:18.

12. Petersson GH, Twetman S. Caries risk assessment in young adults: a 3 year validation of the Cariogram model. BMC Oral Health 2015;15:17.

13. Grossi JA, Cabral RN, Leal SC. Caries Experience in children with and without molar-incisor hypomineralisation: a case-control study. Caries Res 2017;51(4):419–24.

14. Carvalho JC, Dige I, Machiulskiene V, et al. Occlusal caries: biological approach for its diagnosis and management. Caries Res 2016;50(6):527–42.

15. Dige I, Gronkjaer L, Nyvad B. Molecular studies of the structural ecology of natural occlusal caries. Caries Res 2014;48(5):451–60.

16. Cianetti S, Lombardo G, Bravi M, et al. Is pit and fissure sealing of buccal surfaces useful in reducing incidence of caries of first permanent molars? Eur J Paediatr Dent 2016;17(3):193–6.

17. Teixeira R, Andrade NS, Queiroz LCC, et al. Exploring the association between genetic and environmental factors and molar incisor hypomineralization: evidence from a twin study. Int J Paediatr Dent 2018;28(2):198–206.

18. Schwendicke F, Elhennawy K, Reda S, et al. Global burden of molar incisor hypomineralization. J Dent 2018;68:10–8.

19. Jeremias F, de Souza JF, Silva CM, et al. Dental caries experience and Molar-Incisor Hypomineralization. Acta Odontol Scand 2013;71(3–4):870–6.

20. Mathu-Muju K, Wright JT. Diagnosis and treatment of molar incisor hypomineralization. Compend Contin Educ Dent 2006;27(11):604–10 [quiz: 611].

21. Tewari A, Chawla HS, Utreja A. Comparative evaluation of the role of NaF, APF & Duraphat topical fluoride applications in the prevention of dental caries–a 2 1/2 years study. J Indian Soc Pedod Prev Dent 1991;8(1):28–35.

22. Contreras V, Toro MJ, Elias-Boneta AR, et al. Effectiveness of silver diamine fluoride in caries prevention and arrest: a systematic literature review. Gen Dent 2017;65(3):22–9.

23. Chestnutt IG, Hutchings S, Playle R, et al. Seal or Varnish? A randomised controlled trial to determine the relative cost and effectiveness of pit and fissure sealant and fluoride varnish in preventing dental decay. Health Technol Assess 2017;21(21):1–256.

24. Ahovuo-Saloranta A, Forss H, Hiiri A, et al. Pit and fissure sealants versus fluoride varnishes for preventing dental decay in the permanent teeth of children and adolescents. Cochrane Database Syst Rev 2016;(1):CD003067.

25. Buonocore MG. A simple method of increasing the adhesion of acrylic filling materials to enamel surfaces. J Dent Res 1955;34(6):849–53.

26. Buonocore MG. Caries prevention in pits and fissures sealed with an adhesive resin polymerized by ultraviolet light: a two-year study of a single adhesive application. J Am Dent Assoc 1971;82(5):1090–3.

27. Horowitz HS, Heifetz SB, Poulsen S. Adhesive sealant clinical trial: an overview of results after four years in Kalispell, Montana. J Prev Dent 1976;3(3 Pt 2):38–9, 44, 46–7 passim.

28. Brooks JD, Mertz-Fairhurst EJ, Della-Giustina VE, et al. A comparative study of two pit and fissure sealants: three-year results in Augusta, Ga. J Am Dent Assoc 1979;99(1):42–6.
29. Mertz-Fairhurst EJ, Fairhurst CW, Williams JE, et al. A comparative clinical study of two pit and fissure sealants: 7-year results in Augusta, GA. J Am Dent Assoc 1984;109(2):252–5.
30. Houpt M, Fuks A, Shapira J, et al. Autopolymerized versus light-polymerized fissure sealant. J Am Dent Assoc 1987;115(1):55–6.
31. Wright JT, Crall JJ, Fontana M, et al. Evidence-based clinical practice guideline for the use of pit-and-fissure sealants: a report of the American Dental Association and the American Academy of Pediatric Dentistry. J Am Dent Assoc 2016; 147(8):672–82.e12.
32. Ahovuo-Saloranta A, Hiiri A, Nordblad A, et al. Pit and fissure sealants for preventing dental decay in the permanent teeth of children and adolescents. Cochrane Database Syst Rev 2008;(4):CD001830.
33. Wright JT, Tampi MP, Graham L, et al. Sealants for preventing and arresting pit-and-fissure occlusal caries in primary and permanent molars: a systematic review of randomized controlled trials-a report of the American Dental Association and the American Academy of Pediatric Dentistry. J Am Dent Assoc 2016;147(8): 631–45.e18.
34. Mickenautsch S, Yengopal V. Caries-preventive effect of high-viscosity glass ionomer and resin-based fissure sealants on permanent teeth: a systematic review of clinical trials. PLoS One 2016;11(1):e0146512.
35. McKinney C, Rue T, Sathyanarayana S, et al. Dental sealants and restorations and urinary bisphenol A concentrations in children in the 2003-2004 national health and nutrition examination survey. J Am Dent Assoc 2014;145(7):745–50.
36. McCafferty J, O'Connell AC. A randomised clinical trial on the use of intermediate bonding on the retention of fissure sealants in children. Int J Paediatr Dent 2016; 26(2):110–5.
37. Askarizadeh N, Heshmat H, Zangeneh N. One-year clinical success of embrace hydrophilic and helioseal-f hydrophobic sealants in permanent first molars: a clinical trial. J Dent (Tehran) 2017;14(2):92–9.
38. Griffin SO, Wei L, Gooch BF, et al. Vital signs: dental sealant use and untreated tooth decay among U.S. school-aged children. MMWR Morb Mortal Wkly Rep 2016;65(41):1141–5.
39. Gooch BF, Griffin SO, Gray SK, et al. Preventing dental caries through school-based sealant programs: updated recommendations and reviews of evidence. J Am Dent Assoc 2009;140(11):1356–65.
40. Lam A. Increase in utilization of dental sealants. J Contemp Dent Pract 2008;9(3): 81–7.
41. O'Donnell JA, Modesto A, Oakley M, et al. Sealants and dental caries: insight into dentists' behaviors regarding implementation of clinical practice recommendations. J Am Dent Assoc 2013;144(4):e24–30.
42. Makhija SK, Shugars DA, Gilbert GH, et al. Surface characteristics and lesion depth and activity of suspicious occlusal carious lesions: findings from the National Dental Practice-Based Research Network. J Am Dent Assoc 2017; 148(12):922–9.

Oral Health Disparities in Children
A Canary in the Coalmine?

Richard G. Watt, PhD[a],*, Manu Raj Mathur, PhD[b], Jun Aida, PhD[c],
Marcelo Bönecker, PhD[d], Renato Venturelli, MSc[e],
Stuart A. Gansky, DrPH[f]

KEYWORDS

• Oral health • Disparities • Inequalities • Social determinants • Health policy

KEY POINTS

• Oral diseases in children remain a major global public health problem with significant negative impact on quality of life. However, oral diseases are largely preventable and now disproportionately affect more disadvantaged populations.

• Oral health disparities are caused by the broad conditions in which people are born, grow, live, work, and age; the so-called social determinants.

• Dental treatment and clinical prevention alone will not eliminate oral health disparities, and may even widen inequalities. Instead a radical, multifaceted, integrated approach that addresses the underlying root cause of oral diseases in childhood is urgently required.

BACKGROUND

The values of equal opportunity and equality have a long and distinguished political history across the democratic nations of the world. These values are embedded at the core of many national constitutions as the foundations of modern societies. The founding fathers of the US Constitution highlighted that all people are created equal

[a] Epidemiology and Public Health, University College London, 1-19 Torrington Place, London WC1E 6BT, UK; [b] Department of Dental Public Health, Public Health Foundation of India, Plot No. 47, Sector 44, Institutional Area Gurgaon, Gurgaon, Haryana 122002, India; [c] Department of International Health, Graduate School of Dentistry, Tohoku University, 4-1, Seiryo-machi, Aoba-ku, Sendai, Miyagi 980-8575, Japan; [d] Dental Faculty, Av. Prof Lineu Prestes 2227 - University of Sao Paulo, Sao Paulo 05508-900, Brazil; [e] Epidemiology and Public Health, University College London, 1-19 Torrington Place, London WC1E 6BT, UK; [f] Division of Oral Epidemiology and Dental Public Health, Center to Address Disparities in Children's Oral Health (Known As CAN DO), Philip R. Lee Institute for Health Policy Studies, University of California, San Francisco, Box #1361, San Francisco, CA 94143, USA
* Corresponding author.
E-mail address: r.watt@ucl.ac.uk

Pediatr Clin N Am 65 (2018) 965–979
https://doi.org/10.1016/j.pcl.2018.05.006
0031-3955/18/© 2018 Elsevier Inc. All rights reserved.

pediatric.theclinics.com

with the right to life, liberty and the pursuit of happiness. However, across the globe, many communities and populations are facing huge challenges that severely limit their future opportunities and life chances. Increasingly, the world is becoming a deeply divided and polarized place with escalating economic and social differences evident both within and among countries.[1,2] One stark manifestation of economic and social inequalities is the disparities that exist in health, including oral health status. Tackling health inequalities to promote health equity therefore has now become a major policy priority around the world.[3,4]

DEFINITIONS OF HEALTH DISPARITIES AND HEALTH INEQUALITIES

Many different definitions of health disparities and health inequalities exist depending on the context, discipline, and policy arena. However, a common theme across different definitions is the recognition of population-specific health differences in prevalence of disease, health outcomes, or access to health care, particularly those that are avoidable, unjust, and unfair when considered from a social justice, ethics, and human rights perspective.[3] Health disparities have been defined as differences that exist among specific population groups in the attainment of full health potential and in incidence, prevalence, mortality, burden of disease, and other adverse health conditions.[5] Health equity is the state in which everyone has the opportunity to attain their full health potential and no one is disadvantaged from achieving this potential because of their social position or other socially defined circumstance. An underlying concept across the various definitions is the recognition that health inequalities and disparities stem from systematic differences in society that are preventable (something can be done to change them) and unjust (these differences are collectively considered as unacceptable and unfair) among groups and communities occupying unequal positions of power in society.[6] Based on historical and political differences across the world, different health disparities research foci have been emphasized. In the United States, for example, particular emphasis in research and policy is placed on exploring racial and/or ethnic health disparities, whereas, in many other Organization of Economically Developed Countries (OEDCs), socioeconomic health inequalities are the main focus of attention. In addition to race/ethnicity and socioeconomic status, sexual orientation, gender identity, primary language, geographic location, and various forms of disability are also included in health disparities research.

HEALTH DISPARITIES IN US CHILDREN AND ADULTS: AN OVERVIEW

A healthy childhood provides the foundation and opportunities for life. However, not all groups in society have the best start in life. In the United States, for example, stark racial/ethnic inequalities exist in early life for various health outcomes. Although overall infant mortalities have decreased since 2005, sharp racial/ethnic disparities persist. In 2013, infant mortality among African Americans (11.1 per 1000 live births) was more than double the rate among white people (5.06 per 1000 live births).[7] Among US adults, life expectancy was recently found to be directly related to income levels.[8] Between the top 1% and bottom 1% of the income distribution, life expectancy differed by 15 years for men and 10 years for women. The analysis also revealed that the life expectancy gap had widened in recent years. Between 2001 and 2014, the individuals in the top 1% of the income distribution gained approximately 3 years of life expectancy, whereas individuals in the bottom 1% experienced no gains.

How does the United States compare in terms of health outcomes with other similar OEDC members? A recent National Research Council and Institute of Medicine report compared health outcomes among 16 high-income countries.[9] Despite spending more on health care as percentage of gross domestic product than any other country, the United States fared worse in 9 health domains, including important areas of child and maternal health such as:

- Adverse birth outcomes: higher rates of infant mortality and low birth weight
- Injuries and homicides: deaths from motor vehicle accidents, non–transport-related injuries, and violence, which are the leading cause of death in US children, adolescents, and young adults
- Adolescent reproductive health: adolescent pregnancies and sexually transmitted infections are highest in the United States
- Obesity and diabetes: US obesity rates in children, adolescents, and young adults are highest among the 16 comparable countries

WIDER CONSEQUENCES OF HEALTH DISPARITIES

Concerns about health disparities are not merely a theoretic or ethical issue; they have profound social, political, and economic consequences for society. Children raised in poverty, food insecurity, or poor housing, or who lack of access to high-quality early-years education, are more likely to experience chronic adult illnesses and the intergenerational perpetuation of poverty and poor health; the spiral of disadvantage across generations.[10] The economic effects of health inequalities are the consequence of both increased health expenditure and the broader diminished economic productivity in society. In the United States, eliminating health disparities for racial/ethnic minorities between 2003 and 2006 would have reduced indirect costs associated with illness and premature death by an estimate of more than $1 trillion.[11] In the European Union, inequality losses related to health have been estimated to account for 15% of the costs of social welfare systems and 20% of health care costs.[12]

Oral diseases in children and young people are a major public health problem in many parts of the world. This article analyzes oral diseases through the lens of health disparities. Oral diseases in childhood are early markers of social disadvantage and can be used as social indicators of patterns of systemic disease in populations. The authors argue that action to combat oral health disparities requires a radical multifaceted strategy and integrated approach that addresses the underlying root causes of oral diseases in childhood.

ORAL HEALTH DISPARITIES: AN OVERVIEW

Globally, oral diseases remain highly prevalent chronic conditions that have a significant negative impact on quality of life across the life course from early childhood, through adulthood, to older age.[13] Increasingly, however, oral diseases disproportionately affect socially disadvantaged groups in society. Stark disparities in clinical outcomes, subjective oral health measures, and oral health–related behaviors exist across a range of different indicators of socioeconomic position, including educational status, income, occupation, and geographic area–based measures of deprivation.[14–16] Oral health disparities are not merely the differences between the rich and poor in society. As is the case with most other health conditions, a consistent, stepwise, graded relationship exists across the entire social spectrum, with oral health being worse at each point down the social hierarchy, the so-called social gradient. The social gradient in oral health is a universal phenomenon found at all points across the life course and in different populations around the world.[17–19] Oral health disparities also exist across certain racial/ethnic groups in society, reflecting socioeconomic disadvantage and cultural differences.

Systematic reviews of the international literature have highlighted the considerable body of epidemiologic evidence on oral health disparities in children and adults.[20–23] Various large-scale studies have also reported that children from deprived neighborhoods had higher dental caries levels and greater dental pain experience than their counterparts from more affluent neighborhoods.[24–29]

The evidence on disparities in oral health specifically in low-income and middle-income countries (LMICs) is still sparse. Da Silveira Moreira[30] showed that 70% to 90% of children attending school experience dental caries, with highest rates in LMICs such as India, Thailand, and Indonesia. Recent studies have also shown socioeconomic gradients in prevalence of dental caries, self-rated oral health, and oral health–related behaviors of children and adolescents from LMICs.[19,31–35] A systematic review of Brazilian epidemiologic studies between 1999 and 2008 showed poor socioeconomic conditions were associated with adverse adult periodontal outcomes.[36]

The effect of oral health disparities is not just confined to childhood. Thomson and colleagues[37] (2000) showed that childhood socioeconomic position has a significant influence on the lifelong trajectories of oral health. Nicolau and colleagues[38] (2005) showed that adolescents with poor material conditions, both at birth and 13 years of age, have poorer oral health outcomes than those having better standard of living at either life stage.

ORAL HEALTH DISPARITIES IN CHILDREN IN THE UNITED STATES

In the United States, oral health disparities exist in children for cleft lip, cleft lip and palate,[39] and gingivitis,[40] but the largest population health impact of disparities is on dental caries. Dr. Vivek Murthy, the previous US Surgeon General, recently summarized progress in the 15 years since the first and only *Surgeon General's Report* on oral health. Children's dental insurance coverage and dental sealant use have increased, whereas caries experience and untreated caries have decreased.[41] For example, based on the US National Health and Nutrition Examination Survey (NHANES), prevalence of caries experience in primary dentition decreased from 28% in 2004 to 2011 to 23% in 2011 to 2014.[42] Mean number of decayed or filled primary tooth surfaces (DFS) increased in children 3 to 5 years old from 2.1 in 1988 to 1994 to 2.6 in 1999 to 2004 and 2011 to 2014, but mean number of decayed, missing, or filled permanent tooth surfaces (DMFSs) decreased in children 12 to 17 years old from 4.4 in 1988 to 1994 to 3.5 in 1999 to 2004 and 2004 to 2011.[43]

Nevertheless, children's oral health disparities persist based on families' economic, educational, linguistic, immigration, racial/ethnic, and geographic characteristics. Despite overall reductions in prevalence of children's caries experience and untreated caries comparing NHANES from 1999 to 2004 with 2011 to 2014, economic disparities across the household income percentage federal poverty level (FPL) gradient remain essentially unchanged over time.[44] Primary dentition caries experience for children 2 to 8 years old in 1999 to 2004 with less than 100% FPL was 52% compared with 27% in those greater than or equal to 200% FPL, corresponding with a relative risk (RR) of 1.92; in 2011 to 2014, prevalences were 48% and 27%, respectively, for an RR of 1.78; primary dentition untreated caries RR for children 2 to 8 years old of less than 100% FPL to greater than or equal to 200% FPL in 1999 to 2004 of 2.34 and in 2011 to 2014 of 2.28. Disparities in severe caries in the primary dentition (3 or more decayed surfaces) seems to have decreased substantially over time: prevalences for children 2 to 8 years old in 1999 to 2004 were 16% for less than 100% FPL and 5% for greater than or equal to 200% FPL in 1999 to 2004 with RR = 3.16; in 2011 to 2014 prevalences were 8% and 4% respectively with RR = 2.00.

Compared with non-Hispanic white people with untreated caries in the primary dentition, disparities for racial/ethnic minorities increased from 1999 to 2004 to 2011 to 2014.[42] NHANES analyses from 1988 to 1994, to 1999 to 2004, to 2011to 2014 showed mean DFS and DMFS for 3 child age groups along a consistent 4-category poverty-income ratio gradient over time.[43]

County-level untreated caries rates in children 6 to 9 years old from a small-area estimation NHANES 2005 to 2010 model varied significantly by individual-level, tract-level, and county-level variables,[45] so incorporating a multilevel approach is important. Accounting for child-level, family-level, and community-level/state-level socioeconomics and other factors, racial/ethnic disparities in the 2007 National Survey of Children's Health for parent reports of children's fair/poor oral health rating, preventive care, and delayed care/unmet need attenuated or disappeared.[46]

DISPARITIES IN ACCESS TO ORAL HEALTH CARE SERVICES

In much of the world, particularly in many LMICs, coverage, availability, and access to oral health care services, including early diagnosis, prevention, and basic treatment of children and adolescents, are grossly inadequate or completely lacking.[47–50] Studies in high-income countries, including the United States, demonstrate inequalities in access to oral health care services for young children[51,52] based on family income,[53,54] race/ethnicity,[55] and caregiver education.[56,57] Similar challenges in inequalities to those seen in the United States are also being faced by the children and adolescents from LMICs in South America,[58] Africa,[59] and Asia.[32]

Access to oral health care services in pregnant women[60] and children with special health care needs[61,62] has also been well researched in high-income countries.[63,64] However, there is a lack of evidence from many LMICs.

IMPACT OF ORAL HEALTH DISPARITIES

Oral diseases have many adverse consequences for individuals, families, and society. For example, dental caries can have negative impacts on quality of life, such as pain and discomfort, impaired chewing, decreased appetite, sleep problems, poor self-esteem, reduced social interaction, and poor school and work performance.[65] The social gradient in oral diseases means that people from the most disadvantaged backgrounds are affected disproportionately. Children from poorer backgrounds have higher caries rates and consequently often experience dental pain and its consequences, leaving them at a substantial disadvantage compared with their wealthier and healthier peers. Children with poor oral health are almost 3 times more likely to miss school days from dental pain and have poorer subsequent school examination performance and job attainment.[66] In the United Kingdom, extracting carious teeth is the most common reason for admitting children less than the age of 11 years for surgery under general anesthesia, a psychologically traumatic and costly procedure.[67] In several countries, including the United Kingdom[68] and Korea,[69] children from disadvantaged and poorer backgrounds are far more likely to be admitted to hospital to have carious teeth extracted.[68,69] A recent Health Policy Institute survey showed almost one-third of low-income US adults, twice the rate of their high-income counterparts, reported that the appearance of their teeth and mouth affected their ability to interview for a job.[70] Dental treatment is often costly and in many countries is not included in the mainstream health care system or is excluded from many health insurance plans. Thus, dental treatment costs are often incurred by individuals covered through personal out-of-pocket expenditures, a major challenge for low-income individuals. Across 41 LMICs, 7% of households reported that personal expenditures for dental treatment significantly affected family budgets, limiting their ability to purchase essential daily necessities.[71] The disproportionate impact of oral diseases on poor school performance, reduced employment opportunities, and financial burden for dental treatment on the poorest segments of communities perpetuates and reinforces social and economic inequalities in society.

UNDERSTANDING THE CAUSES: SOCIAL DETERMINANTS AGENDA

Contemporary analysis of the underlying causes of these unfair, unjust, and unacceptable differences in oral health status across populations must inform action to address oral health disparities. Perhaps a good starting point is the need to dispel and dismiss certain commonly held views on health disparities, such as:

- Poor people behave badly: that is their choice
- People cannot all be equal; differences in society will always exist
- It is too difficult to change society for the better

Over the last 30 years or so, a considerable body of scientific research has explored the range of interacting factors that cause health disparities. Poverty, unemployment, poor housing, low educational attainment, violence, loneliness, and discrimination all influence the health of children and families, and ultimately determine health disparities.[72] These overriding social, economic, environmental, and societal factors, known as the social determinants of health (SDOH), create the unequal conditions in society that ultimately cause health inequities among and within countries.[3] Marmot[73] (2007) described SDOH as the "fundamental structures of social hierarchy and the socially determined conditions these create in which people grow, live, work and age"[73]; the inequitable distribution of power, money, and resources are the root causes of inequality in society.

Families living in disadvantaged communities have limited choices available to them. Their daily lives are governed by a constant struggle to do the best they can for their children. Health-related behaviors, such as tobacco use, poor diets, and drug and alcohol misuse, are important influences on health, but these behaviors are largely determined by the social and physical conditions in which people live and are often used as coping strategies to deal with stress and hardship.

International comparative studies have shown that health disparities are much worse in countries such as the United States and United Kingdom that have the widest socioeconomic inequalities between rich and poor. In contrast, in more egalitarian countries such as the Nordic nations and Japan, where the economic differences are much smaller, health disparities are less pronounced. More equal and socially cohesive societies have healthier populations.[74]

An SDOH perspective has been applied to better understand inter-relationships between the proximal (biological and behavioral) influences on child oral diseases and how these are largely determined and driven by the broader distal (social, community, economic, and political) factors in society. Researchers have developed various SDOH conceptual models and frameworks to describe the range of influences, interconnections, and pathways leading to oral health disparities.[75–80] These models provide valuable insights to inform developing interventions to tackle oral health disparities and highlight the need for joint collaborative action at different levels and across sectors; the common risk factor approach.[79] Action focusing solely on the proximal biological and behavioral factors are ineffective at achieving sustained improvements in oral health and may widen oral health disparities.[81] A good example to illustrate this was a school-based health education program in Scotland that significantly increased oral health disparities; children from more advantaged social backgrounds appreciably improved their oral hygiene behaviors as a result of the program, whereas their contemporaries from poorer households had minimal benefit, widening the oral health gap.[82]

TIME FOR ACTION TO TACKLE ORAL HEALTH DISPARITIES

The universal and pervasive nature of the social gradient in oral and general health outcomes has profound implications for action to tackle health disparities. Reducing health disparities is therefore everybody's business, affecting the whole of society, not just the poorest and most marginalized. Politicians, policy makers, clinicians, professional organizations, commercial sector, civil society, and the wider community all have an important role to play. The US Department of Health and Human Services[83] (DHHS) (2016) recently developed an oral health framework with 5 goals, including increasing access to oral health care and eliminating disparities, which had 8 suggested strategies:

- Expand the number of health care settings that provide oral health care, including diagnostic, preventive, and restorative services in federally qualified health centers, school-based health centers, Ryan White human immunodeficiency virus/acquired immunodeficiency syndrome–funded programs, and Indian Health Service (IHS)-funded health programs.
- Strengthen the oral health workforce, expand capabilities of existing providers, and promote models that incorporate other clinicians.
- Improve the knowledge, skills, and abilities of providers to serve diverse patient populations.
- Promote health professionals' training in cultural competency.
- Assist individuals and families in obtaining oral health services and connecting with a dental home.
- Align dental homes and oral health services for children.
- Create local, regional, and statewide partnerships that bridge the aging population and oral health systems.
- Support the collection of data stratified by sex and race/ethnicity pertaining to oral health.

To reduce the social gradient in health, actions must be universal but with scale and intensity proportionate to the level of disadvantage and need to correct the imbalance.[84] The traditional clinical high-risk approach, solely focusing on individuals and families at greatest risk of disease, alone cannot tackle the broader root causes of oral health disparities. The inter-related and shared underlying causes of both oral and general health disparities require coordinated and integrated upstream action, including healthy public policy, the creation of supportive environments, and strengthened grass roots community action for good health. However, health care systems, particularly primary care and pediatric services, also have an important contribution to make to promote greater oral health equity.

ROLE OF HEALTH SERVICES

Giving every child the best start in life is one of the key recommendations from a strategic review of actions needed to promote health equity.[84] Clinicians working in pediatrics are therefore in a unique position to support and empower children and families to attain their full health potential, including good oral health. DHHS[83] (2016) suggested strategies to achieve this goal, including interprofessional collaboration, providing oral health training to primary care providers (who then provide care to patients, including fluoride varnish), developing policies/practices that reconnect the mouth to the rest of the body, and creating programs that support a systems change approach that promotes a unified patient-centered model of care.[83] For example, providing evidence-based support, without victim blaming, on breastfeeding and healthy-eating advice, including ways to reduce sugar consumption, is important for both oral and general good health.[79] Working in partnership with clinical colleagues in primary dental care settings is critical to ensure that children and families receive additional dental support on such things as the appropriate use of fluoride toothpastes and access to dental treatment and preventive care from an early age. Rather than working in isolated and compartmentalized professional silos, providing more integrated care in colocated premises offers opportunities for more effective and coordinated joint care.

Collaborative work across clinical boundaries is important, but collaboration can be extended more broadly to other essential sectors, such as social and welfare services, education services, employment opportunities, housing support, debt management and financial planning advice, immigration support, and community groups. Signs in everyday language and linking with these other sectors and agencies to provide warm handoffs can help vulnerable families access key support and potentially avoid future problems.

UPSTREAM ACTION TO PROMOTE ORAL HEALTH EQUITY

Although more than 40 years have passed since John McKinlay[85] first proposed the need for upstream action to tackle underlying root causes of poor health, this approach still remains highly relevant in promoting health equity. Reviews of the public health literature indicate that interventions to effectively reduce health inequalities include[86,87]:

- Structural changes in the environment (such as improvements in quality of social housing)
- Legislation and regulation (such as tighter controls on the marketing of sugary foods and drinks to young children)
- Fiscal policy (such as sugar levy on sugary foods and drinks)
- Programs that focus on early childhood (such as improved access to high quality preschool education and care)
- Community action (such as community engagement on road safety in neighborhoods)
- Programs that prioritize disadvantaged population groups (such as nutrition programs targeted at low-income families)

Many of the interventions discussed earlier can tackle oral health disparities at both local and national levels. For example, food policies in early-life settings and schools can be implemented to create healthier environments for infants and children.[88] At the local level in the United States, Berkeley, California, starting in 2015 and Philadelphia, Pennsylvania, starting in 2016 enacted sugar taxes; this was followed by Albany, California; Oakland, California; San Francisco, California; Boulder, Colorado; Cook County (Chicago), Illinois; Portland, Oregon; and Seattle, Washington. At the national level, fiscal policies can be introduced with even greater impact to promote healthier and more affordable food and drink choices. Norway and Denmark enacted sugar taxes in the 1920s and 1930s. More recently, additional countries have enacted sugar taxes, such as Samoa (1984), French

Polynesia (2002), Nauru (2007), Hungary (2011), France (2012), and Mexico (2013). Evaluations have shown that such taxes decreased sugar-sweetened beverage consumption in Mexico[89–91] and Berkeley, California.[92] In the United Kingdom, a national 20% sugar tax will commence in 2018 on sugar-sweetened beverages with total sugar content more than 5 g per 100 mL.[93] Legislation and regulation can also be used to improve food labeling and control the marketing and advertising of high-sugar foods and drinks that are specifically targeted at young children. Such measures will substantially reduce both dental caries and obesity levels in children.[94]

Specific oral health community-based population-level interventions include fluoridation of public water supplies, as well as fluoride varnish and fissure sealant programs. Community water fluoridation was first introduced in Grand Rapids, Michigan, in 1945 and is now implemented in many countries around the world, including Australia, Ireland, and Brazil. Water fluoridation has been described as one of the top 10 public health achievements of the twentieth century,[4] and systematic reviews have demonstrated its effectiveness in preventing dental caries.[95–97] The most recent Cochrane Review applying stringent selection criteria found insufficient evidence to determine whether water fluoridation had an effect in reducing socioeconomic inequalities in caries outcomes.[97] In contrast, an Australian National Health and Medical Research Council review concluded that consistent evidence existed that water fluoridation reduced caries levels across socioeconomic groups and reduced inequalities, despite study quality often being poor.[95] A recent Australian study has shown that fluoridation reduced absolute inequalities in childhood caries but did not eliminate them.[98]

Topically applied fluoride varnish is a highly concentrated form of fluoride that has been used extensively as a clinician-applied caries preventive intervention in infants, children, and adolescents for many decades (please see Howard Pollick's article, "The Role of Fluoride in the Prevention of Tooth Decay," in this issue). Because of its adherent nature, fluoride varnish stays in contact with the tooth surface for several hours. A Cochrane systematic review concluded that fluoride varnish is effective in both permanent and primary teeth,[15] but it is unclear whether fluoride varnish reduces disparities in caries levels. Dental sealants are effective in preventing dental caries mainly in the pits and fissures of occlusal permanent tooth surface. They provide a physical barrier to protect natural tooth surfaces and grooves, inhibiting buildup of bacteria and food trapped within such fissures and grooves. A Cochrane systematic review on dental sealants found moderate-quality evidence that resin-based sealants applied on occlusal surfaces of permanent molars are effective in preventing caries in children and adolescents, but it is unclear whether fissure sealant programs promote oral health equity.[99]

WIDER SIGNIFICANCE OF SOCIAL PATTERNING OF ORAL DISEASES: CANARY IN COALMINE

Children's oral epidemiologic surveillance data are an inexpensive and noninvasive way to identify early-marker evidence of early-life social disadvantage manifesting in health effects. Not only is poor children's oral health itself an important health problem that leads to reduced quality of life but it is also a precursor for other clinical conditions with the same common causes of early-life social disadvantage. Thus, childhood caries and other oral health problems can be viewed as sentinel health problems that should alert health providers to potential additional health sequelae.

SUMMARY

Oral health disparities in children are a major public health problem across the world. Oral diseases and their effects on quality of life have a disproportionate impact on socially disadvantaged groups and contribute to and reinforce wider social and economic inequity in society. Oral health disparities in children are caused by a complex array of interconnected biological, behavioral, social, economic, and political factors: the social determinants. Future action to promote oral health equity in children requires a radical multistrategy and integrated approach that addresses the underlying root causes of oral disparities.

REFERENCES

1. Piketty T, Saez E. Income inequality in Europe and the United States. Science 2014;344(6186):838–43.
2. Sen A. Reason, freedom and well-being. Utilitas 2006;18(1):80–96.
3. World Health Organization Commission on Social Determinants of Health. Closing the gap in a generation: health equity through action on the social determinants of health. Final report of the Commission on Social Determinants of Health. Geneva (Switzerland): World Health Organization; 2008.
4. Centers for Disease Control and Prevention. Healthy People 2020 (US). 2011. Available at: https://www.cdc.gov/nchs/healthy_people/hp2020.htm. Accessed January 7, 2018.
5. National Institutes of Health. NIH announces Institute on Minority Health and Health Disparities 2010. 2010. Available at: https://www.nih.gov/news-events/news-releases/nih-announces-institute-minority-health-health-disparities. Accessed January 7, 2018.
6. Graham H, East T. Social determinants and their unequal distribution: clarifying policy understandings. Milbank Q 2004;82(1):101–24.
7. Mathews TJ, MacDorman MF, Thomas ME. Infant mortality statistics from the 2013 period linked birth/infant death data set. Natl Vital Stat Rep 2015;64(9):1–30.
8. Chetty R, Stepner M, Abraham S, et al. The association between income and life expectancy in the United States, 2001-2014. J Am Med Assoc 2016;315(16):1750–66.
9. Institute of Medicine and National Research Council. U.S. health in international perspective: shorter lives, poorer health. Washington, DC: The National Academic Press; 2013.
10. American Academy of Pediatrics. Health equity and children's rights. Pediatrics 2010;125(4):838–49.
11. LaVeist TA, Gaskin DJ, Richard P. The economic burden of health inequalities in the United States. Washington, DC: Join Center for Political and Economic Studies; 2009.
12. Mackenbach JP, Meerding WJ, Kunst AE. Economic costs of health inequalities in the European Union. J Epidemiol Community Health 2011;65:412–9.
13. Marcenes W, Kassebaum NJ, Bernabé E, et al. Global burden of oral conditions in 1990-2010: a systematic analysis. J Dent Res 2013;97(7):592–7.
14. Watt R, Sheiham A. Inequalities in oral health: a review of the evidence and recommendations for action. Br Dent J 1999;187(1):6–12.
15. Sisson KL. Theoretical explanations for social inequalities in oral health. Community Dent Oral Epidemiol 2007;35(2):81–8.

16. Locker D. Deprivation and oral health: a review. Community Dent Oral Epidemiol 2000;28(3):161–9.
17. Sanders AE, Slade GD, Turrell G, et al. The shape of the socioeconomic-oral health gradient: implications for theoretical explanations. Community Dent Oral Epidemiol 2006;34(4):310–9.
18. Sabbah W, Tsakos G, Chandola T, et al. Social gradients in oral and general health. J Dent Res 2007;86(10):992–6.
19. Mathur MR, Tsakos G, Millett C, et al. Socioeconomic inequalities in dental caries and their determinants in adolescents in New Delhi, India. BMJ Open 2014;4: e006391.
20. Reisine ST, Psoter W. Socioeconomic status and selected behavioural determinants as risk factors for dental caries. J Dent Educ 2001;65(10):1009–16.
21. Boillot A, El Halabi B, Batty GD, et al. Education as a predictor of chronic periodontitis: a systematic review with meta-analysis population-based studies. PLoS One 2011;6(7):e21508.
22. Schwendicke F, Dörfer CE, Schlattmann P, et al. Socioeconomic inequality and caries. J Dent Res 2015;94(1):10–8.
23. Costa SM, Martins CC, Bonfim Mde LC, et al. A systematic review of socioeconomic indicators and dental caries in adults. Int J Environ Res Public Health 2012;9(10):3540–74.
24. Conway DI, Quarrell I, McCall DR, et al. Dental caries in 5-year-old children attending multi-ethnic schools in Greater Glasgow - The impact of ethnic background and levels of deprivation. Community Dent Health 2007;24(3):161–5.
25. McMahon AD, Blair Y, McCall DR, et al. The dental health of three-year-old children in greater Glasgow, Scotland. Br Dent J 2010;209(4):E5.
26. Levin KA, Davies CA, Douglas GVA, et al. Urban-rural differences in dental caries of 5-year old children in Scotland. Soc Sci Med 2010;71(11):2020–7.
27. Gatou T, Koletsi Kounari H, Mamai-Homata E. Dental caries prevalence and treatment needs of 5- to 12-year-old children in relation to area-based income and immigrant background in Greece. Int Dent J 2011;61(3):144–51.
28. Enjary C, Tubert-Jeannin S, Manevy R, et al. Dental status and measures of deprivation in Clermont-Ferrand, France. Community Dent Oral Epidemiol 2006;34(5): 363–71.
29. Da Rosa P, Nicolau B, Brodeur J-M, et al. Associations between school deprivation indices and oral health status. Community Dent Oral Epidemiol 2011;39(3): 213–20.
30. Da Silveira Moreira R. Epidemiology of dental caries in the world. In: Virdi M, editor. Oral health care - Pediatric, research, epidemiology and clinical practices. In Tech; 2012. p. 149–69. https://doi.org/10.5772/31951.
31. Delgado-Angulo EK, Hobdell MH, Bernabé E. Poverty, social exclusion and dental caries of 12-year-old children: a cross-sectional study in Lima, Peru. BMC Oral Health 2009;9:16.
32. Perera I, Ekanayake L. Influence of oral health-related behaviours on income inequalities in oral health among adolescents. Community Dent Oral Epidemiol 2011;39(4):345–51.
33. Perera I, Ekanayake L. Social inequality in perceived oral health among Sri Lankan adolescents. Community Dent Health 2010;27(1):29–34.
34. Keller Celeste R, Nadanovsky P, Ponce De Leon A, et al. The individual and contextual pathways between oral health and income inequality in Brazilian adolescents and adults. Soc Sci Med 2009;69:1468–75.

35. Do LG. Distribution of caries in children: variations between and within populations. J Dent Res 2012;91(6):536–43.
36. Bastos JL, Boing AF, Peres KG, et al. Periodontal outcomes and social, racial and gender inequalities in Brazil: a systematic review of the literature between 1999 and 2008. Cad Saude Publica 2011;27(2):141–53.
37. Thomson WM, Poulton R, Kruger E, et al. Socio-economic and behavioural risk factors for tooth loss from age 18 to 26 among participants in the Dunedin multidisciplinary health and development study. Caries Res 2000;34(5):361–6.
38. Nicolau B, Marcenes W, Bartley M, et al. Associations between socio-economic circumstances at two stages of life and adolescents' oral health status. J Public Health Dent 2005;65(1):14–20.
39. Lupo PJ, Danysh HE, Symanski E, et al. Neighborhood-based socioeconomic position and risk of oral clefts among offspring. Am J Public Health 2015;105(12):2518–25.
40. Rizk SP, Christen AG. Falling between the cracks: oral health survey of school children ages five to thirteen having limited access to dental services. ASDC J Dent Child 2018;61(5–6):356–60.
41. Murthy VH. Oral health in America, 2000 to present: progress made, but challenges remain. Public Health Rep 2016;131(2):224–5.
42. Rozier RG, White A, Slade G. Trends in oral diseases in the U.S. population. J Dent Educ 2017;81(8s):e97–109.
43. Slade GD, Sanders AE. Two decades of persisting income-disparities in dental caries among U.S. children and adolescents. J Public Health Dent 2017. https://doi.org/10.1111/jphd.12261.
44. Dye BA, Mitnik GL, Iafolla TJ, et al. Trends in dental caries in children and adolescents according to poverty status in the United States from 1999 through 2004 and from 2011 through 2014. J Am Dent Assoc 2017;148(8):550–65.e7.
45. Lin M, Zhang X, Holt JB, et al. Multilevel model to estimate county-level untreated dental caries among US children aged 6-9years using the National Health and Nutrition Examination Survey. Prev Med 2018;111:291–8.
46. Fisher-Owens SA, Isong IA, Soobader M-J, et al. An examination of racial/ethnic disparities in children's oral health in the United States. J Public Health Dent 2013;73(2):166–74.
47. Nash DA, Nagel RJ. Confronting oral health disparities among American Indian/Alaska Native children: the pediatric oral health therapist. Am J Public Health 2005;95(8):1325–9.
48. Roberts RZ, Erwin PC. Pediatricians and the oral health needs of children: one potential means for reducing oral healthcare inequities. J Tenn Dent Assoc 2015;95(2):23–7 [quiz: 28–9].
49. Fine JI, Isman RE, Grant CB. A comprehensive school-based/linked dental program: an essential piece of the California access to care puzzle. J Calif Dent Assoc 2012;40(3):229–37.
50. Flores G, Tomany-Korman SC. Racial and ethnic disparities in medical and dental health, access to care, and use of services in US children. Pediatrics 2008;121(2):e286–98.
51. Edelstein BL. Disparities in oral health and access to care: findings of national surveys. Ambul Pediatr 2002;2(2 Suppl):141–7.
52. Edelstein BL. Dental care considerations for young children. Spec Care Dentist 2002;22(3 Suppl):11S–25S.

53. Edelstein BL, Manski RJ, Moeller JF. Pediatric dental visits during 1996: an analysis of the Federal Medical Expenditure Panel Survey. Pediatr Dent 2000;22(1): 17–20.
54. Valencia A, Damiano P, Qian F, et al. Racial and ethnic disparities in utilization of dental services among children in Iowa: the Latino experience. Am J Public Health 2012;102(12):2352–9.
55. Lazarus Z, Pirutinsky S, Korbman M, et al. Dental utilization disparities in a Jewish context: reasons and potential solutions. Community Dent Health 2015;32(4): 247–51.
56. Edelstein BL, Chinn CH. Update on disparities in oral health and access to dental care for America's children. Acad Pediatr 2009;9(6):415–9.
57. Bernstein J, Gebel C, Vargas C, et al. Integration of oral health into the well-child visit at federally qualified health centers: study of 6 clinics, August 2014-March 2015. Prev Chronic Dis 2016;13:E58.
58. Junqueira SR, Pannuti CM, Rode Sde M. Oral health in Brazil - Part I: public oral health policies. Braz Oral Res 2008;22(suppl 1):8–17.
59. Petersen P. Improvement of oral health in Africa in the 21st century - the role of the WHO Global Oral Health Programme. Dev Dent 2004;1(5):9–20.
60. Silk H, Douglass AB, Douglass JM, et al. Oral health during pregnancy. Am Fam Physician 2008;77(8):1139–44.
61. Anders PL, Davis EL. Oral health of patients with intellectual disabilities: a systematic review. Spec Care Dentist 2010;30(3):110–7.
62. Hartnett E, Haber J, Krainovich-Miller B, et al. Oral health in pregnancy. J Obstet Gynecol Neonatal Nurs 2016;45(4):565–73.
63. Le M, Riedy C, Weinstein P, et al. Barriers to utilization of dental services during pregnancy: a qualitative analysis. J Dent Child (Chic) 2009;76(1):46–52.
64. Newacheck PW, McManus M, Fox HB, et al. Access to health care for children with special health care needs. Pediatrics 2000;105(4 Pt 1):760–6.
65. Sheiham A. Dental caries affects body weight, growth and quality of life in pre-school children. Br Dent J 2006;201(10):625–6.
66. Jackson SL, Vann WF, Kotch JB, et al. Impact of poor oral health on children's school attendance and performance. Am J Public Health 2011;101(10):1900–6.
67. Royal College of Surgeons. Faculty of Dental Surgery. The state of children's oral health in England. London: Royal College of Surgeons; 2015.
68. Health and Social Care Information Centre. Provisional monthly hospital episode statistics for admitted patient care, outpatients and accident and emergency data - April 2012 to November 2012. 2013. Available at: http://www.hscic.gov.uk/catalogue/PUB10466. Accessed January 20, 2018.
69. Park J-B, Han K, Park Y-G, et al. Association between socioeconomic status and oral health behaviors: the 2008-2010 Korea National Health and Nutrition Examination Survey. Exp Ther Med 2016;12(4):2657–64.
70. American Dental Association. Health Policy Institute. Oral Health and Well-Being in the United States. Available at: https://www.ada.org/~/media/ADA/Science and Research/HPI/OralHealthWell-Being-StateFacts/US-Oral-Health-Well-Being.pdf?la=en. Accessed January 24, 2018.
71. Masood M, Sheiham A, Bernabé E. Household expenditure for dental care in low and middle income countries. PLoS One 2015;10(4):e0123075.
72. National Academics of Sciences, Engineering and Medicine. Communities in action: pathways to health equity. Washington, DC: The National Academies Press; 2017. https://doi.org/10.17226/24624.

73. Marmot M, For the Commission on Social Determinants of Health. Achieving health equity: from root causes to fair outcomes. Lancet 2007;370(9593): 1153–63.
74. Wilkinson RG, Pickett K. The spirit level: why more equal societies almost always do better. London: Allen Lane; 2009.
75. Newton JT, Bower EJ. The social determinants of oral health: new approaches to conceptualizing and researching complex causal networks. Community Dent Oral Epidemiol 2005;33(1):25–34.
76. Fisher-Owens SA, Gansky SA, Platt LJ, et al. Influences on children's oral health: a conceptual model. Pediatrics 2007;120(3):e510–20.
77. Petersen PE, Kwan S. Equity, social determinants and public health programmes - the case of oral health. Community Dent Oral Epidemiol 2011;39(6):481–7.
78. Tomar SL. Social determinants of oral health and disease in U.S. men. J Mens Health 2012;9(2):113–9.
79. Watt RG, Sheiham A. Integrating the common risk factor approach into a social determinants framework. Community Dent Oral Epidemiol 2012;40(4):289–96.
80. Lee JY, Divaris K. The ethical imperative of addressing oral health disparities. J Dent Res 2014;93(3):224–30.
81. Public Health England. Local authorities improving oral health: commissioning better oral health for children and young people. London: Public Health England; 2014.
82. Schou L, Wight C. Does dental health education affect inequalities in dental health? Community Dent Health 1994;11(2):97–100.
83. US Department of Health and Human Services Oral Health Coordinating Committee. U.S. Department of Health and Human Services Oral Health Strategic Framework, 2014-2017. Public Health Rep 2016;131(2):242–57.
84. Marmot M, Allen J, Goldblatt P, et al. Fair societies, healthy lives: strategic review of health inequalities in England post-2010. London: The Marmot Review; 2010.
85. McKinlay J. A case for refocusing upstream: the political economy of illness. In: Gartley J, editor. Patients, physicians and illness: a sourcebook in behavioral science and health. New York: Free Press; 1979. p. 9–25.
86. Macintyre S. Inequalities in health in Scotland: what are they and what can we do about them? Glasgow: MRC Social and Public Health Sciences Unit; 2007.
87. Bambra C, Gibson M, Sowden A, et al. Tackling the wider social determinants of health and health inequalities: evidence from systematic reviews. J Epidemiol Community Health 2010;64(4):284–91.
88. Watt RG, Rouxel PL. Dental caries, sugars and food policy. Arch Dis Child 2012; 97(9):769–72.
89. Batis C, Rivera JA, Popkin BM, et al. First-year evaluation of Mexico's tax on nonessential energy-dense foods: an observational study. PLoS Med 2016; 13(7):e1002057.
90. Mendoza A, Pérez AE, Aggarwal A, et al. Energy density of foods and diets in Mexico and their monetary cost by socioeconomic strata: analyses of ENSANUT data 2012. J Epidemiol Community Health 2017;71(7):713–21.
91. Guerrero-López CM, Molina M, Colchero MA. Employment changes associated with the introduction of taxes on sugar-sweetened beverages and nonessential energy-dense food in Mexico. Prev Med 2017;105:S43–9.
92. Ibarra S, Taillie LS, Induni M, et al. Changes in prices, sales, consumer spending, and beverage consumption one year after a tax on sugar-sweetened beverages in Berkeley, California, US: a before-and-after study. PLoS Med 2017;14(4): e1002283.

93. Public Health England. Sugar reduction: achieving the 20%. A technical report outlining progress to date, guidelines for industry, 2015 baseline levels in key foods and next steps. London: Public Health England; 2015.

94. Cecchini M, Sassi F, Lauer JA, et al. Tackling of unhealthy diets, physical inactivity, and obesity: health effects and cost-effectiveness. Lancet 2010; 376(9754):1775–84.

95. National Health and Medical Research Council. Information paper – Water fluoridation: dental and other human health outcomes. Canberra (Australia): National Health and Medical Research Council; 2017.

96. McDonagh MS, Whiting PF, Wilson PM, et al. Systematic review of water fluoridation. BMJ 2000;321(7265):855–9.

97. Iheozor-Ejiofor Z, Worthington HV, Walsh T, et al. Water fluoridation for the prevention of dental caries. Cochrane Database Syst Rev 2015;(6):CD010856.

98. Spencer J, Do L, Ha D. Fluoride and oral health inequalities; childhood caries. In: Peres M, Watt RG, editors. Policy solutions for oral health inequalities. Melbourne (Australia): International Centre for Oral Health Inequalities Research and Policy; 2017. p. 11–4.

99. Jaafar N, Hakim H, Mohd Nor NA, et al. Is the burden of oral diseases higher in urban disadvantaged community compared to the national prevalence? BMC Public Health 2014;14(Suppl 3):S2.

Oral Health for US Children with Special Health Care Needs

Donald L. Chi, DDS, PhD

KEYWORDS

- Children with special health care needs (CSHCN) • Access to dental care
- Unmet dental care needs • Tooth brushing • Diet
- Behavioral determinants of oral health • Oral health promotion interventions

KEY POINTS

- One-in-five US children have a special health care need but there are no comprehensive studies on the clinical oral health of children with special health care needs (CSHCN).
- The lack of high-quality data on tooth decay prevalence, oral health behaviors, and evidence-based interventions is a barrier to oral health promotion in CSHCN.
- Oral health researchers should work with other health care providers and behavioral and social scientists to develop, implement, evaluate, and refine clinical interventions for CSHCN.
- Pediatric health care providers are well positioned to help promote the oral health of CSHCN in clinical practice.

INTRODUCTION

One-in-five children in the United States have a special health care need,[1] which is equivalent to nearly 15 million children nationwide. The US Maternal and Child Health Bureau defines children with special health care needs (CSHCN) as "those who have or are at increased risk for a chronic physical, developmental, behavioral, or emotional condition and who also require health and related services of a type or amount beyond that required by children generally."[2]

Anecdotal evidence suggests CSHCN are at increased risk for poor oral health. However, research supporting this assertion is sparse. To date, there are no known comprehensive studies on the clinical oral health of CSHCN. Only a few studies have documented tooth decay rates in CSHCN, most of which focus on use of professional dental care services and caregiver-reported unmet dental care need. Even less

Disclosure Statement: The author has no disclosures.
Department of Oral Health Sciences, University of Washington, School of Dentistry, Box 357475, B509f Health Sciences Building, Seattle, WA 98195-7475, USA
E-mail address: dchi@uw.edu

Pediatr Clin N Am 65 (2018) 981–993
https://doi.org/10.1016/j.pcl.2018.05.007
0031-3955/18/© 2018 Elsevier Inc. All rights reserved.

pediatric.theclinics.com

is known about oral hygiene behaviors, fluoride exposure, and dietary risk factors, particularly sugar intake, which is one of the main behavioral determinants of oral health in this pediatric population. The dearth of research is a barrier to progress and prevents the field from generating scalable evidence-based interventions, clinical practice guidelines, and health policies that could prevent dental disease and promote the oral health of CSHCN.

This article focuses on the oral health of CSHCN with the goal of providing insight on what is currently known and the barriers to progress. First, a brief update will be presented on tooth decay epidemiology, oral health status, and the behavioral determinants of oral health for CSHCN. Next, the limitations of research to date will be highlighted, with an emphasis on problems associated with the current conceptualization of special health care needs and other methodologic challenges. Cystic fibrosis (CF) and autism spectrum disorders (ASD) will be used as case studies to elucidate problems, solutions, and lessons learned. Broader recommendations will be made on ways to improve future research. Finally, drawing on the best available scientific evidence, clinical recommendations will be made to help guide pediatricians and other health care providers committed to the oral health of CSHCN. The goal is to advance the field through high-quality science, evidence-based standards of clinical care, and behavior change strategies that promote the oral and systemic health of CSHCN.

TOOTH DECAY EPIDEMIOLOGY

Tooth decay (dental caries) is the most significant oral health problem in children, including CSHCN. Dentists spend most of their practice time treating tooth decay. However, there are no national or state-level data on dental caries epidemiology in CSHCN. A pilot study from Washington State focused on enrollees in 2 Head Start centers, a school readiness program for preschool-aged children aged 3 to 5 years from low-income households. The mean number of decayed, missing, and filled primary tooth surfaces for Head Start children was 5.8 ± 11.2 surfaces compared with the US mean of 2.6 surfaces.[3,4] Head Start children with a developmental delay were 1.26 times as likely to have tooth decay compared with those without a developmental delay ($P = .04$). Similarly, clinical studies have focused on small subgroups of CSHCN identified by medical condition or diagnosis, with mixed findings on tooth decay rates compared to children without special health care needs.[5–12]

ORAL HEALTH STATUS AND UNMET DENTAL CARE NEEDS

In the absence of comprehensive tooth decay data for CSHCN, relevant studies focus on caregiver-reported measures of dental disease, oral health status, or unmet dental care needs. The main source of US data on CSHCN is the National Survey of CSHCN, which includes caregiver-reported oral health measures. Dental care was first documented as the most common unmet health care need for CSHCN in 2000, a finding replicated a decade later.[13,14]

Based on the 2007 National Survey of CSHCN, 22.8% of caregivers reported having a child younger than 18 years with any cavities in the previous 6 months.[15] About 15% to 18.7% of caregivers of CSHCN reported their child as having a toothache in the previous 6 months.[16] At least 4 studies have documented higher levels of caregiver-reported unmet dental care needs for CHSCN when compared with their medically unremarkable peers.[17–19] However, a study from West Virginia found comparable rates of caregiver-reported unmet preventive and orthodontic dental care needs by special needs status.[20]

Several factors are associated with unmet dental care needs for CSHCN. These include living in low-income households or rural area, failure to receive medical care, increased special needs severity and lower degree of functioning, and poor psychological adjustment.[21–26] Caregiver factors such as depression and low levels of functioning are also associated with unmet dental care need for CSHCN.[26,27]

Although it is encouraging that oral health measures are part of the National Survey of CSHCN, there are at least 3 main limitations with caregiver-reported measures: (1) no verification of dental needs by an oral health professional; (2) inability to capture dental disease severity; and (3) lack of specificity on the type of unmet need (eg, preventive, restorative, orthodontic). Previous work indicates high consistency between caregiver- and dentist-reported oral health status for children,[28] but validity studies have not been conducted on CSHCN, which is relevant given the difficulty of assessing oral health status and needs when there is limited child cooperation secondary to poor behavior or cognitive deficit.

ORAL HEALTH BEHAVIORS

There are 3 main oral health behaviors that help to prevent tooth decay: preventive dental care use, tooth brushing with fluoride toothpaste, and minimizing sugar intake (both volume and frequency).

Preventive dental care use is the most extensively studied behavioral determinant of oral health for CSHCN. National data indicate that 54% of CSHCN used preventive dental care compared with 44.6% for children without special health care needs ($P<.001$).[23] Other studies based on national data indicate preventive care utilization rates are not significantly different by special needs status.[29,30]

At the state-level, significantly larger proportions of Medicaid-enrolled CSHCN aged 3 to 17 years in Iowa used preventive dental care than those without special health care needs ($P<.001$).[31] In this particular study, the association between special needs severity and preventive dental care use was hypothesized to be linear, but the actual associations were curvilinear: utilization was highest for children with moderate

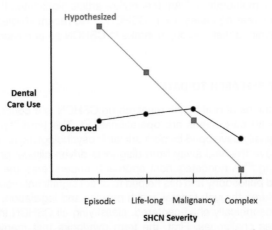

Fig. 1. Hypothesized and observed association between severity of special health care needs (SHCN) and preventive dental care use for Medicaid-enrolled children with special health care needs. (*Data from* Chi DL, Momany ET, Neff J, et al. Impact of chronic condition status and severity on dental utilization for Iowa Medicaid-enrolled children. Med Care 2011;49(2):180–92.)

special needs and lowest for children with lower and higher severity special needs (**Fig. 1**). Barriers to preventive dental care for CSHCN include caregiver burden, not having a family member enrolled in Medicaid, not having a personal dentist, lack of preventive medical care, and the absence of coordination among community-based organizations.[31–34]

In a recent study, Medicaid-enrolled CSHCN younger than 6 years in Washington State's Access to Baby and Child Dentistry (ABCD) program were slightly more likely to use preventive dental care than those without special health care needs (odds ratio: 1.04; 95% confidence interval: 1.03, 1.05; $P<.001$).[35] The ABCD program provides care coordination services to families of preschool-aged children in Medicaid, gives enrollees additional dental benefits (eg, coverage for increased number of checkups and fluoride treatments), and pays dentists enhanced reimbursement rates. Recent legislation in Washington State has passed that will extend the program to Medicaid-enrolled CSHCN aged 6 to 12 years with special needs diagnoses (eg, intellectual and/or developmental disability, cerebral palsy, epilepsy, autism).

Collectively, available studies indicate that preventive dental care utilization for CSHCN is comparable or greater than utilization for children without special health care needs, although unmet dental care needs appear to be higher for CSHCN. The type of unmet dental care need as reported by caregivers of CSHCN is unknown.

Fewer studies have focused on tooth brushing in CSHCN. One study examined barriers to twice daily tooth brushing for young CSHCN aged 23 to 62 months.[36] Inadequate caregiver skills and lack of hygiene supplies were documented as barriers to twice daily tooth brushing. Another study found caregiver tooth brushing was associated with tooth brushing in CSHCN.[33] A pilot program involving oral hygiene instructions for children and young adults with developmental disabilities did not change plaque scores, but improved toothpaste use, which is an important source of topical fluoride.[37]

There is a dearth of research on dietary behaviors in CSHCN. A review article from 1998 discussed nutritional issues in CSHCN with an emphasis on subgroups of CSHCN at risk for malnutrition.[38] Another review article highlighted the role of sugared medications in increasing caries risk in CSHCN.[39] No recent studies from the United States have examined diet and sugar intake in CSHCN as behavioral risk factors for tooth decay.

LIMITATIONS OF RESEARCH TO DATE

One of the limitations of oral health research on CSHCN is a conceptual problem of how special health care needs are operationalized. The term "special health care needs" was originally developed by pediatricians, psychologists, and health policy researchers to move the field away from diagnosis-driven clinical practice, research, and policymaking.[40] A noncategorical approach underscores the importance of a person-centered philosophy and has helped to direct significant resources to affected families and children through federal health policies and legislation.

Although philosophically child-centered, classifying all CSHCN into a single category also creates challenges. First, the term overlooks that many CSHCN are no different from healthy children regarding oral health outcomes and associated behaviors.[41] Methods are needed to identify CSHCN who are similar to healthy children in terms of oral health status and caries risk so that resources can be directed to those in greatest need. Second, it obscures within group heterogeneity. For instance, classifying children with a severe intellectual and/or developmental disability and those with well-controlled asthma into a single category assumes that the barriers to dental visits and tooth brushing are the same for these 2 groups of children. As a result, data generated from this approach may not be helpful in developing interventions tailored to the needs of subgroups of CSHCN.

Third, the noncategorical approach is primary care–focused and is not aligned with the current structure of the health care delivery system or generally with how health research is funded. Although there are demonstration projects involving integrated care models in which patients are treated holistically (eg, accountable and coordinated care organizations), the US health care delivery system continues to be driven by organ-based specialty care. Similarly, the funding agencies that support biomedical research are typically organized along organs and diseases (eg, National Health, Lung, and Blood Institute; National Institute of Dental and Craniofacial Research; National Cancer Institute). One exception is the Eunice Kennedy Shriver National Institute of Child Health and Human Development, which received about 4% of the total US National Institutes of Health budget in fiscal year 2017 and funds some but not all child health research.[42] Thus, the health care delivery system and research funding model are out of sync with a noncategorical approach espoused by the concept of special health care needs.

There are 2 ways to approach this conceptual problem. First, researchers should continue to conduct studies using the Maternal and Child Health Bureau's datasets, however limited these data may be in terms of documenting disease rates and informing clinical intervention development. These studies help drive federal and state health policies and are important in ensuring that oral health is a priority to policymakers.[43] In addition, efforts should be directed toward advocating for inclusion of CSHCN in other datasets such as the National Health and Nutrition Examination Survey (NHANES), which includes dental screenings.

Second, researchers leading primary data collection studies should adopt a diagnosis-based approach to identify subgroups of CSHCN at risk for poor oral health. This approach should account for the pathophysiology of the condition and has the greatest potential to lead to condition-specific knowledge that can be used to design relevant oral health promotion programs. This approach also facilitates the process of identifying research collaborators from medicine as well as clinics through which study participants are recruited for studies.

The current lack of clinical specificity in oral health research on CHSCN presents tremendous opportunities to conduct important research. When adopting a diagnosis-based approach to identify high-risk subgroups of CSHCN, there are at least 6 scientific and study design considerations. First, clinical research begins with a problem, question, and conceptual model. Each component needs to be pre-specified, with the end goal being to solve a clinical problem. Models should be based on the attributes and pathophysiology of the given medical condition. Researchers should work with primary care clinicians, medical specialists, social and behavioral scientists, and basic scientists to develop preliminary models.

Second, the model should include relevant factors that are modifiable to help guide future clinical interventions. Because tooth decay has its cause in oral health behaviors, models should include relevant behavioral risk factors. From a social determinant of health perspective, models should include factors that may not be amenable to direct change but need to be accounted for when planning behavioral interventions.[44] Based on the particular behaviors and social determinants, interventions may need to be tailored rather than targeted.[45] This point underscores the importance of conducting clinical research with translational relevance.[46]

Third, there is a need for high-quality, systematic, condition-specific epidemiologic studies to test disease models in CSHCN. Clinical epidemiologic studies are the mechanism by which models are tested and refined. Case finding is based on medical diagnosis, and relevant information should be collected on subgroups within diagnostic categories (eg, CF genotype or ASD subgroup). Pilot data are important in designing subsequent studies with adequate statistical power.

Fourth, the process by which subgroups of CSHCN are identified and recruited for studies will depend on the prevalence of the condition. For conditions such as CF and ASD, there may be a need to recruit from specialty medical clinics across multiple sites to achieve adequate statistical power. Community-based approaches are feasible for more common conditions. These factors can inform subsequent study design features and how interventions are deployed.

Fifth, careful consideration should be given to the need for a control group consisting of individuals without the condition. Misspecified controls can introduce systematic bias and other problems.[47] Depending on the specific conditions under investigation, it may be more appropriate to include comparison groups rather than controls (eg, children vs adolescents vs young adults with CF).

Sixth, because scientific advances are made and medical therapies improve over time, conceptual models should be revised and updated as needed. Epidemiologic sciences and clinical practice are fluid processes and may undergo significant changes as scientific knowledge grows and progress is made.

CASE STUDY 1: CYSTIC FIBROSIS

Individuals with CF are believed to be at low risk for tooth decay. In fact, caries is considered a negligible disease in CF in 2 of the main pediatric dentistry textbooks.[48,49] The purported reason is that chronic systemic antibiotic use targets cariogenic bacteria and protects individuals with CF from tooth decay. However, the scientific evidence for this hypothesis is weak. In addition, a systemic review, which accounted for age-based heterogeneity in the pathophysiology of CF, suggested that the prevailing clinical paradigm is incorrect.[11] To further test this new hypothesis, an interdisciplinary team of dentists, pulmonologists, microbiologists, chemist, nurses, dental hygienists, and biostatisticians conducted the largest clinical oral health study of CF in the United States in 1980. The pilot study confirmed findings from the earlier systematic review that although children with CF were at lower risk for dental caries, adolescents with CF were not. As part of this study, the team used a historical control group from the US NHANES dataset. The team has proposed a larger multicenter study to further refine the conceptual model and generate the data needed for intervention development[50].

There are 3 lessons learned. First, published models and data pertaining to the oral health of CSHCN should be carefully scrutinized. For decades, the oral health model for CF has been accepted by the field and taught to generations of dentists, but the model is likely to be incorrect. There may be similar problems with the published science pertaining to other subgroups of CSHCN. This not only raises concerns about existing clinical standards of care for CSHCN but also is a reminder to the scientific community of the importance of reevaluating established clinical paradigms.

Second, careful consideration should be devoted to the issue of control groups. The pilot data were consistent with the original hypothesis of age-based heterogeneity in tooth decay by CF status. This underscores the need for CF-focused interventions. Thus, future research should recruit individuals with CF stratified on age. This broadly reinforces the importance of ensuring that study design is aligned with the purpose of the study and helps preserve scare research resources.

Third, this model included oral health behaviors (eg, dental visits, fluoride exposure, sugar intake), which are considered upstream determinants of oral health adapted from behavior change theories, as well as social factors related to tooth decay. Once researchers have a refined sociobehavioral conceptual model in hand, the potential points of intervention should be clearer.

CASE STUDY 2: AUTISM SPECTRUM DISORDERS

Many children with ASD are unable to participate in oral health behaviors because of difficulties cooperating, oral hypersensitivity, and low tolerance for new procedures.[51,52] There are few recent US studies on tooth decay in children with ASD. One study found that children younger than 8 years with ASD had significantly higher caries rates than children aged 8 to 19 years with ASD.[53] A study from 2008 found that caries rates were similar for a population of individuals with and without ASD aged 3 to 28 years.[54] A small study (N = 43) from 1999 reported that 62.8% of children with ASD had less than 5% of decayed teeth, 11.6% with 5% to 20% decayed teeth, and 25.6% with more than 20% decayed teeth.[55] The only other US study was published in 1977.[56] A systematic review based mostly on non-US studies reported high caries rates among children and adolescents with ASD.[57]

Nearly all published dental studies involving children with ASD focus on ways to improve the dental care experience, except for one exploring inconsistent tooth brushing as a risk indicator for caries.[53] Strategies to improve dental chairside management of children with ASD include identifying predictors of poor cooperation; desensitization training and behavior guidance; addressing dental fear; and adapting the physical environment.[58–64] These approaches are generally consistent with documented barriers to dental care for children with ASD, which increases the odds that proposed solutions will be effective.

There are 2 lessons learned. First, there are no population-based dental disease data for US children with ASD, making it impossible to determine the extent to which tooth decay is a problem in children with ASD. A large number of highly functioning children with ASD are likely to have similar caries risk as developmentally unremarkable children. Large-scale epidemiologic studies would help to clarify heterogeneity within the ASD population regarding the ability to cooperate, specific barriers to oral health, and other factors. In addition, studies should continue to follow children with ASD longitudinally through adolescence and adulthood to assess which risk factors for dental disease change with age.

Second, nearly all documented oral health-related interventions for US CSHCN are for young children with ASD. Efforts are focused entirely on dental care use, with no attention devoted to other oral health-related behaviors such as diet and tooth brushing. This is surprising given the absence of strong evidence that dental care prevents dental disease coupled with anecdotal data on caregivers' use of sweet foods as rewards and reports of difficulties enforcing regular hygiene in children with ASD. Only one exploratory study has examined the potential links between diet and behavioral patterns that could ease routines for children with ASD.[65] Future behavior change interventions should address diet and hygiene and could be implemented within dental and home settings. Biopsychosocial approaches could be used to develop comprehensive models to help guide intervention development for children with ASD, as previous researchers have done for childhood obesity.[66] From a health equity perspective, it is also important to consider how socioeconomic status and poverty influence biopsychosocial approaches for children with ASD[67] and other special health care needs.

CLINICAL RECOMMENDATIONS FOR PEDIATRIC HEALTH CARE PROVIDERS

Although researchers continue to grow the scientific knowledge needed to improve the oral health of CSHCN, there are 5 key clinical recommendations for pediatric health care providers. These recommendations are applicable to all children but are especially important for CSHCN.

1. *Conduct a caries risk assessment at each visit and provide tailored anticipatory guidance based on risk.* Anticipatory guidance should incorporate known risk factors associated with the child's medical condition, comorbidities, and medications. Previous work indicates that up to 1 in 2 pediatricians conduct caries risk assessments,[68] a rate that is likely to be lower in underserved areas. In addition to examining the teeth for gross caries and restorations, health care providers should assess the child's diet and fluoride exposure, with special attention to sugar intake and fluoride toothpaste use. The relative balance between sugar intake and fluoride exposure will form the basis for the child's risk for developing tooth decay. Advice should be kept simple, health providers should follow-up with caregivers on progress at subsequent visits, and anticipatory guidance may change based on progress and new risk factors.

2. *Determine whether patients have a dental home and refer those without a dental home to a dentist.* The American Academy of Pediatric Dentistry and the American Academy of Pediatrics recommend that all children see a dentist by age 12 months. Low-income children in Medicaid are more likely to see a physician for well-baby visits than to see a dentist by age 1 year.[69] However, children with more well-baby visits before age 1 year are significantly more likely to have a delayed first dental visit.[70] This suggests physicians are not referring children as recommended, which is consistent with previous work indicating low dentist referrals by pediatricians.[71] All CSHCN should be referred to a dentist by age 12 months to ensure the child has a dentist who can provide anticipatory guidance, preventive care, and restorative care as needed.

3. *Recommend appropriate use of fluoride and advocate for community water fluoridation.* Fluoride is one of the few evidence-based strategies available to prevent tooth decay.[72] The persistence of oral health inequalities indicates that fluoride will continue to play an important role in caries prevention.[73] Twice daily tooth brushing with fluoride toothpaste should be encouraged.[74,75] There is also a need to address potential fluoride hesitancy expressed by caregivers, which has been documented among caregivers of children with ASD.[76,77] Pediatric health care providers also play an important role in advocating for public health strategies such as community water fluoridation, talking to caregivers about the importance of fluoride, organizing community health events to educate the public about fluoride, and writing op-eds in support of fluoride.

4. *Identify dietary sugar sources and find ways to reduce excess sugar intake.* Previous work suggests that fluoride alone is insufficient in preventing tooth decay in high-risk children.[78] For these children, excess sugar intake is likely to be the driving cause of tooth decay. One predictor of sugar intake is availability of sugary foods and beverages within the home environment.[79] In addition, caregivers may not be aware of hidden sugars in the child's diet, especially in fruit drinks like Tang and Kool-Aid that are marketed as healthy.[80] Many medications used by CSHCN contain sugars or caregivers may add sweeteners to improve palatability

and some medications lead to xerostomia that exacerbate the effects of a high-sugar diet.[81] Strategies are needed to reduce caregivers' use of sugary food items and drinks as treats or rewards.[82]

5. *Facilitate dental care transitions as CSHCN enter adolescence and young adult-hood.* Many CSHCN fail to transition from child-to adult-centered dental care as they age.[83,84] Pediatric health care providers should discuss dental care transitions in the context of broader health care transitions.[85] Special attention should be given to CSHCN with a functional limitation because this subgroup of CSHCN is not likely to undergo a dental care transition even though they transition to adult-centered medical care.[86] Adolescent and caregiver perspectives should be incorporated into the transition process.[87]

In conclusion, there are many CSHCN in the United States who may be at increased risk for poor oral health, including tooth decay, but little is known about the epidemiology of dental disease in CSHCN. These critical knowledge gaps underscore the importance of high-quality research that will help the field to assess dental disease rates and identify modifiable risk factors. More importantly, there is the possibility of using this knowledge to develop clinical interventions to prevent disease and promote oral health, which is expected to eventually lead to evidence-based practice guidelines and health policies. These steps will help to protect oral and systemic health of a medically vulnerable pediatric population and help reduce persisting oral health disparities within subgroups of CSHCN.

REFERENCES

1. Child and Adolescent Health Measurement Initiative (CAHMI). Who are children with special health care needs (CSHCN). Data Resource Center for Child and Adolescent Health. Available at: http://childhealthdata.org/. Accessed March 1, 2018.

2. McPherson M, Arango P, Fox H, et al. A new definition of children with special health care needs. Pediatrics 1998;102(1 Pt 1):137–40.

3. Chi DL, Rossitch KC, Beeles EM. Developmental delays and dental caries in low-income preschoolers in the USA: a pilot cross-sectional study and preliminary explanatory model. BMC Oral Health 2013;13:53.

4. Dye BA, Hsu KL, Afful J. Prevalence and measurement of dental caries in young children. Pediatr Dent 2015;37(3):200–16.

5. Barnett ML, Press KP, Friedman D, et al. The prevalence of periodontitis and dental caries in a Down's syndrome population. J Periodontol 1986;57(5):288–93.

6. Hicks MJ, Flaitz CM, Carter AB, et al. Dental caries in HIV-infected children: a longitudinal study. Pediatr Dent 2000;22(5):359–64.

7. Shulman JD. Is there an association between low birth weight and caries in the primary dentition? Caries Res 2005;39(3):161–7.

8. Macek MD, Mitola DJ. Exploring the association between overweight and dental caries among US children. Pediatr Dent 2006;28(4):375–80.

9. Kopycka-Kedzierawski DT, Auinger P, Billings RJ, et al. Caries status and overweight in 2- to 18-year-old US children: findings from national surveys. Community Dent Oral Epidemiol 2008;36(2):157–67.

10. Oberoi S, Huynh L, Vargervik K. Velopharyngeal, speech and dental characteristics as diagnostic aids in 22q11.2 deletion syndrome. J Calif Dent Assoc 2011; 39(5):327–32.

11. Chi DL. Dental caries prevalence in children and adolescents with cystic fibrosis: a qualitative systematic review and recommendations for future research. Int J Paediatr Dent 2013;23(5):376–86.
12. Sunderji S, Acharya B, Flaitz C, et al. Dental caries experience in Texan children with cleft lip and palate. Pediatr Dent 2017;39(5):397–402.
13. Newacheck PW, Hughes DC, Hung YY, et al. The unmet health needs of America's children. Pediatrics 2000;105(4 Pt 2):989–97.
14. Lewis CW. Dental care and children with special health care needs: a population-based perspective. Acad Pediatr 2009;9(6):420–6.
15. Wiener RC. Children with special health care need's association of passive tobacco smoke exposure and dental caries: 2007 National Survey of Children's Health. J Psychol Abnorm Child 2013;1 [pii:1000104].
16. Lewis C, Stout J. Toothache in US children. Arch Pediatr Adolesc Med 2010;164(11):1059–63.
17. Nelson LP, Getzin A, Graham D, et al. Unmet dental needs and barriers to care for children with significant special health care needs. Pediatr Dent 2011;33(1):29–36.
18. Paschal AM, Wilroy JD, Hawley SR. Unmet needs for dental care in children with special health care needs. Prev Med Rep 2015;3:62–7.
19. McManus BM, Chi D, Carle A. State Medicaid eligibility criteria and unmet preventive dental care need for CSHCN. Matern Child Health J 2016;20(2):456–65.
20. Wiener RC, Wiener MA. Unmet dental and orthodontic need of children with special healthcare needs in West Virginia. Rural Remote Health 2012;12:2069.
21. Skinner AC, Slifkin RT, Mayer ML. The effect of rural residence on dental unmet need for children with special health care needs. J Rural Health 2006;22(1):36–42.
22. Kane D, Mosca N, Zotti M, et al. Factors associated with access to dental care for children with special health care needs. J Am Dent Assoc 2008;139(3):326–33.
23. Iida H, Lewis C, Zhou C, et al. Dental care needs, use and expenditures among U.S. children with and without special health care needs. J Am Dent Assoc 2010;141(1):79–88.
24. Sarkar M, Earley ER, Asti L, et al. Differences in health care needs, health care utilization, and health care outcomes among children with special health care needs in Ohio: a comparative analysis between Medicaid and private insurance. J Public Health Manag Pract 2017;23(1):e1–9.
25. Weil TN, Inglehart MR. Three- to 21-year-old patients with autism spectrum disorders: parents' perceptions of severity of symptoms, oral health, and oral health-related behavior. Pediatr Dent 2012;34(7):473–9.
26. Gaskin DJ, Mitchell JM. Health status and access to care for children with special health care needs. J Ment Health Policy Econ 2005;8(1):29–35.
27. Petrova EG, Hyman M, Estrella MR, et al. Children with special health care needs: exploring the relationships between patients' level of functioning, their oral health, and caregivers' oral health-related responses. Pediatr Dent 2014;36(3):233–9.
28. Talekar BS, Rozier RG, Slade GD, et al. Parental perceptions of their preschool-aged children's oral health. J Am Dent Assoc 2005;136(3):364–72.
29. Kenney MK, Kogan MD, Crall JJ. Parental perceptions of dental/oral health among children with and without special health care needs. Ambul Pediatr 2008;8(5):312–20.
30. Beil H, Mayer M, Rozier RG. Dental care utilization and expenditures in children with special health care needs. J Am Dent Assoc 2009;140(9):1147–55.

31. Chi DL, Momany ET, Neff J, et al. Impact of chronic condition status and severity on dental utilization for Iowa Medicaid-enrolled children. Med Care 2011;49(2): 180–92.
32. Chi DL, McManus BM, Carle AC. Caregiver burden and preventive dental care use for US children with special health care needs: a stratified analysis based on functional limitation. Matern Child Health J 2014;18(4):882–90.
33. Huebner CE, Chi DL, Masterson E, et al. Preventive dental health care experiences of preschool-age children with special health care needs. Spec Care Dentist 2015;35(2):68–77.
34. Cruz S, Chi DL, Huebner CE. Oral health services within community-based organizations for young children with special health care needs. Spec Care Dentist 2016;36(5):243–53.
35. Craig M. Dental care utilization for children with special health care needs in Washington State's access to baby and child dentistry program [master's thesis]. Seattle (WA): University of Washington; 2017.
36. Campanaro M, Huebner CE, Davis BE. Facilitators and barriers to twice daily tooth brushing among children with special health care needs. Spec Care Dentist 2014;34(4):185–92.
37. Shin CJ, Saeed S. Toothbrushing barriers for people with developmental disabilities: a pilot study. Spec Care Dentist 2013;33(6):269–74.
38. Boyd LD, Palmer C, Dwyer JT. Managing oral health related nutrition issues of high risk infants and children. J Clin Pediatr Dent 1998;23(1):31–6.
39. Bigeard L. The role of medication and sugars in pediatric dental patients. Dent Clin North Am 2000;44(3):443–56.
40. Chi DL. The impact of chronic condition status, chronic condition severity, and other factors on access to dental care for Medicaid-enrolled children in Iowa [dissertation]. Iowa City (IA): University of Iowa; 2009.
41. Glassman P. Interventions focusing on children with special health care needs. Dent Clin North Am 2017;61(3):565–76.
42. U.S. Department of Health and Human Services (USDHHS). HHS FY 2017 budget in brief – NIH. 2018. Available at: http://www.hhs.gov/about/budget/fy2017/budget-in-brief/nih/index.html. Accessed March 13, 2018.
43. Kenney MK. Oral health care in CSHCN: state Medicaid policy considerations. Pediatrics 2009;124(Suppl 4):S384–91.
44. Knighton AJ, Stephenson B, Savitz LA. Measuring the effect of social determinants on patient outcomes: a systematic literature review. J Health Care Poor Underserved 2018;29(1):81–106.
45. Schmid K, Rivers SE, Latimer AE, et al. Targeting or tailoring? Mark Health Serv 2008;28(1):32–7.
46. Galea S. An argument for a consequentialist epidemiology. Am J Epidemiol 2013; 178(8):1185–91.
47. Wacholder S, McLaughlin JK, Silverman DT, et al. Selection of controls in case-control studies. I. Principles. Am J Epidemiol 1992;135(9):1019–28.
48. Cameron A, Widmer R. Handbook of pediatric dentistry. 3rd edition. London: Mosby-Wolfe; 2008.
49. McDonald RE, Avery DR, Dean JA. Dentistry for the child and adolescent. Maryland Heights (MO): Mosby Elsevier; 2011.
50. Chi DL, Rosenfeld M, Mancl L, et al. Age-related heterogeneity in dental caries and associated risk factors in individuals with cystic fibrosis ages 6-20 years: a pilot study. Journal of Cystic Fibrosis, in press.

51. Klein U, Nowak AJ. Autistic disorder: a review for the pediatric dentist. Pediatr Dent 1998;20(5):312-7.
52. Gandhi RP, Klein U. Autism spectrum disorders: an update on oral health management. J Evid Based Dent Pract 2014;14(Suppl):115-26.
53. Marshall J, Sheller B, Mancl L. Caries-risk assessment and caries status of children with autism. Pediatr Dent 2010;32(1):69-75.
54. Loo CY, Graham RM, Hughes CV. The caries experience and behavior of dental patients with autism spectrum disorder. J Am Dent Assoc 2008;139(11):1518-24.
55. Klein U, Nowak AJ. Characteristics of patients with autistic disorder (AD) presenting for dental treatment: a survey and chart review. Spec Care Dentist 1999;19(5):200-7.
56. Kopel HM. The autistic child in dental practice. ASDC J Dent Child 1977;44(4):302-9.
57. da Silva SN, Gimenez T, Souza RC, et al. Oral health status of children and young adults with autism spectrum disorders: systematic review and meta-analysis. Int J Paediatr Dent 2017;27(5):388-98.
58. Marshall J, Sheller B, Williams BJ, et al. Cooperation predictors for dental patients with autism. Pediatr Dent 2007;29(5):369-76.
59. Loo CY, Graham RM, Hughes CV. Behaviour guidance in dental treatment of patients with autism spectrum disorder. Int J Paediatr Dent 2009;19(6):390-8.
60. Marshall J, Sheller B, Mancl L, et al. Parental attitudes regarding behavior guidance of dental patients with autism. Pediatr Dent 2008;30(5):400-7.
61. Nelson T, Chim A, Sheller BL, et al. Predicting successful dental examinations for children with autism spectrum disorder in the context of a dental desensitization program. J Am Dent Assoc 2017;148(7):485-92.
62. Nelson TM, Sheller B, Friedman CS, et al. Educational and therapeutic behavioral approaches to providing dental care for patients with Autism Spectrum Disorder. Spec Care Dentist 2015;35(3):105-13.
63. Isong IA, Rao SR, Holifield C, et al. Addressing dental fear in children with autism spectrum disorders: a randomized controlled pilot study using electronic screen media. Clin Pediatr (Phila) 2014;53(3):230-7.
64. Cermak SA, Stein Duker LI, Williams ME, et al. Sensory adapted dental environments to enhance oral care for children with autism spectrum disorders: a randomized controlled pilot study. J Autism Dev Disord 2015;45(9):2876-88.
65. Harris C, Card B. A pilot study to evaluate nutritional influences on gastrointestinal symptoms and behavior patterns in children with Autism Spectrum Disorder. Complement Ther Med 2012;20(6):437-40.
66. Goetz DR, Caron W. A biopsychosocial model for youth obesity: consideration of an ecosystemic collaboration. Int J Obes Relat Metab Disord 1999;23(Suppl 2):S58-64.
67. Anderson NB, Armstead CA. Toward understanding the association of socioeconomic status and health: a new challenge for the biopsychosocial approach. Psychosom Med 1995;57(3):213-25.
68. Weatherspoon DJ, Horowitz AM, Kleinman DV. Maryland physicians' knowledge, opinions, and practices related to dental caries etiology and prevention in children. Pediatr Dent 2016;38(1):61-7.
69. Chi DL, Momany ET, Jones MP, et al. An explanatory model of factors related to well baby visits by age three years for Medicaid-enrolled infants: a retrospective cohort study. BMC Pediatr 2013;13:158.
70. Park S, Momany ET, Jones MP, et al. The effects of medical well baby visits in promoting earlier first dental visits for children. JDR Clin Trans Res 2018;3(1):91-100.

71. Long CM, Quinonez RB, Beil HA, et al. Pediatricians' assessments of caries risk and need for a dental evaluation in preschool aged children. BMC Pediatr 2012; 12:49.
72. Weyant RJ, Tracy SL, Anselmo TT, et al. Topical fluoride for caries prevention: executive summary of the updated clinical recommendations and supporting systematic review. J Am Dent Assoc 2013;144(11):1279–91.
73. Milgrom P, Reisine S. Oral health in the United States: the post-fluoride generation. Annu Rev Public Health 2000;21:403–36.
74. Buda LV. Ensuring maintenance of oral hygiene in persons with special needs. Dent Clin North Am 2016;60(3):593–604.
75. Horst JA, Tanzer JM, Milgrom PM. Fluorides and other preventive strategies for tooth decay. Dent Clin North Am 2018;62(2):207–34.
76. Chi DL. Parent refusal of topical fluoride for their children: clinical strategies and future research priorities to improve evidence-based pediatric dental practice. Dent Clin North Am 2017;61(3):607–17.
77. Rada RE. Controversial issues in treating the dental patient with autism. J Am Dent Assoc 2010;141(8):947–53.
78. Fontana M, Eckert GJ, Keels MA, et al. Fluoride use in health care settings: association with children's caries risk. Adv Dent Res 2018;29(1):24–34.
79. Schneider S, Jerusalem M, Mente J, et al. Sweets consumption of preschool children–extent, context, and consumption patterns. Clin Oral Investig 2013;17(5): 1301–9.
80. Chi DL, Hopkins S, O'Brien D, et al. Association between added sugar intake and dental caries in Yup'ik children using a novel hair biomarker. BMC Oral Health 2015;15(1):121.
81. Clark SA, Vinson LA, Eckert G, et al. Effect of Commonly Prescribed Liquid Medications on Streptococcus mutans Biofilm. An in vitro study. J Clin Pediatr Dent 2017;41(2):141–6.
82. Eli K, Hörnell A, Etminan Malek M, et al. Water, juice, or soda? Mothers and grandmothers of preschoolers discuss the acceptability and accessibility of beverages. Appetite 2017;112:133–42.
83. Nowak AJ, Casamassimo PS, Slayton RL. Facilitating the transition of patients with special health care needs from pediatric to adult oral health care. J Am Dent Assoc 2010;141(11):1351–6.
84. Bayarsaikhan Z, Cruz S, Neff J, et al. Transitioning from pediatric to adult dental care for adolescents with special health care needs: dentist perspectives–part two. Pediatr Dent 2015;37(5):447–51.
85. Lotstein DS, McPherson M, Strickland B, et al. Transition planning for youth with special health care needs: results from the national survey of children with special health care needs. Pediatrics 2005;115(6):1562–8.
86. Chi DL. Medical care transition planning and dental care use for youth with special health care needs during the transition from adolescence to young adulthood: a preliminary explanatory model. Matern Child Health J 2014;18(4):778–88.
87. Cruz S, Neff J, Chi DL. Transitioning from pediatric to adult dental care for adolescents with special health care needs: dentist perspectives–part one. Pediatr Dent 2015;37(5):442–6.

Orthodontics in Children and Impact of Malocclusion on Adolescents' Quality of Life

Lucas Guimarães Abreu, PhD, MSc, DDS*

KEYWORDS

- Adolescent • Malocclusion • Orthodontics • Quality of life • Pediatrician
- Family physician • Primary care

KEY POINTS

- Malocclusion exerts an adverse effect on oral health and has a negative impact on adolescents' quality of life.
- The timely referral of children/adolescents to orthodontic treatment is a concern that the pediatric provider should have.
- Pediatricians and physicians in primary care have an important role on the anticipatory guidance of children/adolescents and their parents/caregivers regarding children/adolescents' oral health, particularly for orthodontic outcomes.

INTRODUCTION

Orthodontics is the dental specialty that is concerned with treating malocclusion, which is characterized by the presence of misaligned teeth and/or maxilla and mandible discrepancies. Tooth malposition and inadequacies in the growth of the craniofacial bones may adversely affect the dentition by means of the stress imposed to teeth and surrounding tissues.[1] In this sense, the early diagnosis of malocclusion during childhood and adolescence is acknowledged in the literature.[2] The pediatric provider should know what the dentist is looking for and basics about referral, even if the details will be managed by the dentist. The practitioner who is concerned and able to recognize malocclusion and to refer his or her patients to orthodontic treatment in their early ages is indeed providing comprehensive pediatric health care.[3] Moreover, orthodontics and other oral health outcomes hold a major impact on oral health-related quality of life (OHRQoL), which has been defined as the functional and psychosocial repercussions of oral outcomes on people's lives.[4]

Disclosure Statement: The author has nothing to disclose.
Department of Pediatric Dentistry and Orthodontics, School of Dentistry, Universidade Federal de Minas Gerais, Maranhão, Belo Horizonte, Minas Gerais 30150-331, Brazil
* Rua Maranhão, 1447/1101, Funcionários, Belo Horizonte, Minas Gerais 30150-331, Brazil.
E-mail address: lucasgabreu01@gmail.com

Pediatr Clin N Am 65 (2018) 995–1006
https://doi.org/10.1016/j.pcl.2018.05.008
0031-3955/18/© 2018 Elsevier Inc. All rights reserved.

pediatric.theclinics.com

Studies evaluating OHRQoL have become viable through the use of psychometric quality-of-life instruments that have been developed to reliably assess such impact.[5,6]

Results of OHRQoL studies have been extensively reported in the literature.[7,8] Oral health conditions, such as dental caries and dental trauma, may have a significant impact on adolescents' quality of life. Mostly, adolescents affected by severe dental caries and those with dental fractures involving dentin/pulp show poorer OHRQoL than their peers with no dental caries and those with no dental trauma or only minor fractures.[9,10] For dental caries, particularly, quality of life deteriorates considerably when symptoms emerge, oral functioning is impaired, or caries affect psychosocial issues.[11] The consequences go beyond the adolescent. In the face of severe disease, parents/caregivers may feel guilty because of their sons'/daughters' oral health condition. The number of those reporting family disagreements and time off work due to their children's/adolescents' oral health issues cannot be overlooked.[9]

Other craniofacial issues, such as malocclusion, have also been a matter of concern. Severe discrepancies may be experienced as unattractive by adolescents, which may lead to episodes of embarrassment and distress depending on the individuals' parameters.[12] This article aims to discuss the impact of malocclusion and orthodontic treatment on adolescents' OHRQoL and to comment on the role of the pediatrician in adolescents' oral health, especially for orthodontic outcomes.

Adolescence and the Impact of Malocclusion on Oral Health-Related Quality of Life

Quality of life has many dimensions covering physical, functional, and emotional well-being.[13] In this regard, OHRQoL research evaluates the effects of oral outcomes on oral symptoms, functional limitations, emotional well-being, and social well-being.[14] The literature has comprehensively recognized that severe malocclusion presents a more negative impact on the quality of life of adolescents than a slight malocclusion or none at all.[15–17] The major repercussions of malocclusion are on an individual's emotional and social well-being.[16] Detrimental impact on oral functions (eating and speaking) has also been observed.[18]

Adolescence is a period of life in which social relations shift from the family environment to that of friends. Therefore, physical appearance and concerns with self-image are issues of great significance for the adolescent, who seeks endorsement of his or her characteristics when those characteristics come under peers' scrutiny.[19] The main concerns related to body features usually center on body weight and facial features. Particularly, an individual with unaesthetic occlusal traits faces more challenges with quality of life than his or her peers with no or slight orthodontic treatment needs.[20] In fact, those with unattractive occlusal traits may become targets of teasing or even harassment by his or her peers.[16]

Bullying Among Adolescents and the Association with Malocclusion

Malocclusion has been scientifically linked to bullying as well.[21] Bullying, as described previously, is a peculiar type of hostile behavior, through which an individual continuously exposes another individual to the ridicule.[22] Although both are regarded as hostile practices, teasing and bullying have different meanings. While teasing has no harmful intent toward the victim, bullying is a more aggressive behavior resulting in harm and even violence toward the individual being bullied.[23] An adolescent with severe discrepancy may be peer victimized by other adolescents who are aggressive to the victim because of his or her occlusal traits. Because of the physical and verbal aggressions, bullied adolescents usually show up as apprehensive, reticent, and withdrawn individuals. There is an important role for pediatricians in this regard, involving the identification of adolescents with malocclusion (or any dental disorder for that matter) at risk for bullying and its effects. Such children and their parents/caregivers need appropriate counseling and support.[24]

Orthodontic Treatment Associated with Improvement in Adolescents' Oral Health-Related Quality of Life

As mentioned, malocclusion deteriorates the quality of life of adolescents.[15–18] Orthodontic treatment, however, in general improves young individuals' OHRQoL.[25,26] Longitudinal studies have demonstrated that an adolescent's OHRQoL after orthodontic treatment is much improved when compared with OHRQoL before treatment.[27–29] Likewise, cross-sectional research that evaluated the quality of life of individuals who had already finished fixed appliance therapy showed that these individuals had better OHRQoL scores than those who had not undergone any orthodontic treatment.[30] There has been a consensus in the current literature regarding the benefits and gains that orthodontic treatment provides to an adolescent individual. However, much debate still exists regarding the OHRQoL of adolescents during orthodontic treatment. Some researchers have advocated that shortly after fixed appliances' placement, adolescents experience a worsening in their quality of life due to the deterioration of oral symptoms and functional limitations domains.[27–29] Pain and chewing impairment usually take place as a result of the presence of the orthodontic devices, such as orthodontic brackets, wires, and ligatures. The most challenging period encompasses the first months following fixed appliances' bonding.[28]

More recently, however, research has demonstrated that adolescents experience nonsignificant pain and chewing impairment at orthodontic treatment onset but improvement in the emotional and the social well-being, which, ultimately, enhances the overall quality of life.[31,32] The emotional benefit might be related to the recognition that dealing with malocclusion is a priority and to the fortuity for being able to treat such a disorder or, more simply, the desire to improve their own appearance. The social gain comes after the orthodontic treatment, which allows the treated individual to have improved social interaction with his or her peers.[33] Perhaps this seeming contradiction can be explained by the improvements in quality of life have to do not only with experiences of what has already happened but also expectations about what will come.[34,35]

The Role of the Pediatrician in Adolescents' Oral Health

During consultation with a pediatrician, adolescents with or without their parents or caregivers are usually carefully interviewed about their general health. It is suggested that special attention be geared toward obtaining information that would suggest the diagnosis of any tooth or skeletal discrepancies. The physician/pediatrician should be aware whether the adolescent has a history of permanent tooth loss during childhood or any deleterious oral habits, such as non-nutritive sucking habits or mouth breathing. Adolescents should also undergo a comprehensive physical examination, including assessment of growth and development. The pediatrician should not only evaluate the patients' height, weight, and other anthropometric measures but also investigate the growth pattern of craniofacial structures and tooth eruption order.[36] In fact, the author suggests that a comprehensive health care examination of adolescents should include anticipatory guidance on facial bone growth as well as on tooth eruption and the consolidation of the permanent teeth.

Maxilla and mandible growth issues may have substantial effects on the face. Therefore, the pediatric provider should be able to conduct facial analysis, examining patients from the side. For preschoolers, a slight convex profile is adequate. Severe facial convexity (upper incisors excessively forward beyond the lower incisors or mandible positioned backwards) is a matter of concern at any age. Likewise, severe concavity (constriction of the maxilla or large mandible growth) also denotes craniofacial growth problems.[37,38] With regard to the development of the dentition, the first primary teeth to erupt are the mandibular central incisors between 5 and 8 months of age. The primary dentition is completed between 20 and 30 months of age, when the primary second molars erupt. The eruption of the first permanent tooth takes place between 5 and 7 years of age (permanent first molars or the permanent mandibular central incisors after the exfoliation of the primary mandibular central incisors). By 14 years of age, all deciduous teeth will have been lost and the permanent teeth (except the third molars) erupted. **Tables 1** and **2** display the development of primary and permanent dentition.[39] The premature loss of posterior primary teeth may have detrimental effects on the arch length, which, in turn, may affect the eruption of posterior permanent teeth.[40] Accurate diagnosis of facial growth inadequacies or tooth position disorders and immediate referral to the orthodontist for malocclusion treatment can have short- and long-term benefits for patients on their way to achieve a harmonic occlusion.[41]

For an accurate malocclusion diagnosis, the pediatrician should be familiar with what normal occlusion looks like. In the sagittal plane, the correct relationship between maxilla and mandible is featured by the position of the permanent upper first molar in relation to the permanent lower first molar. The former should be half a tooth behind the latter (**Fig. 1**).[42] For the anterior teeth, the vertical relationship between upper and lower incisors is denominated overbite (vertical overlap of incisors); the sagittal relationship is denominated overjet (horizontal overlap of incisors). The upper incisors usually cover one-third of the lower incisors' crowns. If the upper incisors cover the entire crown of the lower incisors, patients have an increased overbite (**Fig. 2**). If no vertical relationship exists, patients have an anterior open bite (**Fig. 3**). The upper incisors are also 2 or 3 mm ahead of the lower incisors.[43] Patients with an anterior crossbite show up with the lower incisors ahead of the upper incisors (**Fig. 4**). In the transverse plane, all upper teeth should be wider than the lower teeth. Otherwise, patients have a posterior crossbite unilateral or bilateral. Posterior crossbite may be associated with anterior open bite (**Fig. 5**). Teeth should present no rotation. Crowding or the lack of space for all teeth to fit within the maxilla or the mandible is a condition of abnormality (**Fig. 6**).[42] Any deviation from the norm should be understood as a potential discrepancy that is worth investigating (**Table 3**).

Table 1
Development of the primary dentition

	Maxillary Arch			Mandibular Arch	
Tooth	Erupt (mo)	Exfoliation (y)	Tooth	Erupt (mo)	Exfoliation (y)
Central incisor	6–10	7–8	Central incisor	5–8	6–7
Lateral incisor	8–12	8–9	Lateral incisor	7–10	7–8
Canine	16–20	11–12	Canine	16–20	9–11
First molar	11–18	9–11	First molar	11–18	10–12
Second molar	20–30	9–12	Second molar	20–30	11–13

Data from Logan WHG, Kronfeld R. Development of the human jaws and surrounding structures from birth to the age of fifteen years. J Am Dent Assoc 1933;20:379–427.

Table 2
Development of the permanent dentition

Maxillary Arch		Mandibular Arch	
Tooth	Erupt (y)	Tooth	Erupt (y)
Central incisor	7–8	Central incisor	6–7
Lateral incisor	8–9	Lateral incisor	7–8
Canine	11–12	Canine	9–11
First premolar	10–11	First premolar	10–12
Second premolar	10–12	Second premolar	11–13
First molar	5–7	First molar	5–7
Second molar	12–14	Second molar	12–14

Data from Logan WHG, Kronfeld R. Development of the human jaws and surrounding structures from birth to the age of fifteen years. J Am Dent Assoc 1933;20:379–427.

Alertness to the presence of hypertrophied adenoids or tonsils during the physical examination is also relevant. Such changes may have harmful long-term effects on the normal position of teeth and on adequate growth of the maxilla and mandible.[44] Hypertrophic adenoids or tonsils may cause upper airway obstruction, which, ultimately, alters the individual's breathing pattern. Among mouth-breather children, changes in maxilla and mandible are observed intraorally, in the form of posterior crossbite, a high palatal vault, narrowing of the maxillary arch, and increased overbite and overjet.[45] Facial consequences also take place with individuals presenting an increase in lower facial height, narrow alar base, and lip apart posture. Those children have been described as having adenoidal facies. The pediatric provider has an important role in the early diagnosis of enlarged adenoids and tonsils. If the nasal obstruction is diagnosed and adequately treated during childhood or adolescence, a combination of orthodontic and orthopedic treatment may resolve the dental and the skeletal problems. In nongrowing individuals, however, dentofacial orthopedics are not indicated at all and orthodontic treatment combined with orthognathic surgery may be necessary.[46]

The consequences of malocclusion may be far beyond psychosocial issues. Individuals with excessive growth of the maxilla or those with prominent maxillary incisors are

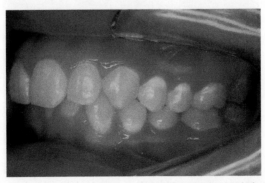

Fig. 1. Relationship between the permanent upper first molar and the permanent lower first molar. The former should be half a tooth behind the latter.

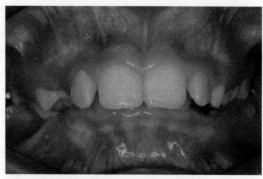

Fig. 2. Individual with an increased overbite. Upper incisors cover the entire crown of the lower incisors.

more likely to report traumatic dental injuries.[47] Indeed, increased overjet or the projection of more than 3 mm of the upper incisors in front of the lower incisors (**Figs. 7** and **8**) and inappropriate lip coverage of upper incisors are determinant factors for dental trauma.[48] In terms of overjet reduction, the literature has recognized that providing interceptive orthodontic treatment of adolescents with excessive growth of maxilla or prominent incisors in the mixed dentition is less efficacious in terms of costs and treatment duration than providing orthodontic treatment when the individual is a young adult. However, outcomes, such as the psychosocial impact and the mitigation of the likelihood of dental trauma, must be discussed with the parent/caregiver when referring his or her son or daughter to early orthodontic treatment.[49] In addition, arch irregularities may be associated with periodontal outcomes. Individuals affected by tooth crowding are more likely to present retained dental plaque and gingival inflammation than those with aligned and leveled teeth.[50]

The interest of the pediatrician should not be restricted to malocclusion, but dental caries and gingival diseases also need to be investigated. Adolescents may be unable to perform adequate oral cleaning or to seek dental treatment because of their dependence on parents/caregivers. Therefore, the pediatrician may be an advisor to the adolescent and his or her family regarding the importance of preventive measures

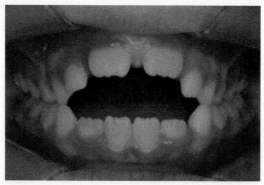

Fig. 3. Individual with anterior open bite. No vertical relationship between the upper and lower incisors.

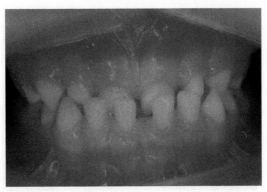

Fig. 4. Individual with anterior crossbite. Lower incisors ahead of the upper incisors.

for dental caries or any other oral health issue. The recommendations should fit to the needs of the patients. Adequate information on dietary practices, tooth brushing with fluoridated dentifrices and flossing will unequivocally have a positive effect on oral health and, therefore, prevent or reduce the risk for oral health disease. Plaque and calculus accumulation, tooth cavities, pain, and tooth color alterations may indicate oral health issues. This indication should alert the pediatrician to refer the adolescent to a dentist.[51] Although most pediatricians are not experts on oral health issues and/or on how to diagnosis and treat these properly, oral health should be, at least, a concern in his or her daily practice, as with other body systems.[52]

The information presented herein may be useful for pediatric providers. Primary health care providers should be aware that malocclusion and other oral outcomes have a negative impact on adolescents' quality of life. Awareness of such information may contribute to the improvement of the counseling that pediatricians or family physicians may provide to adolescents and their guardians regarding young individuals' oral health problems. Alertness on oral health issues would also allow pediatricians to be more assertive on these issues and increase the likelihood of appropriate and timely referral to dental care services.[53] Adequate communication between the health care provider and patients may have a substantial influence on the quality of health

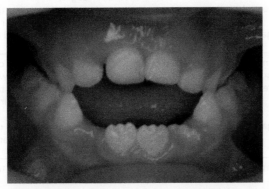

Fig. 5. Individuals with bilateral posterior crossbite. Posterior lower teeth wider than the posterior upper teeth. This individual also presents an anterior open bite.

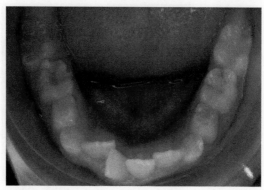

Fig. 6. Crowding or lack of space for the lower incisors.

care delivery as a whole. A physician's basic knowledge of oral and craniofacial health and disease greatly contributes to adequate communication, which, ultimately, improves physician–patient/family rapport and mitigates noncompliance with recommendations.[52]

Future research should evaluate the current knowledge and skills of pediatricians and family physicians regarding topics on children's and adolescents' oral health[54] and also assess the attention provided to oral health in the medical school curriculum.[52] Medical education has been split into 3 different stages: undergraduate programs (medical school), graduate programs (residency), and continued education

Table 3		
Description of the clinical aspects of the relationship between the upper and the lower teeth		
Plane	**Clinical Situation**	**Description**
Sagittal	Normal permanent first molars relationship	Permanent upper first molar half a tooth behind the permanent lower first molar.
	Normal overjet (horizontal overlap of incisors)	Upper incisors 2 or 3 mm ahead of the lower (upper incisors ahead of the lower by the thickness of their incisal edges)
	Increased overjet	Upper incisors more than 2 or 3 mm ahead of the lower
	Negative overjet (anterior crossbite)	Lower incisors ahead of the upper incisors
Vertical	Normal overbite (vertical overlap of incisors)	Upper incisors cover one-third of the lower incisors' crowns
	Increased overbite	Upper incisors cover the entire (or almost the entire) lower incisors' crowns
	Negative overbite (open bite)	No overlap between upper and lower incisors; a space between upper and lower incisors
Transverse	Normal relationship	The posterior upper teeth wider than the lower teeth
	Posterior crossbite	The posterior lower teeth wider than the upper teeth

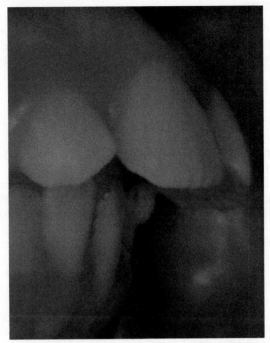

Fig. 7. Lateral view of an individual with increased overjet. Projection of more than 3 mm of the upper incisors in front of the lower incisors.

(for physicians already in practice). Adequate training in oral health would be uncomplicated if elementary expertise was introduced to medical students at the undergraduate level. For physicians who are interested in allied specialties, such as pediatrics and family medicine, oral health education should be expanded and included in residency programs. Finally, for those who have already been in daily practice, changes in practice standards may be challenging but attainable if continued education programs are faithfully implemented. Pediatric providers will be more successful when they are aware of how to deal with oral health, including awareness of the importance of conducting oral examinations to assess for many conditions, including malocclusion; using skills to promote preventive behaviors; and referring patients for dental care.[55]

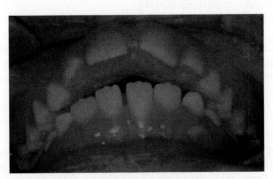

Fig. 8. Occlusal view of an individual with increased overjet.

ACKNOWLEDGMENTS

Support from the Pró-Reitoria de Pesquisa da Universidade Federal de Minas Gerais (UFMG) and FAPEMIG is highly acknowledged. The author would also like to thank Dr Rodrigo Xavier Silveira de Souza. There are no financial conflicts of interest to disclose.

REFERENCES

1. Davies SJ, Gray RM, Sandler PJ, et al. Orthodontics and occlusion. Br Dent J 2001;191:539–42.
2. Proffit WR. The timing of early treatment: an overview. Am J Orthod Dentofacial Orthop 2006;129:S47–9.
3. Starnbach HK, Gellin ME. What should the physician know about orthodontics? An overview for the pediatrician. Clin Pediatr (Phila) 1977;16:552–5.
4. Sischo L, Broder HL. Oral health-related quality of life: what, why, how, and future implications. J Dent Res 2011;90:1264–70.
5. Slade GD, Spencer AJ. Development and evaluation of the Oral Health Impact Profile. Community Dent Health 1994;11:3–11.
6. Travess HC, Newton JT, Sandy JR, et al. The development of a patient-centered measure of the process and outcome of combined orthodontic and orthognathic treatment. J Orthod 2004;31:220–34.
7. Kragt L, Dhamo B, Wolvius EB, et al. The impact of malocclusions on oral health-related quality of life in children-a systematic review and meta-analysis. Clin Oral Investig 2016;20:1881–94.
8. Zaror C, Martínez-Zapata MJ, Abarca J, et al. Impacto f traumatic dental injuries on quality of life in preschoolers and schoolchildren: a systematic review and meta-analysis. Community Dent Oral Epidemiol 2018;46:88–101.
9. Bendo CB, Paiva SM, Abreu MH, et al. Impact of traumatic dental injuries among adolescents on family's quality of life: a population-based study. Int J Paediatr Dent 2014;24:387–96.
10. Martins MT, Sardenberg F, Bendo CB, et al. Dental caries remains as the main oral condition with the greatest impact on children's quality of life. PLoS One 2017;12:e0185365.
11. Alsumait A, ElSalhy M, Raine K, et al. Impact of dental health on children's oral health-related quality of life: a cross-sectional study. Health Qual Life Outcomes 2015;13:98.
12. Abreu LG, Melgaço CA, Abreu MH, et al. Agreement between adolescents and parents/caregivers in rating the impact of malocclusion on adolescents' quality of life. Angle Orthod 2015;85:806–11.
13. Cella DF. Quality of life: concepts and definition. J Pain Symptom Manage 1994;9:186–92.
14. Jokovic A, Locker D, Stephens M, et al. Validity and reliability of a questionnaire for measuring child oral-health-related quality of life. J Dent Res 2002;81:459–63.
15. Liu Z, McGrath C, Hagg U. The impact of malocclusion/orthodontic treatment need on the quality of life. A systematic review. Angle Orthod 2009;79:585–91.
16. Dimberg L, Arnrup K, Bondemark L. The impact of malocclusion on the quality of life among children and adolescents: a systematic review of quantitative studies. Eur J Orthod 2015;37:238–47.
17. Sun L, Wong HM, McGrath CP. Relationship between the severity of malocclusion and oral health related quality of life: a systematic review and meta-analysis. Oral Health Prev Dent 2017;15(6):503–17.

18. Bernabé E, Sheiham A, de Oliveira CM. Impacts on daily performances attributed to malocclusions by British adolescentes. J Oral Rehabil 2009;36:26–31.
19. Vannucci A, Ohannessian CM. Body image dissatisfaction and anxiety trajectories during adolescence. J Clin Child Adolesc Psychol 2017;1–11 [Epub ahead of print].
20. Johal A, Cheung MY, Marcenes W. The impact of two different malocclusion traits on quality of life. Br Dent J 2007;202:E2.
21. Bullying scientifically linked to malocclusion. Br Dent J 2011;211:587.
22. Olweus D. Bullying at school. Basic facts and an effective intervention programme. Promot Educ 1994;1:27–31.
23. Seehra J, Newton JT, Dibiase AT. Bullying in schoolchildren – its relationship to dental appearance and psychosocial implications: an update for GDPs. Br Dent J 2011;210:411–5.
24. Seehra J, Fleming PS, Newton T, et al. Bullying in orthodontic patients and its relationship to malocclusion, self-esteem and oral health-related quality of life. J Orthod 2011;38:247–56.
25. Zhou Y, Wang Y, Wang X, et al. The impact of orthodontic treatment on the quality of life a systematic review. BMC Oral Health 2014;14:66.
26. Javidi H, Vettore M, Benson PE. Does orthodontic treatment before the age of 18 years improve oral health-related quality of life? A systematic review and meta-analysis. Am J Orthod Dentofacial Orthop 2017;151:644–55.
27. Zhang M, McGrath C, Hagg U. Changes in oral health-related quality of life during fixed orthodontic appliance therapy. Am J Orthod Dentofacial Orthop 2008; 133:25–9.
28. Chen M, Wang DW, Wu LP. Fixed orthodontic appliance therapy and its impact on oral health-related quality of life in Chinese patients. Angle Orthod 2010;80: 49–53.
29. Johal A, Fleming PS, AlJawad FA. A prospective longitudinal controlled assessment of pain experience and oral health-related quality of life in adolescents undergoing fixed appliance therapy. Orthod Craniofac Res 2014;17:178–86.
30. de Oliveira CM, Sheiham A. Orthodontic treatment and its impact on oral health-related quality of life in Brazilian adolescents. J Orthod 2004;31:20–7.
31. Abreu LG, Lages EM, Abreu MH, et al. Preadolescent's oral health-related quality of life during the first month of fixed orthodontic appliances. J Orthod 2013;40: 218–24.
32. Abreu LG, Melgaço CA, Lages EM, et al. Parents' and caregivers' perceptions of the quality of life of adolescents in the first four months of orthodontic treatment with a fixed appliance. J Orthod 2014;41:181–7.
33. Abreu LG, Melgaço CA, Abreu MH, et al. Effect of year one orthodontic treatment on the quality of life of adolescents, assessed by the short form of the child Perceptions Questionnaire. Eur Arch Paediatr Dent 2014;15:435–41.
34. Sajobi TT, Brahmbatt R, Lix LM, et al. Scoping review of response shift methods: current reporting practices and recommendations. Qual Life Res 2018;27(5): 1133–46.
35. Weldring T, Smith SM. Patient-reported outcomes (PROs) and patient-reported outcomes measures (PROMs). Health Serv Insights 2013;6:61–8.
36. Ditto MR, Jones JE, Sanders B, et al. Pediatrician's role in children's oral health: an Indiana survey. Clin Pediatr (Phila) 2010;49:12–9.
37. Fields HW. Craniofacial growth from infancy through adulthood. Background and clinical implications. Pediatr Clin North Am 1991;38:1053–88.

38. Bishara SE, Jakobsen JR, Hession TJ, et al. Soft tissue profile changes from 5 to 45 years of age. Am J Orthod Dentofacial Orthop 1998;114:698–706.
39. Logan WHG, Kronfeld R. Development of the human jaws and surrounding structures from birth to the age of fifteen years. J Am Dent Assoc 1933;20:379–427.
40. Davies SJ, Gray RJ, Mackie IC. Good occlusal practice in children's dentistry. Br Dent J 2001;191:655–9.
41. American Academy on Pediatric Dentistry Clinical Affairs Committee-Developing Dentition Subcommittee, American Academy on Pediatric Dentistry Council on Clinical Affairs. Guideline on management of the developing dentition and occlusion in pediatric dentistry. Pediatr Dent 2009;30:184–95.
42. Salzmann JA. The Angle classification as a parameter of malocclusion. Am J Orthod 1965;51:465–6.
43. Smith RJ. Identifying normal and abnormal development of dental occlusion. Pediatr Clin North Am 1991;38:49–71.
44. Moimaz SA, Garbin AJ, Lima AM, et al. Longitudinal study of habits leading to malocclusion development in childhood. BMC Oral Health 2014;14:96.
45. Zhu Y, Li J, Tang Y, et al. Dental arch dimensional changes after adenoidectomy or tonsillectomy in children with airway obstruction: a meta-analysis and systematic review under PRISMA guidelines. Medicine (Baltimore) 2016;95:e4976.
46. Vig KW. Nasal obstruction and facial growth: the strength of evidence for clinical assumptions. Am J Orthod Dentofacial Orthop 1998;113:603–11.
47. Kramer PF, Pereira LM, Ilha MC, et al. Exploring the impact of malocclusion and dentofacial anomalies on the occurrence of traumatic dental injuries in adolescents. Angle Orthod 2017;87:816–23.
48. Kindelan SA, Day PF, Kindelan JD, et al. Dental trauma: an overview of its influence on the management of orthodontic treatment. Part 1. J Orthod 2008;35: 68–78.
49. Flores-Mir C. Clinical significance of early treatment of overjet is questionable. At what age should orthodontic treatment for prominent upper teeth be carried out? Evid Based Dent 2007;8:103–4.
50. Ngom PI, Diagne F, Benoist HM, et al. Intraarch and interarch relationships of the anterior teeth and periodontal conditions. Angle Orthod 2006;76:236–42.
51. Sedrak MM, Doss LM. Open up and let us in: an interprofessional approach to oral health. Pediatr Clin North Am 2018;65:91–103.
52. Cohen LA. Expanding the physician's role in addressing the oral health of adults. Am J Public Health 2013;103:408–12.
53. Lewis CW, Grossman DC, Domoto PK, et al. The role of the pediatrician in the oral health of children: a national survey. Pediatrics 2000;106:E84.
54. Rabiei S, Mohebbi SZ, Patia K, et al. Physicians' knowledge of and adherence to improving oral health. BMC Public Health 2012;12:855.
55. Douglass AB, Douglass JM, Krol DM. Educating pediatricians and family physicians in children's oral health. Acad Pediatr 2009;9:452–6.

Recognizing the Relationship Between Disorders in the Oral Cavity and Systemic Disease

Paul S. Casamassimo, DDS, MS[a],*, Catherine M. Flaitz, DDS, MS[a],
Kimberly Hammersmith, DDS, MPH, MS[a], Shilpa Sangvai, MD, MPH[b],
Ashok Kumar, DDS, MS[a]

KEYWORDS

- Oral cavity • Oral disorder • Systemic disease • Trauma • Pediatric dentistry

KEY POINTS

- Systemic disease may present with signs in the oral cavity. Its recognition contributes to the diagnosis of that illness during clinical examination.
- Medical and dental providers collaborate in the care and management of children with systemic illness that involves the oral cavity.
- When acute-onset oral cavity symptoms that families do not attribute to primarily dental conditions occur, children may present at their pediatrician office, an urgent care facility, or an emergency department. These providers then need to provide first-line interventions for dental conditions.

INTRODUCTION

The mouth as the portal to the rest of the body has long justified the link between oral and systemic health. Today, the expansion of interdisciplinary care as a means to provider better care has reemphasized the need to have once-siloed disciplines, at a minimum, be aware of key health indicators traditionally outside their realm. More focused to this article, provision of simpler services, in the past restricted to peculiar providers, are now shared among providers. Examples include blood pressure monitoring by dental providers and the application of fluoride varnish by pediatric providers. This emerging crossover of service provision demands better understanding of how oral and systemic health relate to one another; can be synergistic in patient health; or, if ignored, can lead to potential problems.

Oral conditions can affect or be a manifestation of systemic health. For example, children with multiple decayed teeth (caries) can have difficulty with learning, have

[a] The Ohio State University College of Dentistry, Nationwide Children's Hospital, Columbus, OH, USA; [b] The Ohio State University College of Medicine, Nationwide Children's Hospital, Columbus, OH, USA
* Corresponding author.
E-mail address: Casamassimo.1@osu.edu

Pediatr Clin N Am 65 (2018) 1007–1032
https://doi.org/10.1016/j.pcl.2018.05.009
0031-3955/18/© 2018 Elsevier Inc. All rights reserved.

Table 1
Infectious diseases

Systemic Disease	Orofacial Lesions/Conditions	Location	Significance
Primary herpetic gingivostomatitis HSV-1	Diffuse swelling and erythema Multifocal vesicles and superficial ulcers Acute pharyngitis Lymphadenopathy Keratoconjunctivitis	Gingiva, oral mucosa, lip vermilion Gingiva, oral mucosa, lip vermilion, perioral skin Oropharynx Cervical, submandibular nodes Eyes	May be very painful and interfere with nutrition and hydration Fever, malaise, irritability are common findings Oral hygiene is important to prevent secondary bacterial infection and delayed healing Risk of disseminated disease in neonates and immunocompromised Recurrent HSV is common; occurs on lip vermilion, gingiva, palate
Varicella Varicella-zoster virus	Single to multiple, mildly tender, oral vesicles, ulcers Widespread, pruritic macules, vesicles, pustules, crusting of skin Rhinitis Pharyngitis Tender, erythematous gingivitis (uncommon)	Oral mucosa Face and trunk that spreads to extremities Nasal skin, mucosa Oropharynx Generalized gingivae	Fever, malaise, headache are common findings Oral and lip vermilion lesions precede widespread skin lesions Risk for bacterial skin infections, pneumonia, encephalitis Herpes zoster (recurrent varicella-zoster virus) is uncommon in children
Infectious mononucleosis Epstein-Barr virus	Exudative pharyngitis Tonsillar hyperplasia Necrotizing ulcerative gingivitis Necrotizing pericoronitis Palatal petechiae Lymphadenopathy Rhinitis	Oropharynx Pharyngeal and lingual tonsils Generalized gingivae Mandibular molar operculum Hard and soft palate Cervical, submandibular nodes Nose, nasal mucosa	Fever, malaise, fatigue, headache, myalgia, hepatosplenomegaly are common findings Complications include thrombocytopenia, splenic rupture, autoimmune hemolytic anemia, aplastic anemia, myocarditis Latent virus associated with malignancies

Disease (Virus)	Oral Findings	Location	Systemic Features
Hand-foot-mouth disease Enteroviruses (Coxsackie A, echovirus, Enteroviridae)	Multiple vesicles and ulcers Pharyngitis Dysphagia	Tongue, buccal, labial mucosa Oropharynx Oropharynx	Maculopapular, vesicular, pustular lesions on hands, feet, buttocks, genitals, and legs Oral lesions precede cutaneous lesions Fever, cough, coryza, diarrhea, myalgia, and headache are common Complications include pneumonia, encephalitis, meningitis, carditis
Herpangina Enteroviruses (Coxsackie A, B, echovirus, Enteroviridae)	Several small erythematous macules, vesicles Pharyngitis Dysphagia	Soft palate, tonsillar pillars Oropharynx Oropharynx	Fever, coryza, vomiting, diarrhea, myalgia, headache are common Complications include pneumonia, encephalitis, meningitis, carditis Systemic symptoms resolve before oral ulcers heal
Measles Paramyxoviridae	Koplik spots (clusters of tiny, white necrotic papules) Lingual and pharyngeal lymphoid hyperplasia Candidiasis, angular cheilitis Necrotizing ulcerative gingivitis Necrotizing stomatitis Enamel hypoplasia Morbilliform rash	Buccal, labial mucosa Oropharynx, posterior tongue Buccal mucosa, tongue, lip commissures Generalized gingivae Buccal mucosa, tongue, soft palate complex Permanent teeth Starts on face and moves to trunk, extremities	Classic signs include coryza, cough, conjunctivitis Koplik spots are often presenting sign Complications include pneumonia, croup, keratoconjunctivitis, appendicitis, encephalitis
Human immunodeficiency virus	Linear gingival erythema Necrotizing ulcerative gingivitis/periodontitis Candidiasis, angular cheilitis Oral hairy leukoplakia Recurrent herpes simplex infection Tonsillar hyperplasia Cervical lymphadenopathy Parotid enlargement Aphthous ulcers Dry mouth Purpura Delayed dental development	Anterior gingiva Generalized gingivae, alveolar bone Oral mucosa, lip commissures Lateral tongue Lip vermilion, oral mucosa Oropharynx Bilateral neck Bilateral face Buccal, labial mucosa, soft palate Oral cavity Oral mucosa Primary, permanent teeth	Less common in US children because of decreased vertical transmission rates Oral candidiasis may be first presenting sign Impaired hemostasis and cytopenias Problem with partial airway obstruction Painful mouth interferes with oral hygiene Multiple adverse drug reactions May require antibiotic prophylaxis for invasive dental treatment

Data from Refs. [17–22]

Table 2
Gastrointestinal diseases

Systemic Disease	Orofacial Lesions/Conditions	Location	Significance
Celiac disease (gluten-sensitive enteropathy)	Enamel hypoplasia Enamel discoloration Delayed eruption of teeth Aphthous ulcers Gingivitis Lichen planus Atrophic glossitis Decreased salivary flow Mucosal pallor Burning mouth Decreased bone density	Permanent teeth Permanent teeth Permanent teeth Labial, buccal mucosa, tongue Generalized gingivae Buccal mucosa, tongue Dorsal tongue Oral cavity Oral mucosa Tongue and lips Jaws	Comorbidities include osteoporosis, vitamin deficiencies, diabetes mellitus, type 1, Sjögren syndrome, and lymphoma, all of which have oral manifestations
GERD	Difficult or painful swallowing Gingivitis Aphthous ulcers Hypersalivation, drooling Palatal erythema and petechiae Coated, discolored tongue Halitosis Sour taste Dental erosion Tooth sensitivity	Oropharynx Generalized gingivae Soft palate, buccal mucosa Oral cavity Hard, soft palate Dorsal tongue Oral cavity Dorsal tongue Primary, permanent teeth Teeth with erosion	Common comorbidities include obesity, neurodevelopmental disorders Contributing factors include poor dietary habits Chronic cases may result in significant tooth destruction
Inflammatory bowel disease Ulcerative colitis Crohn disease	Aphthous and linear ulcers Tissue tags Mucosal erythema Spontaneous gingival bleeding Diffuse gingival and labial enlargement (orofacial granulomatosis) Cobblestone swellings Atrophic glossitis Bacterial infection, abscesses Candidiasis Angular cheilitis Multifocal fissuring Linear pustules (pyostomatitis vegetans) Periodontitis Burning mouth Tonsillar enlargement	Nonkeratinized mucosa Vestibular mucosa Palatal, buccal mucosa Generalized gingivae Generalized gingivae and lips Buccal, labial mucosa Dorsal tongue Oral mucosa, jaws Oral mucosa Lip vermilion Lip vermilion, dorsal tongue Diffuse buccal mucosa, soft palate Alveolar bone loss Tongue, lips, soft palate Oropharynx	Nutritional deficiencies are common, which may have oral manifestations Drug-induced lesions include oral ulcers, nonspecific stomatitis, candidiasis, dry mouth, angioedema, erythema multiforme, altered taste

(continued on next page)

| | Orofacial Lesions/ | | |
Systemic Disease	Conditions	Location	Significance
Eating disorders	Sore throat	Oropharynx	Comorbidities include
Anorexia nervosa	Painful swallowing	Oropharynx	psychiatric,
Bulimia nervosa	Oropharyngeal	Palatal complex, tonsils	endocrine,
Binge eating	erythema, ulcers	Soft palate	metabolic, cardiac,
disorder	Palatal petechiae	Lip commissures	and nutritional
Eating disorder;	Angular cheilitis	Oral cavity	disorders
not elsewhere	Dry mouth	Permanent teeth	Binge eating may occur
classified	Dental erosion	Permanent teeth	with substance abuse
	Tooth sensitivity	Oral mucosa	disorders, which
	Mucosal pallor, if	Oral mucosa, tongue	increases risk for oral
	anemic	Jaws	diseases
	Atrophic mucosa,	Face	Antidepressant/
	glossitis	Permanent teeth	antianxiety drug oral
	Osteopenia	Generalized gingivae	side effects include
	Parotid enlargement	Alveolar bone loss	dry mouth, taste
	Dental caries		alterations,
	Gingivitis		hypersalivation,
	Periodontitis		stomatitis, glossitis,
			erythema
			multiforme, bruxism,
			paresthesia
Peutz-Jeghers	Multiple brown	Lips, buccal mucosa,	Autosomal dominant
syndrome	macules evident	periorificial facial	condition with
	in early childhood	skin	hamartomatous
			polyps of the GI tract
			Increased risk for
			several cancers

Table 2
(continued)

Data from Refs.[17–22]

their growth and development (directly and through nutrition) affected, and be affected by chronic pain and its consequences.[1] In contrast, systemic illness can affect oral health by compromising dentofacial development, affecting oral physiology, and altering a patient's ability to maintain oral health.[2] Previously simple manifestations of the oral-systemic connection have now been altered by new medications, survivorship, and dependence on technology.

This article attempts to break down the oral-systemic link into 3 clinically useful areas in which dental and medical providers interact on a regular basis. It also offers several guidelines on how to optimize care delivery for the different disciplines. Readers should consider this a primer because the relationship between oral and systemic health is vast and constantly changing. This article begins with a review of the oral manifestations of systemic disease and its correlate of the effect of oral disease and its management on systemic health. The interaction of dental and medical providers in on-going care is the next focus, and then the importance of oral health considerations in the emergency department, beyond traumatic dental injury, is reviewed.

Oral-Systemic Manifestations of Disease

The connection between oral health and overall general health has received significant attention for the past 2 decades. In particular, the potential links between health outcomes and periodontal status in several diseases or health conditions, including

Table 3
Respiratory diseases

Systemic Disease	Orofacial Lesions/ Conditions	Location	Significance
Broncho-pulmonary dysplasia	Cyanotic mucosa Enamel defects Enamel erosion Discolored teeth Delayed tooth eruption Increased caries risk Microdontia Hypodontia Class II malocclusion Increase plaque, gingivitis Decreased salivary flow Palatal groove Traumatic lesions (purpura, erosions, ulcers) Candidiasis	Lips, tongue Primary, permanent teeth Primary teeth Primary, permanent teeth Primary, permanent teeth Primary teeth Permanent teeth Permanent teeth Mandible Generalized gingivae Oral cavity Hard palate Labial, buccal mucosa, soft palate Oral mucosa, tongue	The orodental findings can be generalized to very low birth weight infants Comorbidities may be present Oral dryness and candidal infections caused by disease management Traumatic oral lesions and palatal groove caused by nutritional and airway support
Asthma	Decrease salivary flow Increased caries risk Dental erosion Increase gingivitis, calculus Constricted, narrow palate Malocclusion; posterior crossbite Tongue enlargement Candidiasis Traumatic lesions (purpura, erosions, ulcers) Sore, burning mouth and throat	Oral cavity Primary, permanent teeth Primary, permanent teeth Anterior gingivae Hard palate Maxilla Generalized tongue Oral mucosa, tongue Labial, buccal mucosa, soft palate Oropharyngeal mucosa	Many oral lesions are drug induced, especially candidiasis, sore throat and mouth, and oral dryness Traumatic lesions are caused by severe coughing, reflux disease, and inhaler devices Dental treatment and materials may trigger attacks
Obstructive sleep apnea	Adenotonsillar hypertrophy Open mouth facies Mouth breathing Anterior tongue position Retrognathic mandible Increase plaque, gingivitis Dental erosion Oral dryness Coated tongue Halitosis Traumatic lesions (purpura, erosions, ulcers) Temporomandibular joint pain	Oropharyngeal region Lower face Oral cavity Anterior mouth, lips Anterior mouth Anterior gingivae Primary, permanent teeth Oral cavity Dorsal tongue Oropharyngeal region Oropharyngeal region, labial, buccal mucosa, tongue tip Face, temporal region	Oral findings are associated with changes in the upper airway and obligate mouth breathing Traumatic lesions and temporomandibular joint pain are caused by oral appliances Dental treatment is challenging in obligate mouth-breathers

(continued on next page)

Table 3 (continued)			
Systemic Disease	Orofacial Lesions/ Conditions	Location	Significance
Cystic fibrosis	Enamel defects Dental erosion Increased salivary pH Decreased salivary flow Parotid enlargement Gingivitis, increased calculus Halitosis Decreased bone density (bisphosphonates) Candidiasis Traumatic lesions (purpura, erosions, ulcers) Sinusitis with referred pain	Primary, permanent teeth Primary, permanent teeth Major salivary glands Major salivary glands Parotid gland Generalized gingivae Oropharyngeal region Jaws Oral mucosa, lips Labial, buccal mucosa, palate Posterior maxilla, face	Disease management, including antibiotics, steroids, decongestants, bisphosphonates, pulmonary devices are responsible for many oral lesions Multiple comorbidities with this disease

Data from Refs.[17–22]

cardiovascular disease, ischemic stroke, diabetes, pulmonary disease, low birth weight and prematurity, dementia, and several cancers, have been investigated.[3–5] Microbial infection, immune cross-reactivity, and inflammatory mediators are hypothesized to be the contributing factors for increased disease risk.[3] Furthermore, it has been shown that systemic diseases, such as diabetes and cyclic neutropenia, significantly increase the risk for developing periodontitis.[6,7] A compromised immune system is a critical risk factor for developing both gingivitis and periodontitis, in addition to several oral infections, such as candidiasis. Because of this important mutual relationship, there is general agreement that individuals cannot enjoy good overall health and quality of life unless they can maintain a disease-free orodental environment.

Other potential associations with systemic and organ diseases to the oral cavity are the result of direct extension of the gastrointestinal (GI) tract to the mouth or the introduction of pathogens and allergens through the aerodigestive tract. Diseases such as Crohn disease and oral ulcers and tooth erosion associated with gastroesophageal reflux disease (GERD) are good examples of oral lesions that are a direct extension of digestive tract disorders. Multiple childhood infectious diseases, such as primary herpetic gingivostomatitis, are the result of spread by oral secretions. Most oral problems linked to systemic conditions are indirectly related to hematologic, immunologic, endocrine, and neoplastic disease and their therapeutic management.

The value of evaluating the oral cavity is that it is easy to visualize, is directly accessible to palpation, and allows less invasive tissue sampling, imaging, and culturing. In addition, in several of these systemic diseases, the oral manifestations are the initial presentation. Because of the high number of diseases that occur in the mouth, extensive outlines have been developed to highlight oral manifestations of important childhood diseases. The most common oral manifestations of systemic disease depend on the primary organ system that is affected and the medications used to manage the disease. Oral ulcers, gingival bleeding, gingival enlargement, mucosal purpura, candidiasis, recurrent herpes simplex virus (HSV) infection, salivary hypofunction, glossitis, and lymphadenopathy account for most of the soft tissue findings. Periodontitis, enamel hypoplasia, dental caries, discolored teeth, premature loss or delayed

Table 4
Cardiovascular diseases and potential medication side effects

Systemic Disease	Orofacial Lesions/ Conditions	Location	Significance
Cyanotic congenital heart disease	Violaceous mucosa Dental caries Enamel hypoplasia	Gingivae, tongue, lips Primary, permanent teeth Primary, permanent teeth	Risk for infectious endocarditis with invasive dental treatment Drug-induced oral lesions
Noncyanotic congenital heart disease	Dental caries Enamel hypoplasia	Primary, permanent teeth Primary, permanent teeth	Risk for infectious endocarditis with invasive dental treatment Drug-induced oral lesions
Hypertension	Gingival enlargement Facial paralysis (rare with severe disease)	Widespread gingivae Unilateral face and mouth	Drug-induced oral lesion Delay dental treatment if hypertensive
Cardiovascular drug side effects	Dry mouth Dental caries Gingival overgrowth Lichenoid reaction Angioedema Aphthouslike ulcers Necrotizing gingivitis/ periodontitis Taste disturbances Burning mouth Bleeding gingivae Mucosal purpura Exfoliative cheilitis Erythema multiforme	Oral cavity, lips Primary, permanent teeth Multifocal gingivae Buccal mucosa, tongue Lips, tongue, face Nonkeratinized mucosa Multifocal gingivae Dorsal tongue Tongue and lips Multifocal gingivae Occlusal plane, soft palate Lip vermilion Widespread oral mucosa, lips, skin	Oral side effects are common for management of cardiovascular disease Increased dental caries risk caused by high cariogenic potential of sweeteners in medications

Data from Refs.[17–22]

eruption of teeth, decreased bone density of the jaws, and temporomandibular joint disorders account for most of the hard tissue findings. **Tables 1–9** offer a selected summary of the relation between oral disorders and systemic disease and/or the effects of systemic treatment.

Care Coordination Between Dental and Medical Providers

Historically, the interaction between physicians and dentists around the care of children was infrequent and often necessitated by a serious or urgent need. Dentists would contact physicians to determine whether general anesthesia was justified for certain interventions. In addition, dentists would ask their help to assess the readiness of a child for general anesthesia, because dentists traditionally did not have this medical staff privilege (and many still do not). Antibiotic coverage for children with heart and other conditions requiring infectious endocarditis prophylaxis/protection or bacteremia mitigation was another frequent reason for communication. In contrast, physicians would refer patients to a dentist usually related to a facial swelling from dental caries or simply a dentition devastated by caries noted on physical examination. The periodicity schedule of the American Academy of Pediatrics only recently

Table 5
Endocrine diseases and vitamin deficiencies

Systemic Disease	Orofacial Lesions/ Conditions	Location	Significance
Diabetes mellitus, types 1, 2	Increased gingivitis, periodontitis Bacterial infections Candidiasis Dry mouth Sialadenosis Delayed wound healing Burning mouth Taste disorder Odontalgia (microangiopathy) Lichen planus (DM 1) Acetone breath (DM 1) Acanthosis nigracans (DM 2)	Generalized gingivae Gingiva, perioral skin Oral mucosa, tongue, lips Oral cavity Parotid glands Oral mucosa, jaws Tongue, lips Tongue Permanent teeth Buccal mucosa, tongue Oropharynx Lip vermilion, neck	Comorbidities include thyroid disease (DM 1), celiac disease (DM 1), Addison disease (DM 1), metabolic syndrome (DM 2), obstructive sleep apnea (DM 2) Control of periodontal health is important for diabetes management Major medication side effects include hypoglycemia, nausea, vomiting, and allergic reactions
Hypothyroidism	Macroglossia Facial edema Dry skin Dry mouth Parotid enlargement Husky voice Delayed eruption of teeth despite normal root development Lichen planus Tongue nodule (lingual thyroid)	Tongue Face, lips, periorbital region Face Oral cavity Face Larynx Primary, permanent teeth Buccal mucosa, gingiva Posterior midline dorsal tongue	Delayed development and intellectual deficiencies in infant, young children Adverse drug effects of levothyroxine therapy include craniosynostosis, premature closure of the epiphyses in young children and allergic reactions
Hyperthyroidism	Exophthalmia Accelerated development of teeth Premature loss of teeth Periodontal disease Osteopenia Warm, moist skin Neck enlargement Craniosynostosis (infant)	Eyes Primary, permanent teeth Primary teeth Alveolar bone loss Jaw bones Face Midline neck Skull	Serious complication is thyrotoxic crisis Following surgical removal, the same adverse drug effects for managing hypothyroidism may occur
Adrenal insufficiency Addison disease Cushing syndrome	Bronzing of the sun-exposed skin (Addison disease) Patchy bluish-black pigmentation (Addison disease) Periodontal disease Candidiasis Bacterial infections Delayed would healing Osteopenia/ osteoporosis Moon facies	Face Lips, buccal mucosa, palate Alveolar bone loss Oral mucosa, tongue, lips Gingivae and alveolar bone Oral mucosa, jaws Jaws Face	May require corticosteroid supplementation before invasive dental treatment to prevent adrenal crisis Except for pigmentary changes in Addison disease, most orofacial findings are associated with long-term use of corticosteroids or Cushing syndrome

(continued on next page)

Table 5 *(continued)*			
Systemic Disease	**Orofacial Lesions/ Conditions**	**Location**	**Significance**
Vitamin D deficiency	Delayed eruption of teeth Caries Enamel defects	Primary, permanent teeth	Rickets, bone deformities
Vitamin C deficiency (scurvy)	Gingival discoloration and swelling Early tooth Loss Petechial hemorrhage	Generalized gingivae Primary teeth Oral mucosa	Easy bruising, petechiae, limb swelling, malaise

Abbreviation: DM, diabetes mellitus.
Data from Refs.[17–22]

incorporated mandated dental referral and often that was left to the parent, not facilitated by the medical provider.[8]

Table 10 provides some contemporary interactions between dental and pediatric providers related to health maintenance and overall child health. A primary relationship of oral and systemic health revolves around well-child primary care, which is described more fully elsewhere in this issue. The importance of collaborative engagement, especially for at-risk populations, is well established, with recognition of common social determinants of health, and it afforded opportunity with combined electronic health records. On an on-going basis, medical and dental providers should be communicating and ensuring that established preventive factors (fluoride adequacy, diet, habits, and care seeking) are in play in children's health. In the current complex (and often changing) world of health coverage, interaction between medical and dental providers requires communication, minimally as a check on availability and access to respective services. Two specific examples are consideration of the oral health of a child with special needs and consideration of oral aspects of sleep apnea and mouth breathing.[9] Some care sources optimize the potential for this type of collaboration, such as federally qualified health centers with collocated medical and dental services.

However, too many children still require hospitalization for dental treatment and sedation or general anesthesia. A recent study suggested that the need for dental care in operating rooms for children is increasing in some populations.[10] Consequently, dentists will more often need assistance in determining readiness of children for these services, beginning with clearance from a primary care provider (PCP) that the child is healthy enough to undergo an advanced procedure. However, the assistance may extend to situations in which a child's routine medications may need to be altered, such as the use of anticoagulants in chronic cardiac disease or steroids in immune-related disorders. Some children benefit from postanesthesia care management and the DDS (Doctor of Dental Surgery) may engage a PCP or hospitalist to admit and oversee the child's progress after a dental surgical procedure under general anesthesia. Critical to success in the recovery is preoperative communication and planning.

In addition, the recognition of oral and systemic interactions in chronic and acute illnesses prompts the need for collaborative care for children with those conditions. For example, child abuse and neglect can require 2 mandated reporters (DDS and PCP) to share concerns and take appropriate action. Up to 50% of such cases include oral manifestations of abuse or neglect. Another common situation is the opportunity

Table 6
Rheumatologic diseases

Systemic Disease	Orofacial Lesions/ Conditions	Location	Significance
Juvenile rheumatoid arthritis and juvenile idiopathic arthritis	TMJ pain	Preauricular face	During dental treatment, decreased extension or pain of cervical spine and mouth opening may restrict access
	Restricted maximum opening	Anterior mouth Mandible	
	Deviation of jaw with opening	Condyle, mandibular ramus	
	Jaw growth asymmetry	Mandible	Oral hygiene compromised by affected joints of hand
	Micrognathia (bird facies)	Ears, sinus, temporal region	
	Referred pain; headache	Oral cavity Anterior mouth	
	Compromised function; eating, speaking	Generalized gingivae Alveolar bone loss	Some of oral lesions caused by adverse drug effect from steroids, NSAIDs, cyclosporine, methotrexate, and other immuno-suppressive agents
	Open-bite malocclusion	Maxilla, mandible	
	Gingivitis	Salivary glands	
	Periodontitis	Oral mucosa	
	Decreased bone density (osteoporosis)	Generalized gingivae Oral mucosa, tongue, lip commissures	
	Compositional changes of saliva	Oral cavity	Early diagnosis of TMJ involvement is important to decrease craniofacial growth abnormalities
	Oral ulcers, stomatitis (ADR)	Gingiva, surgical site Oral mucosa, jaws	
	Gingival overgrowth (ADR)		
	Candidiasis (ADR)		
	Infection (ADR)		
	Bleeding (ADR)		
	Delayed wound healing (ADR)		
Systemic lupus erythematosus	Oral erosions/ulcers	Hard palate, buccal mucosa, lip	Comorbidities include hematologic, cardiac, renal, neuropsychiatric, musculoskeletal diseases
	Perinasal erosions/ulcers		
	White lichenoid lesions	Nasal skin, mucosa	
	Atypical gingivitis	Hard palate, buccal mucosa, lip, tongue	
	Cheilitis		Concurrent rheumatologic diseases. Some of oral lesions/conditions represent ADRs, similar to juvenile rheumatoid arthritis
	Malar rash	Generalized gingivae	
	Annular red patches	Lip vermilion, commissures	
	Alopecia	Midface skin, nose	
	Purpura	Face and scalp	
	Gingival bleeding	Face and scalp	
	Dry mouth and eyes	Oral mucosa	
	Periodontitis	Generalized gingivae	Hydroxychloroquine causes oral pigmentation
	Increased caries risk	Oral and ocular region	
	Candidiasis	Alveolar bone loss	
	Postsurgical bleeding	Permanent teeth	Bleeding disorders may be disease or drug related and need to be assessed before treatment
	Temporomandibular joint pain	Oral mucosa, tongue, lips	
	Headache	Oral mucosa	
	Mucosal pigmentation (ADR)	Temporal region, earache, sinus	Steroid supplementation may be needed
	Delayed wound healing (ADR)	Temporal region	Antibiotics needed for some cardiac diseases and for severe neutropenia before treatment
	Osteoporosis (ADR)	Oral mucosa, hard palate	
		Oral mucosa, jaws	
		Maxilla, mandible	

(continued on next page)

Table 6
(continued)

Systemic Disease	Orofacial Lesions/ Conditions	Location	Significance
Juvenile dermatomyositis	Telangiectasia, erythema	Gingiva, oral mucosa Oral mucosa	Comorbidities include pulmonary, musculoskeletal, cardiac disease
	Oral ulcers, erosions	Buccal mucosa, tongue	
	White lichenoid plaques	Orofacial region	
	Orofacial muscle weakness	Midface, upper eyelid, scalp	Overlaps with other rheumatologic diseases
	Malar, eyelid, scalp rash	Periorbital skin and eyelid rim	
	Periorbital edema		During dental treatment, aspiration may be a risk
	Dysphagia	Oropharynx	
	Dysphonia, hoarseness	Laryngeal region	
	Candidiasis (ADR)	Oral mucosa, tongue, lip commissures	Sedation may contribute to respiratory depression
	Stomatitis (ADR)		
	Osteoporosis (ADR)	Oral mucosa	
	Infection (ADR)	Maxilla, mandible	Fatigue in keeping mouth open during dental treatment
	Bleeding (ADR)	Oral cavity	
	Delayed wound healing (ADR)	Gingiva, surgical site Oral mucosa, jaws	
			Some of oral lesions/ conditions represent ADRs, similar to juvenile rheumatoid arthritis
Behçet disease	Aphthous ulcers	Tongue, buccal, labial mucosa, soft palate	Cutaneous lesions, genital ulcers, and ocular lesions are important for diagnosis
	Mucosal erythema		
	Gingivitis	Oral mucosa	
	Poor oral hygiene	Generalized gingivae	
	Purpura	Generalized dentition	
	Dental erosion	Soft palate	Joint pain and oral ulcers are common and interfere with oral hygiene
	Erythema nodosum	Permanent anterior maxillary teeth	
	Papulopustular lesions		
	Acneiform nodules	Face	
	Pseudofolliculitis	Face	Dyspepsia, nausea, vomiting are common GI symptoms and may be associated with dental erosion and tooth sensitivity
	Uveitis	Face	
	Conjunctivitis	Face	
	Candidiasis (ADR)	Eyes	
	Stomatitis (ADR)	Eyes	
	Gingival overgrowth (ADR)	Oral mucosa, tongue, lip commissures	For dental treatment, steroid supplementation may be needed
	Infection (ADR)	Oral mucosa	
	Bleeding (ADR)	Generalized gingivae	
	Delayed wound healing (ADR)	Oral cavity Gingiva, surgical site	Some of oral lesions/ conditions represent ADRs, similar to juvenile rheumatoid arthritis
	Osteoporosis (ADR)	Oral mucosa, jaws Maxilla, mandible	

Abbreviations: ADR, adverse drug reactions; NSAIDs, nonsteroidal antiinflammatory drugs; TMJ, temporomandibular joint.
Data from Refs.[17-22]

Table 7
Hematologic diseases

Systemic Diseases	Orofacial Lesions/ Conditions	Location	Significance
Hemophilia Type A Type B von Willebrand	Spontaneous gingival bleeding Orofacial purpura, especially ecchymosis and hematoma Prolonged bleeding with trauma Epistaxis Liver clots Pseudotumor Hemarthrosis	Generalized gingival sulcus Oral mucosa, especially adjacent to occlusal plane Oral mucosa, jaws Nasal and pharyngeal mucosa Traumatized mucosa, tooth extraction sites Jaws Temporomandibular joint	Coagulation disorders affecting oral cavity and dental treatment Disease severity depends on type and factor level Limited access to dental care Life-threatening bleeding and airway obstruction Important adverse drug effects include thrombosis, development of inhibitors and allergic reactions
Sickle cell anemia	Mucocutaneous pallor Jaundice Gingival enlargement Atrophic glossitis Enamel hypoplasia Delayed tooth eruption Stepladder bone pattern Widened medullary spaces (osteoporosis) Osteomyelitis Orofacial pain Asymptomatic pulpal necrosis Neuropathy of mandibular nerve Hair-on-end pattern of bone Lymphadenopathy	Orofacial sites Soft palate Generalized gingivae Dorsal tongue Primary, permanent teeth Primary, permanent teeth Maxilla, mandible Maxilla, mandible Usually mandible Nonspecific areas Permanent teeth Mandible, lower lip, chin Skull Cervical, submandibular nodes	Comorbidities include infection, osteoporosis, cerebral vascular accidents, acute chest syndrome, chronic renal disease Odontogenic infections need immediate treatment General anesthesia, sedation, nitrous oxide analgesia may trigger crisis Transfusion-associated complications Adverse drug effect with hydroxyurea: neutropenia, thrombocytopenia Bisphosphonates, other drugs associated with drug-related osteonecrosis of jaws
Aplastic anemia Thrombocytopenia Neutropenia Leukopenia	Mucocutaneous purpura Spontaneous gingival bleeding	Orofacial sites Generalized gingival sulcus Trauma, surgical sites	Treatment with chemotherapy, antibiotics, steroids increase risk for oral

(continued on next page)

Table 7
(continued)

Systemic Diseases	Orofacial Lesions/ Conditions	Location	Significance
Granulocytopenia Anemia	Prolonged bleeding Oral ulcerations with minimal peripheral erythema Gingival enlargement Mucosal pallor Candidiasis, angular cheilitis Herpetic infections Bacterial infections Aggressive periodontitis Tooth mobility Premature loss of teeth Epistaxis	Multifocal mucosal sites Generalized gingivae Oral, perioral sites Oral mucosa, dorsal tongue and lips commissures Lip vermilion, gingiva, hard palate Gingiva, oropharyngeal sites Alveolar bone loss Primary, permanent teeth Primary teeth Nasal, pharyngeal mucosa	mucositis, oral ulcerations, candidiasis, and recurrent viral infections Gingival enlargement usually associated with cyclosporine For dental treatment, antibiotic prophylaxis for neutropenia, platelet support for thrombocytopenia Frequent dental recare visits to manage aggressive periodontitis May require hematopoietic stem cell transplant
Vitamin deficiency anemia Vitamin B$_{12}$ Folate Iron	Mucocutaneous pallor Atrophic glossitis Patchy erythema Recurrent oral ulcers Angular cheilitis Burning sensation Stained teeth (iron)	Orofacial sites Dorsal tongue Tongue, buccal, labial mucosa Buccal, labial mucosa, ventral tongue, soft palate Lip commissures Tongue, lips, hard palate Primary teeth	Medications and underlying diseases may be the cause Liquid iron supplementation may cause extrinsic staining of teeth
Leukemia Lymphocytic ML	Mucocutaneous pallor Purpura Spontaneous gingival bleeding Diffuse gingival enlargement (ML) Soft tissue mass (ML) Necrotic deep ulcers Herpetic infections Candidiasis Bacterial infections Mobile teeth Aggressive periodontitis Periapical radiolucencies Paresthesia Facial swelling	Orofacial sites Hard, soft palate; orofacial sites Generalized gingivae Generalized gingivae Gingiva, palate Any oropharyngeal site Any oropharyngeal & perioral site Oral mucosa, tongue, lip commissures Oral mucosa, jaws Primary, permanent teeth Alveolar bone Maxilla, mandible Lip and chin, usually Unilateral face	Head and neck complications of chemotherapy and radiation therapy are common with long-term craniofacial and dental problems and most severe if treatment occurs before age of 4 y Dental evaluation and treatment are critical before initiation of chemotherapy to prevent serious odontogenic infections

(continued on next page)

	Orofacial Lesions/		
Systemic Diseases	**Conditions**	**Location**	**Significance**
	(cellulitis) Lymphadenopathy	Generalized head and neck region	May require hematopoietic stem cell transplant Lymphoma and Langerhans cell histiocytosis may have similar oral presentation
Langerhans cell histiocytosis	Precocious loss of teeth or mobile teeth Alveolar bone loss Mandibular pain Gingival swelling, erythema, bleeding Floating-in-air teeth on radiographs Punched-out radiolucencies of bone Seborrheic dermatitis Reddish-brown papules Purpura Orbital swelling	Primary, permanent teeth Jaws Posterior mandible Multifocal gingivae Jaws Skull, other bones Face, scalp Face, other skin surfaces Oral mucosa, skin Eyes	One of just a few causes of precocious loss of otherwise healthy primary teeth. Clinical examination shows mobile teeth or teeth with roots exposed Often have multiorgan involvement Impaired hemostasis and cytopenias

Abbreviation: ML, myeloid leukemia.
Data from Refs.[17–22]

to collaborate when a child presents with oral pain without clear cause. Such pain may be a manifestation of a dental issue (teething, primary herpes infection, unseen trauma) or the manifestation of an otitis media, lymphadenopathy, an upper respiratory infection, or a more serious undiagnosed illness or drug reaction. The DDS and PCP can work collaboratively on differential diagnoses and appropriate tests or advanced examinations to come to a final diagnosis and treatment plan.

Earlier in this article oral manifestations of systemic disease are described. For children so afflicted, oral health becomes a focus of concern from several standpoints, including avoiding exacerbation of the disease and its effects and promoting overall quality of life. Two good examples are juvenile diabetes and refractory seizures. Uncontrolled diabetes is associated with increased risk of periodontal disease and oral inflammation, because of excess sugars, and attention to oral hygiene is paramount.[11] In contrast, control of periodontal disease and oral inflammation improves diabetic control. In contrast, seizure disorders require multiple centrally acting medications that can lead to xerostomia and an increased risk of dental caries.[12] The list of oral-systemic relationships in chronic illness is long and growing. For the sake of brevity, both dental and medical providers should be attentive to (1) the potential for oral manifestations of disease, (2) implications of therapies on oral health and vice versa, and (3) both short-term and long-term changes associated with chronic illness and its management.

Table 8
End-stage kidney and liver disease

Systemic Diseases	Orofacial Lesions/ Conditions	Location	Significance
Chronic kidney disease	Mucosal pallor	Oral mucosa, lips, face	Chronic anemia, platelet dysfunction, hypertension, metabolic acidosis are common
	Gingivitis/periodontitis	Generalized gingivae	
	Gingival bleeding	Generalized gingival sulcus	
	Purpura		
	Increase salivary pH	Soft palate, buccal mucosa, tongue	Hyperparathyroidism results in jaw lesions
	Enamel hypoplasia		
	Pulpal obliteration	Oral cavity	Dialysis with shunts may require antibiotic prophylaxis for invasive dental procedures (controversial)
	Malodor	Permanent teeth	
	Metallic taste	Permanent teeth	
	Glossitis	Oropharyngeal region	
	Burning sensation	Dorsal tongue	
	Dry mouth	Dorsal tongue	Drugs, including antibiotics, may need dose adjustment
	Salivary gland enlargement (sialosis)	Tongue, lips, palate Oral cavity	
	Uremic stomatitis	Parotid, submandibular glands	Bleeding caused by kidney disease and anticoagulants, if dialyzed
	Delayed tooth eruption		
	Hyperplastic dental follicles	Ventral tongue, floor of mouth, buccal mucosa	
	Eruption of rootless teeth	Primary, permanent teeth	Increased risk for infection, if leukopenic
	Renal osteodystrophy	Permanent teeth	
	Radiolucent giant cell lesions	Permanent teeth Maxilla, mandible	Multiple drug side effects depending on cause and comorbidities
	Soft tissue calcifications	Maxilla, mandible	
	Decreased caries rate	Tongue	Comprehensive dental care before organ transplant
	Tooth mobility	Primary, permanent teeth	
	Amelogenesis imperfecta	Permanent teeth Primary, permanent teeth	
Acute/ chronic liver failure	Jaundice	Oral mucosa	Multiple causes, including infectious, metabolic, genetic, vascular, immune dysfunction, drug toxicity, and malignancy
	Pallor	Oral mucosa, lips	
	Green-brown teeth (biliverdin)	Primary, permanent teeth Primary, permanent teeth	
	Enamel hypoplasia	Oral mucosa, soft palate	
	Purpura	Oral mucosa, lips	
	Telangiectasia	Generalized gingivae	Impaired hemostasis and hypertension important in dentistry
	Gingival bleeding	Patchy gingival sites	
	Gingival pigmentation (green-brown, yellow-brown)	Permanent teeth Permanent teeth Oropharyngeal region	Many dental drugs, including local anesthetics, antibiotics, NSAIDs, and sedatives, are metabolized in liver
	Delayed tooth eruption	Buccal mucosa, tongue, lips	
	Enlarged pulp chambers	Dorsal tongue	
	Malodor (sweet, musty)	Buccal mucosa	
	Candidiasis, angular cheilitis	Oral mucosa, tongue	Hepatitis B, C may be transmitted to health care professionals through saliva and blood
	Atrophic glossitis		
	Lichenoid mucositis		
	Stomatitis		Multiple drug side effects depending on cause and comorbidities
			Comprehensive dental care before organ transplant

Data from Refs.[17–22]

Table 9
Developmental and intellectual disorders

Systemic Diseases	Orofacial Lesions/ Conditions	Location	Significance
ADHD	Increased rate of dental caries	Oral mucosa Teeth (caries) Dry oral soft tissues	Relationship is not well understood, may be caused by dietary habits, oral hygiene, side effects of medications
Developmental disabilities (cerebral palsy, autism, developmental delay, intellectual disability)	Caries Gingivitis Periodontal disease Bruxism Calculus	Permanent teeth Gingiva	Limited ability for oral self-care/hygiene Decreased clearance of food from oral cavity Oral aversion Impaired salivary function Limited access and barriers to care
Epilepsy	Increased risk of dental injury Gingival overgrowth	Primary, permanent teeth Generalized gingivae	Gingival hyperplasia may occur as a side effect of antiepileptic drugs

Abbreviation: ADHD, attention-deficit/hyperactivity disorder.
Data from Refs.[17–22]

Nondental Oral Emergency Management by Medical Providers

Aside from going to a dentist, children may present to general pediatricians, urgent care facilities, or emergency departments (EDs) with a variety of oral disorders, including tooth trauma, dental pain, tooth eruption and exfoliation problems, oral burns or ulcers, jaw problems, orthodontic concerns, and concerns about oral appliances. The ED in particular is also a place where oral concerns may uncover a more serious, systemic disease, as discussed earlier, such as heavy, sustained bleeding following a dental extraction, which may indicate an undiagnosed bleeding disorder or an underlying oncologic process such as leukemia.

Between 2008 and 2010, nontraumatic dental complaints for patients of all ages equaled 4 million visits (1%) to US EDs.[13] Dental problems account for roughly 20% of all ED visits by children. In just 1 of those years (2008), more than 215,000 ED visits were for patients aged 21 years and younger. The most common diagnoses for children were dental caries (50%) and pulpal or periapical conditions (41%); 3% had mouth abscess or cellulitis. The mean ED charge was $564. Only 3% of patients aged 21 years and younger were admitted, indicating that most patients could have been managed outside of a hospital setting. The mean charge of hospitalization was $22,865 and mean length of stay was 4.6 days for a total of 33,160 days.[14] Patients seek care in the ED because they lack a dental home or because the ED provides no-scheduling access for the patient. In an ED, however, a dentist may not be present or accessible and medical providers are left to manage dental and oral problems on their own. Most patients receive no dental care other than prescriptions of pain medication and/or antibiotics. Symptom management may help the patient in the short term, but this does not resolve the underlying dental or mouth issue. Most ED visits occur during weekdays, when dental offices are generally open.[15] Patients seen in an ED generally still must

Table 10
Examples of interactions between dentists and primary care providers or specialty medical providers related to oral and systemic health

Area of Interaction	Description of Interaction (Roles, Considerations)
Primary care interactions 1. Dental home establishment 2. Fluoride adequacy 3. Developmental screening referral 4. Assistance with oral health considerations in children with special needs 5. Advisement on child oral health needs, including dental caries 6. Administrative assistance on oral health issues (insurance, follow-up care) 7. Airway assessment in ADHD and sleeping disorders, others	1. Either PCP or DDS provides necessary health maintenance services and referral for every child 2. Children should minimally be drinking fluoridated water, brushing with fluoridated toothpaste, or receiving supplements 3. Dental milestones are being achieved, such as tooth eruption, and problems addressed, such as teething or habits 4. Adjustments in oral health maintenance and special considerations in childhood conditions are addressed 5. Dental referral and/or referral for medical issues relevant to dentistry are facilitated 6. Communication exists between PCP and DDS related to care access and mitigating administrative or social factors, such as program enrollment for coverage or medical provider support for medical necessity or supportive/case management services 7. Communication relative to oral aspects of behavioral conditions, such as airway status or dental caries pain
Hospitalization/specialty interactions 1. Concerns about anesthesia readiness 2. Modification of medication regimen for various purposes (steroids, aspirin) 3. Postanesthesia admission and management	1. In its simplest form, a DDS may request medical clearance vis a vis a presurgical H&P before administration of sedation or general anesthesia 2. Some chronic medical conditions involve on-going medications that alter physiology important to surgical dental care, such as aspirin or other anticoagulants in cardiac disease, steroids in immune-related disorders, and antineoplastic medication in childhood cancers 3. With a DDS's limited admissions and in-house care abilities, the PCP or SMP may be called on to manage postoperative issues, which can include sleep apnea, postanesthesia airway compromise, and nausea
Management of acute or chronic medical illness 1. Child abuse and neglect 2. Ruling out oral causes in nonspecific complaints of pain 3. Alternative medication choices 4. Dietary recommendations	1. Collaboration on findings and appropriate course of action and follow through 2. Thorough examination and assessment of history and laboratory testing if needed 3. Classic interactions have been related to tetracycline (tooth staining) and

(continued on next page)

Table 10	
(continued)	
Area of Interaction	**Description of Interaction (Roles, Considerations)**
5. Dental care in children with immunocompromise 6. Dental care after systemic trauma 7. Collaborative care in chronic illness or syndromes 8. Patient self-abuse (indifference to pain) and other oral/airway management	phenytoin (gingival overgrowth) but may extend to salivary flow interference from centrally acting medications and choices for antirejection medications in children with organ transplants and other conditions 4. Special diets (calories, consistency, frequency) may increase risk of dental caries 5. Immunocompromise can mask dental illness and put children at risk for pain and infection and PCP/SMD-DDS communication should be a part of the child's treatment plan 6. Although infrequent, urgent and emergency care of trauma may involve oral considerations 7. Craniofacial syndromes offer the best example of synergy between the medical and dental communities to ensure the best care 8. Niche care of children with self-abusive behaviors, PICU care, and other situations may require a dentist's experience and skills for things like tongue biting, tube stabilization in severe facial burns, and grinding/tetany preventing intubation or feeding

Abbreviations: DDS, Doctor of Dental Surgery; H&P, history and physical; PCP, primary care provider; PICU, pediatric intensive care unit; SMP, specialty medical provider.

seek follow-up care from a dental provider and the types of care provided by medical and dental providers differ, sometimes greatly (**Table 11**).

Dental conditions, when managed by nondental providers, thus unintentionally result in a considerable cost burden to the health care system and an equally substantial time burden to patients. Only one-quarter of patients seeking care at the ED for dental complaints have private insurance; about half of child patients have Medicaid and one-quarter to one-third are uninsured.[14,15] In only a few instances can dentists not manage all sequelae of dental or oral concerns, in which case referral to a hospital ED following examination by a dentist is warranted. In all cases, a dental home provides more efficient and less costly care than an ED.[13,16]

SUMMARY

Medical and dental providers can work together to better serve children by being attentive to the relationship between the oral cavity and the rest of the body. Many pediatric conditions manifest in the oral cavity and providers skilled in the identification of reciprocal symptoms and signs provide better care, use each other appropriately to maximize respective contributions to the care plan, and minimize confusion for the patient. Medical providers should recognize and be aware of oral manifestations of

Table 11
Management of dental and oral urgencies and emergencies, excluding trauma to teeth

Presentation	Example	Diagnosis/ICD-10 Code	Management by Medical Provider	Management by Dentist
Toothaches (pain) in absence of visible facial swelling		Dental caries K02.9	Manage with pain medication and refer to dentist	Restoration or extraction of carious teeth

Abscess/fistula in gingiva from infected tooth	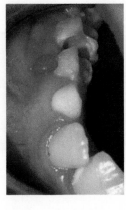	Pulpal necrosis K04.1, periapical abscess without sinus K04.7, periapical abscess with sinus K04.6	Manage with pain medication and/or oral antibiotics (antibiotics are not indicated)	Extraction or pulpal therapy for necrotic tooth
Extraoral swelling from infected tooth	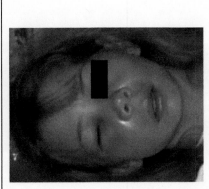	Odontogenic facial cellulitis L03.211	Intravenous antibiotics and possible admission, consult with dentistry	Extraction or pulpal therapy for necrotic tooth, referral to hospital for intravenous antibiotics if drainage not achieved during procedure or if swelling crosses the midline

(continued on next page)

Table 11
(continued)

Presentation	Example	Diagnosis/ICD-10 Code	Management by Medical Provider	Management by Dentist
Mouth or lip sores		Aphthous ulcers (canker sores) K12.0, herpetic lesions (fever blisters/cold sores) B00.1, traumatic ulcers K12.1, postanesthetic soft tissue biting or chewing K13.1, primary herpetic gingivostomatitis B00.2	Palliative care	Palliative care such as crushed ice and popsicles. No treatment or work-up is indicated unless ulcers are large and persistent
Intraoral laceration/soft tissue injury or if any object is embedded into the cheek or palate (eg, a toothbrush or pen)		Open wound of lip and oral cavity S01.5	Remove object, assess laceration for hemostasis and suture requirements. Possible consult with oral surgeon	Same. Difficult lacerations may be referred to an oral surgeon for management

Small bump on the lip		Mucocele K11.6	No treatment needed; standard refer to dentistry	If indicated, dentists can remove small mucoceles or similar lesions in mouth; these may resolve without intervention
Medium to large oral mass		Ranula K11.6; neoplasm of uncertain behavior of lip, oral cavity and pharynx D37.0	Consult oral surgeon	For lesions in floor of mouth, consult oral surgeon
Patient cannot close mouth or jaw		Temporomandibular joint dislocation S03.00XA	Manual maneuver to get condyle into place, administration of muscle relaxants	Same

(continued on next page)

Table 11
(continued)

Presentation	Example	Diagnosis/ICD-10 Code	Management by Medical Provider	Management by Dentist
Tooth eruption or exfoliation problems		Tooth eruption K00.7, abnormal tooth eruption K00.6, failure of exfoliation of primary tooth K00.6	No treatment needed	Encourage patient to wiggle tooth out. Extraction if tooth remains firm and becomes over-retained
Orthodontic concerns: eg, loose brackets, poking wires		Orthodontics Z46.4	Cut loose wires with wire cutter, refer back to orthodontist for emergency care	Replace missing brackets and loose wires

Abbreviation: ICD-10, International Statistical Classification of Diseases and Related Health Problems, 10th Revision.

systemic disease as well as dental disease, and dental providers need to be cognizant of systemic disease effects on the oral cavity and how both the disease and its treatment can affect dental treatment.

REFERENCES

1. Casamassimo PS, Thikkurissy S, Edelstein B, et al. Beyond the dmft: the human and economic costs of early childhood caries. J Am Dent Assoc 2009;140:650–7.
2. Parameters for evaluation and treatment of patients with cleft lip/palate and other craniofacial anomalies. American Cleft Palate-Craniofacial Association. March, 1993. Cleft Palate Craniofac J 1993;(30 Suppl):S1–16.
3. Cullinan MP, Ford PJ, Seymour GJ. Periodontal disease and systemic health: current status. Aust Dent J 2009;54(1 Suppl):S62–9.
4. Michaud DS, Lu J, Peacock-Villada AY, et al. Periodontal disease assessed using clinical dental measurements and cancer risk in the ARIC study. J Natl Cancer Inst 2018. https://doi.org/10.1093/jnci/djx278.
5. Sen S, Giamberardino LD, Moss K, et al. Periodontal disease, regular dental care use, and incident ischemic stroke. Stroke 2018;49. https://doi.org/10.1161/STROKEAHA.117.018990.
6. Lamster IB, Lalla E, Borgnakke WS, et al. The relationship between oral health and diabetes mellitus. J Am Dent Assoc 2008;139(10 Suppl):19s–24s.
7. Khocht A, Albandar JM. Aggressive forms of periodontitis secondary to systemic disorders. Periodontol 2000 2014;65(1):134–48.
8. American Academy of Pediatrics. Recommendations for preventive pediatric health care. Bright Futures. Available at: https://www.aap.org/en-us/Documents/periodicity_schedules.pdf. Accessed January 10, 2018.
9. American Academy of Pediatric Dentistry. Policy on obstructive sleep apnea. Pediatr Dent 2016;39(6):96–8.
10. Bruen BK, Steinmetz E, Bysshe T, et al. Potentially preventable dental care in operating rooms for children enrolled in Medicaid. J Am Dent Assoc 2016; 147(9):702–8.
11. Mealey B. Periodontal disease and diabetes. A two-way street. J Am Dent Assoc 2006;137(10 suppl):26S–31S.
12. Rosenberg SS, Kumar S, Williams NJ. Attention deficit/hyperactivity disorder medication and dental caries in children. J Dent Hyg 2014;88(6):342–7.
13. Allareddy V, Rampa S, Lee MK, et al. Hospital-based emergency department visits involving dental conditions: profile and predictors of poor outcomes and resource utilization. J Am Dent Assoc 2014;145(4):331–7.
14. Allareddy V, Nalliah RP, Haque M, et al. Hospital-based emergency department visits with dental conditions among children in the United States: nationwide epidemiological data. Pediatr Dent 2014;36(5):393–9.
15. Nalliah RP, Allareddy V, Elangovan S, et al. Hospital based emergency department visits attributed to dental caries in the United States in 2006. J Evid Based Dent Pract 2010;10(4):212–22.
16. Mitchell J, Sheller B, Velan E, et al. Managing pediatric dental trauma in a hospital emergency department. Pediatr Dent 2014;36(3):205–10.
17. Chi AC, Neville BW, Krayer JW, et al. Oral manifestations of systemic disease. Am Fam Physician 2010;82(11):1381–8.
18. Thomas DM, Mirowski GW. Nutrition and oral mucosal diseases. Clin Dermatol 2010;28:426–31.

19. Norwood KW Jr, Slayton RL, Council on Children with Disabilities, et al. Oral health care for children with developmental disabilities. Pediatrics 2013;131(3): 614–9.
20. Ramos-Gomez F. Dental considerations for the paediatric AIDS/HIV patient. Oral Dis 2002;8(s2):49–52.
21. Blomqvist M, Ahadi S, Fernell E, et al. Dental caries in adolescents with attention deficit hyperactivity disorder: a population-based follow-up study. Eur J Oral Sci 2011;119(5):381–5.
22. Schroth RJ, Lavelle C, Tate R, et al. Prenatal vitamin D and dental caries in infants. Pediatrics 2014;133(5):e1277–84.

Benign and Malignant Oral Lesions in Children and Adolescents

An Organized Approach to Diagnosis and Management

Brian T. Yuhan, BS[a], Peter F. Svider, MD[a],*, Sean Mutchnick, MD[a], Anthony Sheyn, MD[b,c,d]

KEYWORDS

- Oral cavity • Oral lesion • Benign tumor • Malignant tumor • Vascular lesion
- Hemangioma • Lymphatic malformation • Odontogenic cyst

KEY POINTS

- A greater than 9% incidence of oral mucosal lesions in the pediatric population has been reported in the current literature.
- Although representing less than 10% of oral tumors, malignancies occur in the pediatric population and harbor devastating consequences on quality of life and survival.
- Accurate differentiation between benign and malignant oral lesions mandates an understanding of the possible differential diagnosis as well as optimal diagnostic and therapeutic strategies.

INTRODUCTION

Although many oral cavity lesions encountered in children and adolescents represent benign processes, a small but significant portion may be a sign an impending serious event, underlying systemic illness, or even malignancy. Furthermore,

Financial Disclosures and Conflicts of Interest: None.
[a] Department of Otolaryngology–Head and Neck Surgery, Wayne State University School of Medicine, 4201 Street Antoine, Detroit, MI 48201, USA; [b] Department of Otolaryngology, University of Tennessee Health Science Center, 910 Madison Avenue, Suite 420, Memphis, TN 38163, USA; [c] Department of Pediatric Otolaryngology, LeBonheur Children's Hospital, 848 Adams Avenue, Memphis, TN 38103, USA; [d] Department of Otolaryngology, St. Jude Children's Research Hospital, 262 Danny Thomas Place, Memphis, TN 38105, USA
* Corresponding author. Department of Otolaryngology–Head and Neck Surgery, Wayne State University School of Medicine, Saint Antoine 5E-UHC, Detroit, MI 48201.
E-mail address: psvider@gmail.com

Pediatr Clin N Am 65 (2018) 1033–1050
https://doi.org/10.1016/j.pcl.2018.05.013
0031-3955/18/© 2018 Elsevier Inc. All rights reserved.

numerous seemingly benign entities harbor locally destructive behavior, so the broad differential diagnosis and appropriate work-up of oral lesions are of paramount importance to physicians involved in the care of children and adolescents (**Box 1**). Hence, familiarity with clinical features meriting further work-up may facilitate the identification of troublesome pathologies at an earlier stage. This review encompasses diagnostic and therapeutic strategies for oral lesions, with an emphasis on oral cavity masses.

Box 1
Common pediatric benign and malignant oral lesions

Vascular
  IH
  Lymphangioma
  VM
  Pyogenic granuloma

Cysts and pseudocysts
  Mucocele
  Ranula
  Nonodontogenic
    Epstein pearl
    Bohn nodule
    Foregut duplication cyst
    Dermoid cyst
  Odontogenic
    Radicular (periapical) cyst
    Dentigerous cyst

Salivary gland pathology
  Sialolithiasis
  NS
  Pleomorphic adenoma

Benign tumors
  Nonodontogenic
    Osteoma
    Peripheral giant cell granuloma
    Squamous papilloma
  Odontogenic
    Ameloblastoma
    KCOTs
    Odontomas

Malignant tumors
  Lymphoma
  Rhabdomyosarcoma
  Osteosarcoma
  Squamous cell carcinoma

Miscellaneous
  Aphthous stomatitis
  Mucosal neuromas—multiple endocrine neoplasia type 2B
  Plexiform neurofibromas—neurofibromatosis
  Parulis
  Oral candidiasis
  Herpetic gingivostomatitis
  Strawberry tongue—Kawasaki disease

EPIDEMIOLOGY

Oral cavity lesions encompass a significant yet overlooked clinical concern, because under-appreciation of these lesions has led to a paucity of population-based studies.[1] One analysis of 10,000 children aged between 2 years old and 17 years old in the United States found a greater than 9% incidence of oral mucosal lesions, with the most common site the lip, including lip/cheek bites and aphthous ulcers. More concerning than these seemingly benign entities are oral cavity tumors; in 1 series, the most common benign and malignant tumors included hemangioma and sarcoma, respectively.[2] Although representing less than 10% of oral tumors, malignancies occur in the pediatric population and harbor devastating consequences on quality of life and survival.[3] The age-adjusted incidence for oral cavity malignancies in children and adolescents was 0.24 per 100,000 in 2008, although there is evidence suggesting that the incidence of oral and oropharyngeal cancer has increased in adolescents due to the rising prevalence of oral human papillomavirus (HPV) infection.[4]

PATIENT HISTORY

A thorough patient history is critical for determining which lesions require observation versus further diagnostic work-up. This history should include general questions regarding onset, provoking factors, whether the lesion is painful and how the pain is provoked, the quality of the pain, paresthesias, severity, and onset. In addition to a review of systems, including systemic complaints, patients should be specifically asked about whether a lesion bleeds, is associated with numbness, becomes tender or enlarges during meals, is associated with any foul drainage, or causes trismus. Other considerations for either oral or any other head and neck lesions include asking about dysphonia, dysphagia, odynophagia, neck masses, and respiratory history. A detailed dental, medical, and surgical history should be taken. Furthermore, physicians should inquire about family history, with a focus on immunologic pathologies, syndromes, and head and neck lesions, as well as a social history, including alcohol and smoking (both primary and secondhand exposure).

ORAL CAVITY ANATOMY AND PHYSICAL EXAMINATION

A detailed and targeted physical examination directs the decision to pursue further work-up and intervention. Understanding normal oral cavity anatomy is key for performing an appropriate evaluation (**Fig. 1**). Oral cavity subsites include the oral tongue, floor of mouth, upper and lower lips, hard palate, upper and lower alveolar ridges, buccal mucosa, and retromolar trigone (triangular area in the oral cavity posterior to the upper and lower third molar teeth overlying the ramus of the mandible). The sublingual ducts can be seen in the floor of mouth adjacent to the lingual frenulum, whereas the parotid duct (Stensen duct) opening can be found adjacent to the upper second molar. Oropharyngeal subsites that can be easily viewed in most patients include the soft palate, tonsil/tonsillar pillars, and posterior pharyngeal wall; the base of tongue is another subsite that cannot be directly viewed without direct or mirror laryngoscopy but can be palpated for irregularities during the physical examination.

Proper lighting is crucial for oral cavity evaluation, be it a high-powered flashlight, headlight, or head mirror with a light source, particularly because this examination may be difficult and may have to be done rapidly in a younger or uncooperative patient. In patients with dental appliances, it is important to ask these to be removed

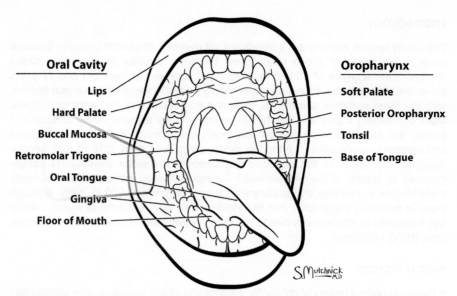

Fig. 1. Structural landmarks of the oral cavity and oropharynx.

for a thorough examination (if feasible). Each of the oral cavity subsites can be directly viewed and palpated, taking note of whether these sites are soft or firm and irregular and whether the mucosa appears moist and of normal color. Additionally, mobile structures, including the oral tongue, can be assessed to see whether there is any diminished movement (ie, the tongue is fixed). A tongue blade applying downward pressure on the oral tongue and base of tongue is usually necessary to complete a more thorough oropharyngeal examination.

Beyond an oral evaluation, any lesions in the oral cavity warrant a further comprehensive head and neck examination. Certain oral lesions, such as ranulas, can have an intraoral (floor of mouth) component extending into the neck, whereas other lesions, such as malignancies and infectious processes, can be associated with cervical lymphadenopathy. Thus, a neck examination, including palpation for lymph nodes, is essential, and further characterization of any palpated nodes based on mobility, softness/firmness, and tenderness is significant. A cranial nerve examination, including evaluation for paresthesias, may provide clues to pathologies.

DIAGNOSTIC CONSIDERATIONS

Detailed information is provided in the sections describing specific diagnoses. Nevertheless, several clinical principles should be followed to avoid missing a diagnosis while also minimizing unnecessary testing. Plain film radiographs have some utility for odontogenic lesions but have a limited role in the diagnosis of other oral cavity lesions. CT, however, is useful in delineating bony involvement of lesions. When used for soft tissue lesions, CT should be performed with intravenous contrast; this modality is invaluable in most straightforward entities (ie, benign nondestructive lesions), such as a ranula or dermoid cyst.[5] On the other hand, MRI is helpful in further characterization of extensive or malignant soft tissue lesions, including sarcoma, and also possesses value in evaluating perineural involvement.[5]

For smaller isolated lesions, tissue sampling may be valuable when a specific diagnosis is not obvious. Smaller soft tissue lesions, removal of which would not cause significant morbidity, can be characterized by simply performing an excisional biopsy or complete excision, whereas more extensive lesions can be evaluated by incisional biopsy. Cystic or fluid-filled lesions can be evaluated using fine needle aspiration. When infectious etiologies are suspected, these lesions and aspirate can be sent for aerobic, anaerobic, mycobacterial, and fungal cultures as well as Gram stain. Vascular-appearing lesions certainly require imaging; biopsy of suspected vascular lesions is usually not recommended due to risk of bleeding. Arterial vascular lesions may also be further categorized using MRI or CT angiography.[5,6]

In patients with oral lesions for which systemic etiologies are suspected, directed viral testing should be considered as appropriate; for example, in patients with risk factors and suspicion for immunosuppression, HIV testing should be considered. Furthermore, laboratory tests, including a basic metabolic panel and complete blood cell count, should be collected for these patients. Patients should also be seen in coordination with pediatric subspecialists who manage the systemic disease considered, that is, pediatric oncology, pediatric infectious disease, or others.

BENIGN LESIONS
Vascular Lesions

Vascular lesions comprise a significant proportion of benign masses occurring in the oral cavity in the pediatric population. The International Society for the Study of Vascular Anomalies has classified vascular lesions into 2 categories: benign vascular tumors and vascular malformations.[7] Because growth characteristics and treatments differ between these 2 groups, accurate diagnosis is of utmost importance.

Infantile hemangioma
Infantile hemangiomas (IHs) are the most common vascular tumors in childhood. Found in approximately 1% of all newborns in the United States, IHs along with lymphangiomas account for up to 30% of oral cavity tumors in the pediatric population and are seen in the lip, cheek, and tongue.[8] They are associated with premature low-birth-weight infants, white ethnicity, and female gender.[9] Classically, IHs are not present at birth but appear within 2 months and undergo a period of rapid proliferation and expansion. Approximately 50% of all IHs gradually involute by 5 years of age.[10] Diagnosis is made with a thorough history and physical examination. Most mucosal hemangiomas present as a raised red lesion that is rubbery on palpation.

Conservative management is recommended for all IHs due to its propensity for involution. The presence of uncontrolled bleeding, ulceration, infection, airway obstruction, or risk of severe cosmetic deformity, however, should warrant active medical and surgical management. The β-adrenergic receptor blocker propranolol, with a target dose of 1 mg/kg/d to 3 mg/kg/d given 3 times daily after a screening EKG for 6 months to 12 months, is appropriate for most cases.[11] Systemic or oral steroids have been shown effective in up to 60% of cases.[12] Surgical management should be considered in cases refractory to medical management or in large IHs and may include carbon dioxide laser treatment, sclerotherapy, or pulse dye laser therapy in addition to surgical excision.[8,12,13]

Lymphatic malformations
Lymphatic malformations (LMs), otherwise known as lymphangiomas or macrocystic LMs (formerly cystic hygromas), involve the presence of low-flow vascular anomalies caused by defective embryologic development.[14] Mucosal lesions appear as small and cystic with a salmon roe appearance.[15] In contrast to hemangiomas, LMs are

typically present at birth, do not regress, and grow in proportion to the child. Rapid expansion of the lesion, however, is associated with 2 common complications: concurrent infection and intralesional hemorrhage.[15] Although diagnosis remains primarily clinical, prenatal ultrasonography is an increasingly popular mode of confirmatory imaging.[16,17]

Management is individualized and often depends on the degree of functional impairment. Conservative management, including proper oral hygiene and regularly scheduled dental prophylaxis, should focus on reducing infectious complications, which have been reported to be as high as 80% in the literature.[14] Both sclerotherapy and surgical excision have been shown equally efficacious although they tend to be more effective in lesions greater than 2 cm in diameter.[9,18]

Venous malformations

Venous malformations (VMs) are present at birth and appear as compressible bluish-purple lesions found on mucosal membranes of the oral cavity and airway, and in certain muscle groups.[19] Dependent drainage of venous blood leading to expansion may be elicited by leaning a child back in Trendelenburg position and on crying.[13] Invasion into adjacent tissue and static blood may lead to acute thrombus formation with calcification and severe pain, which is unique to VMs.[20] Similar to lymphangiomas, VMs grow in proportion with the growth of the patient.

Doppler ultrasonography shows a low-flow lesion with compressible hypoechoic vessels.[21] MRI may be used to distinguish this from other high-flow lesions seen intraorally, such as an arteriovenous malformation, which is rare in children.[22]

Multimodal approaches to treatment, involving a combination of conservative management, sclerotherapy, laser therapy, or surgical excision, depends on proximity to vital structures and depth of involvement. The effectiveness of surgical excision depends on the characteristics of the lesion. Those with poorly defined borders and extensive invasion into normal tissue have the potential for severe blood loss.[8]

Pyogenic granuloma

Pyogenic granulomas involve focal areas of vascular proliferation in response to local trauma.[23] Despite the name, they are not true granulomas but are benign vascular tumors.[24] Described as a lobulated mass, oral pyogenic granulomas are usually red, painless, and slow growing (**Fig. 2**).[25] When seen in a pregnant woman, they are termed *granuloma gravidarum*. Most intraoral lesions are found on the gingiva (75%), may extend between teeth, and are likely due to poor oral hygiene.[26] Because they are friable, bleeding is usually the primary complaint.[23] Treatment involves full-thickness surgical excision. Recurrence occurs in up to 16% of all cases and may necessitate re-excision.[27]

Cysts and Pseudocysts

Mucoceles and ranulas

Cysts and pseudocysts of the minor salivary glands are considered the most prevalent cysts of the oral cavity.[8] In the pediatric population, a majority of mucoceles are seen on the buccal mucosa and palate.[28] Clinically, they present as translucent, fluctuant, smooth masses that are bluish in color when superficial. One study showed spontaneous regression in 43.8% of all cases of mucoceles in their pediatric population.[28] Definitive treatment, however, usually involves complete surgical excision of the underlying minor salivary gland lobules to prevent recurrence.[29]

Mucoceles that develop due to extravasation of mucin from sublingual glands or minor salivary glands in the floor of the mouth are called ranulas. They appear as large blue, fluctuant masses lateral to the midline (**Fig. 3**). Large ranulas that extend through

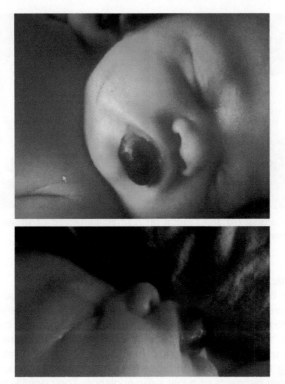

Fig. 2. Frontal (top) and lateral (bottom) images of a pyogenic granuloma in a 1-day-old infant.

the mylohyoid muscle into the neck are called plunging ranulas.[8] CT scanning reveals a low-density cystic lesion involving the sublingual space and may assist with preoperative planning (**Fig. 4**).[5] Marsupialization involves the surgical unroofing of the lesion and is the most conservative approach to treatment.[30]

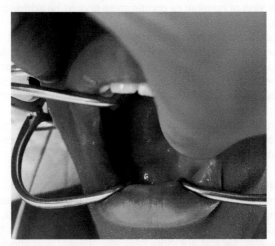

Fig. 3. Palpable lesion in sublingual space with blue hue lateral to midline suggestive of a ranula.

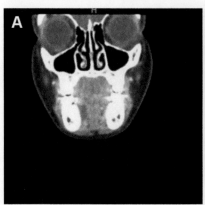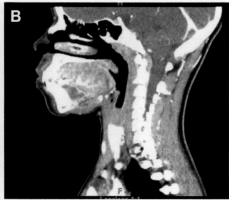

Fig. 4. Ranula. Coronal (*A*) and sagittal (*B*) contrast-enhanced CT showing a low-density cystic lesion involving the sublingual space.

Nonodontogenic cysts

Cysts involving the jaw are often visualized intraorally and are broadly classified as either odontogenic or nonodontogenic depending on the tissue's embryologic origin. Believed to arise from entrapped epithelium, some nonodontogenic cysts were historically known as "fissural" cysts. These cysts usually resolve spontaneously within the first 3 months of life.[25] Epstein pearls, found in up to 80% of all newborns, are observed along the medial palatal raphe.[25] Bohn nodules are true inclusion cysts that develop from remnants of minor salivary glands. They visually present as white papules and may cluster or appear as an isolated nodule.[31] Often appearing between the second and fourth month after birth, most Bohn nodules disappear within a few weeks to months.[31]

Foregut duplication cysts arise from embryologic remnants of the stomach through the second part of the duodenum.[32] Oral involvement is rare, making up 0.3% of all duplication cysts.[33] Children with oral foregut duplication cysts may present with dysphagia or airway obstruction.[34] Although surgical excision remains the mainstay of treatment, any sign of respiratory compromise should be addressed via intubation or, in rare cases, tracheostomy.[32]

Congenitally acquired dermoid cysts are benign neoplasms that may contain hair follicles, sebaceous glands, or sweat glands. Approximately 7% of dermoid cysts occur in the head and neck region, with 23% of those located at the floor of the mouth.[35] Submental swellings result in the characteristic double-chin appearance.[36] Clinically, these lesions are slow growing and most often asymptomatic. They occur in the midline and may display hypoattenuation and a sack-of-marbles appearance on CT scan (**Fig. 5**).[5] Successful extraction is associated with a low rate of recurrence due to the presence of a fibrous capsule that enables ease of enucleation.[37]

Odontogenic cysts

Odontogenic cysts are traditionally subclassified as either inflammatory or developmental depending on their underlying pathogenesis. In 1 study, cystic lesions account for 80% of all odontogenic lesions.[38] There are dozens of different types of odontogenic cysts; however, several are more clinically relevant and should be included in a comprehensive differential diagnosis.

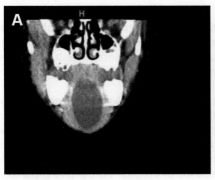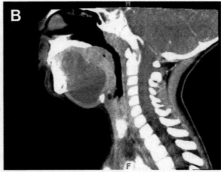

Fig. 5. Dermoid cyst. Coronal (*A*) and sagittal (*B*) contrast-enhanced CT showing a midline cystic lesion.

Radicular (periapical) cysts comprise 62.1% of all odontogenic cysts and 49.6% of all odontogenic lesions.[38] These cysts develop from epithelium of the apical periodontal ligament spaces that undergo inflammatory-mediated proliferation.[39] Considered a direct complication of endodontic infection and subsequent granulation, the chronic inflammatory nature of development results in a lesion that is asymptomatic.[40] Proper oral hygiene and health care habits are essential for prevention.[38] Surgical curettage is usually necessary for successful resolution of true cysts.[40,41]

Dentigerous cysts are the second most frequent odontogenic cysts at 21.5% with a male predilection.[38] Although more well known as a developmental cyst, the inflammatory type presents with pain and swelling within the first and early second decade.[40] Tooth extraction and complete surgical excision of the cyst is the mainstay of treatment and in most cases is curative with an extremely low rate of recurrence.[40]

Nonodontogenic benign masses
Craniofacial presentation of multiple osteomas should raise suspicion for Gardner syndrome, an autosomal dominant disorder with associated familial adenomatous polyposis, epidermoid cysts, desmoid tumors, and supernumerary teeth.[42] Because extraintestinal symptoms occur prior to the development of colon cancer, early identification is of utmost importance. These mandibular osteomas may present as a pedunculated unilateral mass in the lingual molar-premolar area.[42] Surgical excision is appropriate for any symptomatic mass.[43]

Peripheral giant cell granulomas are gingival reactive nodules that are believed to develop secondary to local irritation or trauma. These benign hyperplastic lesions often affect girls and women and are smaller than 2 cm in diameter.[25] Typically asymptomatic, some large lesions may displace adjacent teeth.[29] Treatment involves full-thickness surgical excision.

Squamous papilloma presents as a single whitish pedunculated papule measuring up to 0.5 cm.[29] They appear most often on the larynx; however, they also may be found on the soft palate, tongue, or uvula. Induced by HPV types 6, 11, 14, and 22, squamous papilloma represents approximately 8% of all soft tissue masses in the pediatric population.[44] Treatment involves surgical excision or laser ablation to avoid risk of distal seeding.[8] Importantly, development of the quadrivalent HPV vaccine may lead to reduced rate of infection and decrease in the incidence of squamous papilloma.[45]

Odontogenic benign masses

In comparison to cysts, odontogenic tumors represent approximately 20% of all odontogenic lesions.[38] Although most of these tumors are incidentally found on radiographic imaging, rapid expansion may lead to displacement of teeth and facial asymmetry. These more aggressive benign tumors may require radical ablative surgery with reconstruction.[46]

Ameloblastomas are tumors of epithelial origin and represent the second most aggressive benign odontogenic tumors in the children at 20.8%.[38] Unicystic masses are more common in the pediatric age group.[47] Painless jaw swelling and slow expansion of the jaw are characteristic symptoms. Pathologic diagnosis occurs postenucleation because most unicystic ameloblastomas are often confused initially with dentigerous cysts.[48] Radiographic evidence of irregular border and expansion may indicate the presence of an underlying malignant etiology, specifically ameloblastic sarcoma. Clinicians should be wary of under-treatment that may lead to multiple recurrences of the tumor—the most appropriate treatment is determined by a multidisciplinary team working with a patient's pediatric ear, nose, and throat physician.

Keratocystic odontogenic tumors (KCOTs) were historically called odontogenic keratocysts in an attempt to describe a benign but locally destructive and recurrent odontogenic cyst. Recurrence is attributed to the existence of daughter cysts found between the cystic lining and oral mucosa.[46] They classically present as a syndromic manifestation due to mutations in the patched gene.[49] Therefore, a child with multiple or recurrent KCOTs should be evaluated for associated genetic syndromes; specifically, nevoid basal cell carcinoma syndrome, also known as Gorlin-Goltz syndrome, involves multiple basal cell carcinomas, keratocysts of the jaw, and bifid ribs.[50] Definitive diagnosis of KCOT is made after histologic confirmation obtained after enucleation or curettage. No general consensus has been made regarding the management of KCOT. The goal of treatment, however, should be to initially remove the body of the tumor with subsequent serial surgeries for the removal of residual daughter cells.[51] Simple enucleation alone is not acceptable due to the high rate of recurrence associated with KCOT.[46]

Odontomas are benign tumors of mixed epithelial and mesenchymal origin. They are hamartomatous malformations as opposed to true neoplasms.[52] Composed of dentin and enamel, they are slow growing and are often incidentally diagnosed in the first 2 decades of life by panoramic radiographs.[47] Early detection significantly increases successful preservation of the impacted tooth with simple enucleation and curettage.[46]

Odontogenic abscesses should be considered in the differential diagnosis of pediatric oral lesions. A majority of dental abscesses are restricted to the gingiva around the infected tooth, presenting as an acute-onset localized swelling that is exquisitely tender to palpation. In general, these limited abscesses can be treated with an in-office incision and drainage, although management may require general anesthesia and/or sedation in younger or less cooperative patients. Although anaerobic bacteria are a common culprit, many cases are polymicrobial in origin,[53–55] and familiarity with local resistance patterns is critical in determining whether aminopenicillins, metronidazole, or other antibiotics are sufficient while awaiting culture sensitivities. Far more worrying are the significant potential consequences of an untreated infection spreading into various oral cavity compartments and neck spaces, including submandibular and sublingual abscesses causing floor of mouth swelling (Ludwig angina). Infections in this area can rapidly result in airway obstruction, necessitating emergent intubation and even the need for tracheostomy.[56] Hence, close examination of all oral cavity subsites and palpation of the floor of mouth are critical in recognizing a potential infection and the subsequent need for aggressive treatment and airway intervention. Any stable patients in whom spread of an odontogenic infection is suspected should also undergo CT imaging to identify whether there is any abscesses in the submandibular, sublingual, retropharyngeal, buccal, and masticator spaces.[57]

Salivary Gland Pathology

Although the major salivary glands, which are located in the face and neck, specifically the parotid and submandibular glands, harbor the majority of salivary pathologies and tumors, minor salivary glands are found throughout the oral cavity, in particular the hard palate and mucosal surfaces of the lips, and can present with numerous pathologies.

Sialolithiasis

Pediatric sialolithiasis is rare and occurs in less than 5% of all cases of sialadenitis.[58] Ultrasonography is a useful diagnostic tool that limits the need for radiation and excludes the presence of stones but has low sensitivity for stones less than 2 mm.[59] For the pediatric patient, stimulation of salivary secretion and sialolithotripsy with or without sialendoscopy are appropriate treatments.[59–61] Obstruction or loss of glandular functionality may indicate need for sialadenectomy.[58]

Pleomorphic adenoma

Pleomorphic adenomas account for more than 90% of all benign epithelial salivary gland tumors.[62] Reported in the submandibular gland as well as the hard and soft palate,[63] they present as persistent, slow-growing, painless masses with an average symptom duration for 12 months.[64] Appropriate work-up involves exclusion of any infectious or inflammatory process followed by a fine-needle aspiration biopsy for cytology.[65] Radiographic imaging is a valuable tool used to evaluate the anatomic extent of the tumor. Small calcifications may be seen on CT, with T2-weighted enhancement on MRI.[66]

Necrotizing sialometaplasia

Necrotizing sialometaplasia (NS) is a rare, benign inflammatory disorder of the minor salivary glands that may be confused for a malignant process. There are at most a few documented cases of pediatric NS.[67,68] Seen in glands of the hard palate, NS may present in all other areas where salivary glands exist.[67] It is associated with the chronic self-induced vomiting seen in bulimic patients as well as local trauma, alcohol use, tobacco use, and application of local dental anesthesia.[67–69] Visually, NS appears as a deep ulceration with induration and well-defined edges.[67] Incisional biopsy and analysis by an experienced pathologist is essential to rule out malignancy. NS is self-limiting within 4 weeks to 10 weeks and should be closely followed until complete resolution.[68]

Oral Manifestation of Systemic Disease

Aphthous stomatitis, otherwise known as a canker sore, is the most common inflammatory ulcer diagnosed in North America.[25] Found on the labial or buccal mucosa, it first occurs in childhood and appears with a tan-yellow base and erythematous halo.[30] Although self-limited and spontaneously resolving within a month, it may be extremely painful. Treatment involves topical corticosteroids and analgesics. A thorough history is important due to its association with various nutritional deficiencies (iron, folate, vitamin B_1, vitamin B_2, vitamin B_6, vitamin B_{12}, and zinc) and Behçet syndrome.[25]

Papillomatous lesions of the oral mucosa may be the first signs of Cowden syndrome, a rare autosomal dominant disease. These lesions often appear by the second or third decade.[70] In the case of functional impairment or pain, local excision of the oral lesions may be done with an electric loop. A thorough history and physical examination for early detection are indicated to rule out malignancy every 6 months.

Mucosal neuromas are associated with multiple endocrine neoplasia type 2B, which also presents with medullary thyroid carcinoma, pheochromocytoma, and marfanoid habitus.[70] Affected patients usually present early in childhood with a thyroid mass or vague gastrointestinal symptoms. These masses may be confused with plexiform neurofibromas and underlying neurofibromatosis. To avoid misdiagnosis, immunocytochemistry highlights differing pattern of growth and may be useful in delineating the etiology of these nodules.[71]

Children with vitamin D–resistant rickets may develop spontaneous gingival abscesses, or parulis, in the gingiva. Defects in tooth formation allow invasion by bacteria into the gingiva and subsequent necrosis.[30] These gum boils are fluctuant swellings containing pus.[30] Treatment involves root canal therapy or tooth extraction. Antibiotics are reserved for immunocompromised patients and include penicillins or clindamycin.[25]

Oral candidiasis, or thrush, is a yeast infection seen in milk-fed infants or in children treated with antibiotics or corticosteroids.[8] It is also the second most common AIDS-defining infection and seen in HIV-positive infants and in children treated with chemotherapy or post–bone marrow transplant.[72] Visually, the pseudomembranous form appears as erythematous macules on oral mucosa with a white cottage cheese exudate that may be scraped away.[30] For young children, swabs of oral nystatin or ketoconazole are both acceptable options for primary treatment. For children with a compromised immune system, systemic antifungal therapy is indicated.

Primary herpetic gingivostomatitis is an oral manifestation of acute infection by herpes simplex virus type 1 that presents before 5 years of age.[25] Transmission occurs via saliva or direct contact with a primary or recurrent lesion. Infants and young children often present with vesicles on the distal phalanx, also known as herpetic whitlow, due to their oral habits.[30] These painful vesicles heal spontaneously within 2 weeks. Rinsing and swallowing an acyclovir suspension (15 mg/kg) 5 times per day during the first 3 symptomatic days, however, expedite resolution and decrease pain.[25]

Kawasaki disease, or mucocutaneous lymph node syndrome, is a systemic vasculitis that affects children younger than 5 years of age.[73,74] The American Heart Association published diagnostic criteria in 2004,[75] requiring fever for at least 5 days and at least 4 of 5 of the following symptoms: (1) changes of the oral cavity, including strawberry tongue; (2) polymorphous rash; (3) bilateral nonpurulent conjunctivitis; (4) erythema and desquamation of the hands and feet; and (5) cervical lymphadenopathy. The oral mucosa and lips may be chapped, cracked, crusted, and erythematous.[73] Intravenous immunoglobulin and high-dose aspirin have been the mainstay of treatment.[75]

Malignant lesions

Although exceedingly uncommon, missing a malignant oral cavity lesion can have devastating consequences on functional morbidities, outcomes, and survival. Hence, the authors cannot emphasize enough the importance of pursuing appropriate workup and obtaining a tissue diagnosis for any lesion for which there is not an obvious diagnosis. Persistent masses must be biopsied if conservative management does not resolve these lesions (ie, treating for underlying systemic illness, as detailed previously). Warning signs for malignant lesions include those with irregular borders, friable and bleeding tissue, particularly painful lesions, rapidly enlarging lesions, lesions destructive to adjacent structures, paresthesias, and cranial neuropathies. Furthermore, masses accompanied by systemic symptoms, such as night sweats, fevers, child, and weight loss, should include lymphoma and hematologic malignancies in the differential diagnosis.

Lymphoma

Although lymphoma can be noted in oral cavity subsites, oropharyngeal subsites, including the base of tongue (lingual tonsils) and tonsils (palatine tonsils), are more frequent sites due to the presence of lymphoid tissue. Both Hodgkin and non-Hodgkin lymphomas have been reported, with the greatest incidence in children younger than 5 years and teenagers.[76] In any patients with an easily accessible lesion, such as the oral tongue or elsewhere in the anterior oral cavity, a biopsy can be performed in the clinic if they are cooperative, making sure to send tissue fresh for lymphoma protocol and not in preservative solution. Importantly, patients with oropharyngeal lesions should be referred to an otolaryngologist or oral surgeon because they can undergo flexible laryngoscopy in the clinic to characterize base of tongue involvement and may require biopsy in the operating room. Any patient in whom lymphoma is a consideration should at a minimum have a complete blood cell count and requires consultation with a pediatric oncologic to ensure adequate work-up. On examination, it is important to ensure mirror or flexible laryngoscopy is performed and that the base of tongue and neck are palpated. Specific treatment protocols for lymphoma and hematologic malignancies are beyond the scope of this analysis but are nonsurgical, involving chemotherapy and potentially radiotherapy.

Sarcoma

Rhabdomyosarcoma is the most common soft tissue malignancy of the head and neck in the pediatric population, often involving the oral cavity and pharynx following the orbit. These lesions are fast growing, are locally destructive, and can have distant metastases. Due to the close proximity of critical structures to the oral cavity, missing an early-stage lesion harbors devastating potential consequences. Surgery plays a definitive role in localized lesions, although the decision to pursue surgical resection depends on the expected morbidity of surgical resection, accessibility of the lesion, and whether negative margins can be obtained. Beyond surgery, radiotherapy plays an important potential role in local control, but all patients require adjuvant chemotherapy. Of the histologic subtypes, embryonal rhabdomyosarcoma is seen in younger children and has better survival than alveolar and pleomorphic histologic patterns.[77] Survival is strongly associated with extent of disease rather than primary site.[78]

Osteosarcoma is the most common bone malignancy in the pediatric population,[79] with only 10% localized to the head and neck.[80] Among children, presentation occurs at an average of 15 years of age. These patients present with severe jaw pain and numbness, and CTs are helpful for delineating bony anatomy and involvement. Although there is a 17% rate of distant metastasis for head and neck lesions, survival rates are still superior to cases occurring outside of the head and neck at approximately 80% over 5 years.[81,82] In cases of localized disease, aggressive surgical resection with the ability to obtain negative surgical margins and adjuvant chemotherapy is key for successful therapy, particularly among patients who have positive surgical margins.[80,83,84]

Other Malignant Lesions

There are several other oral cavity malignancies presenting in the pediatric population, although these are even rarer than the uncommon entities described previously. Pediatric head and neck squamous cell carcinoma is particularly rare, although the oral cavity is the most frequently reported location. Oral cavity squamous cell carcinoma has a generally poor survival with median overall survival reported to be 48 months in 1 systematic review of the literature.[80] Syndromes involving defects in DNA repair mechanisms, including Fanconi anemia, are associated with significantly decreased survival. Aggressive multimodality therapy is the treatment of choice. Chemotherapy and radiation are usually the primary modalities with surgery reserved for small lesions or postchemoradiation therapy in cases of persistent or recurrent disease.

Other pediatric malignancies presenting in the oral cavity include histiocytosis as well as salivary gland malignancies arising from the minor salivary glands, including mucoepidermoid carcinoma and adenoid cystic carcinoma. Early identification of oral lesions accompanied by tissue diagnosis is key in facilitating appropriate management.

SUMMARY

The broad range of potential etiologies underlying oral lesions in children mandates an understanding of the differential diagnosis as well as optimal diagnostic and therapeutic strategies. Identifying which lesions require further work-up is necessary for minimizing unnecessary testing and avoiding missed diagnoses of serious entities. A thorough patient history and a detailed and efficient physical examination direct the decision to pursue further work-up and intervention. Understanding normal oral cavity anatomy is crucial for performing an appropriate evaluation.

REFERENCES

1. Shulman JD. Prevalence of oral mucosal lesions in children and youths in the USA. Int J Paediatr Dent 2005;15(2):89–97.
2. Maaita JK. Oral tumors in children: a review. J Clin Pediatr Dent 2000;24(2): 133–5.
3. Childhood Oral Cavity Cancer Treatment. National Cancer Institute. Available at: https://www.cancer.gov/types/head-and-neck/hp/child/oral-cavity-treatment-pdq. Accessed March 26, 2018.
4. Bleyer A. Cancer of the oral cavity and pharynx in young females: increasing incidence, role of human papilloma virus, and lack of survival improvement. Semin Oncol 2009;36(5):451–9.
5. Stern JS, Ginat DT, Nicholas JL, et al. Imaging of pediatric head and neck masses. Otolaryngol Clin North Am 2015;48(1):225–46.
6. Lloyd C, McHugh K. The role of radiology in head and neck tumours in children. Cancer Imaging 2010;10:49–61.
7. Mulliken JB, Glowacki J. Hemangiomas and vascular malformations in infants and children: a classification based on endothelial characteristics. Plast Reconstr Surg 1982;69(3):412–22.
8. Kulbersh BD, Wiatrak BJ. Pediatric lingual and other intraoral lesions. Otolaryngol Clin North Am 2015;48(1):175–90.
9. Buckmiller LM, Richter GT, Suen JY. Diagnosis and management of hemangiomas and vascular malformations of the head and neck. Oral Dis 2010;16(5): 405–18.

10. Margileth AM, Museles M. Cutaneous hemangiomas in children. Diagnosis and conservative management. JAMA 1965;194(5):523–6.

11. Drolet BA, Frommelt PC, Chamlin SL, et al. Initiation and use of propranolol for infantile hemangioma: report of a consensus conference. Pediatrics 2013; 131(1):128–40.

12. Musumeci ML, Schlecht K, Perrotta R, et al. Management of cutaneous hemangiomas in pediatric patients. Cutis 2008;81(4):315–22.

13. Hoff SR, Rastatter JC, Richter GT. Head and neck vascular lesions. Otolaryngol Clin North Am 2015;48(1):29–45.

14. Edwards PD, Rahbar R, Ferraro NF, et al. Lymphatic malformation of the lingual base and oral floor. Plast Reconstr Surg 2005;115(7):1906–15.

15. Sie KC, Tampakopoulou DA. Hemangiomas and vascular malformations of the airway. Otolaryngol Clin North Am 2000;33(1):209–20.

16. Fujita Y, Satoh S, Nakayama H, et al. In utero evaluation and the long-term prognosis of living infants with cystic hygroma. Fetal Diagn Ther 2001;16(6):402–6.

17. Lescale KB, Eddleman KA, Chervenak FA. Prenatal diagnosis of structural anomalies. Curr Opin Obstet Gynecol 1992;4(2):249–55.

18. Balakrishnan K, Menezes MD, Chen BS, et al. Primary surgery vs primary sclerotherapy for head and neck lymphatic malformations. JAMA Otolaryngol Head Neck Surg 2014;140(1):41–5.

19. Glade RS, Richter GT, James CA, et al. Diagnosis and management of pediatric cervicofacial venous malformations: retrospective review from a vascular anomalies center. Laryngoscope 2010;120(2):229–35.

20. Richter GT, Braswell L. Management of venous malformations. Facial Plast Surg 2012;28(6):603–10.

21. Trop I, Dubois J, Guibaud L, et al. Soft-tissue venous malformations in pediatric and young adult patients: diagnosis with Doppler US. Radiology 1999;212(3): 841–5.

22. El-Ghanem M, Kass-Hout T, Kass-Hout O, et al. Arteriovenous malformations in the pediatric population: review of the existing literature. Interv Neurol 2016; 5(3–4):218–25.

23. Bouchard C, Peacock ZS, Troulis MJ. Pediatric vascular tumors of the head and neck. Oral Maxillofac Surg Clin North Am 2016;28(1):105–13.

24. Puttgen KB, Pearl M, Tekes A, et al. Update on pediatric extracranial vascular anomalies of the head and neck. Childs Nerv Syst 2010;26(10):1417–33.

25. Glickman A, Karlis V. Pediatric benign soft tissue oral and maxillofacial pathology. Oral Maxillofac Surg Clin North Am 2016;28(1):1–10.

26. Zain RB, Khoo SP, Yeo JF. Oral pyogenic granuloma (excluding pregnancy tumour)–a clinical analysis of 304 cases. Singapore Dent J 1995;20(1):8–10.

27. Shah SK, Le MC, Carpenter WM. Retrospective review of pediatric oral lesions from a dental school biopsy service. Pediatr Dent 2009;31(1):14–9.

28. Mínguez-Martinez I, Bonet-Coloma C, Ata-Ali-Mahmud J, et al. Clinical characteristics, treatment, and evolution of 89 mucoceles in children. J Oral Maxillofac Surg 2010;68(10):2468–71.

29. Pinto A, Haberland CM, Baker S. Pediatric soft tissue oral lesions. Dent Clin North Am 2014;58(2):437–53.

30. Dilley DH, Blozis GG. Common oral lesions and oral manifestations of systemic illnesses and therapies. Pediatr Clin North Am 1982;29(3):585–611.

31. Mueller DT, Callanan VP. Congenital malformations of the oral cavity. Otolaryngol Clin North Am 2007;40(1):141–60, vii.

32. Hills SE, Maddalozzo J. Congenital lesions of epithelial origin. Otolaryngol Clin North Am 2015;48(1):209–23.
33. Lipsett J, Sparnon AL, Byard RW. Embryogenesis of enterocystomas-enteric duplication cysts of the tongue. Oral Surg Oral Med Oral Pathol 1993;75(5):626–30.
34. Davis PL, Gibson KG, Evans AK. Foregut duplication cysts in siblings: a case report. Int J Pediatr Otorhinolaryngol 2010;74(11):1331–4.
35. Vieira EMM, Borges AH, Volpato LER, et al. Unusual dermoid cyst in oral cavity. Case Rep Pathol 2014;2014:389752.
36. Dillon JR, Avillo AJ, Nelson BL. Dermoid cyst of the floor of the mouth. Head Neck Pathol 2015;9(3):376–8.
37. Jain H, Singh S, Singh A. Giant sublingual dermoid cyst in floor of the mouth. J Maxillofac Oral Surg 2012;11(2):235–7.
38. Soluk Tekkesin M, Tuna EB, Olgac V, et al. Odontogenic lesions in a pediatric population: Review of the literature and presentation of 745 cases. Int J Pediatr Otorhinolaryngol 2016;86:196–9.
39. Lin LM, Huang GT-J, Rosenberg PA. Proliferation of epithelial cell rests, formation of apical cysts, and regression of apical cysts after periapical wound healing. J Endod 2007;33(8):908–16.
40. Arce K, Streff CS, Ettinger KS. Pediatric odontogenic cysts of the jaws. Oral Maxillofac Surg Clin North Am 2016;28(1):21–30.
41. Shetty S, Angadi PV, Rekha K. Radicular cyst in deciduous maxillary molars: a rarity. Head Neck Pathol 2010;4(1):27–30.
42. Basaran G, Erkan M. One of the rarest syndromes in dentistry: gardner syndrome. Eur J Dent 2008;2:208–12.
43. Trosman SJ, Krakovitz PR. Pediatric maxillary and mandibular tumors. Otolaryngol Clin North Am 2015;48(1):101–19.
44. Das S, Das AK. A review of pediatric oral biopsies from a surgical pathology service in a dental school. Pediatr Dent 1993;15(3):208–11.
45. Smith EM, Swarnavel S, Ritchie JM, et al. Prevalence of human papillomavirus in the oral cavity/oropharynx in a large population of children and adolescents. Pediatr Infect Dis J 2007;26(9):836–40.
46. Abrahams JM, McClure SA. Pediatric odontogenic tumors. Oral Maxillofac Surg Clin North Am 2016;28(1):45–58.
47. Perry KS, Tkaczuk AT, Caccamese JF, et al. Tumors of the pediatric maxillofacial skeleton: a 20-year clinical study. JAMA Otolaryngol Head Neck Surg 2015;141(1):40–4.
48. Ord RA, Blanchaert RH, Nikitakis NG, et al. Ameloblastoma in children. J Oral Maxillofac Surg 2002;60(7):762–70 [discussion: 770–1].
49. Todd R, August M. Molecular approaches to the diagnosis of sporadic and nevoid basal cell carcinoma syndrome-associated odontogenic keratocysts. Oral Maxillofac Surg Clin North Am 2003;15(3):447–61.
50. Antonoglou GN, Sándor GK, Koidou VP, et al. Non-syndromic and syndromic keratocystic odontogenic tumors: systematic review and meta-analysis of recurrences. J Craniomaxillofac Surg 2014;42(7):e364–71.
51. Kaczmarzyk T, Mojsa I, Stypulkowska J. A systematic review of the recurrence rate for keratocystic odontogenic tumour in relation to treatment modalities. Int J Oral Maxillofac Surg 2012;41(6):756–67.
52. Shadman N, Ebrahimi SF, Jafari S, et al. Peripheral giant cell granuloma: a review of 123 cases. Dent Res J (Isfahan) 2009;6(1):47–50.

53. Rega AJ, Aziz SR, Ziccardi VB. Microbiology and antibiotic sensitivities of head and neck space infections of odontogenic origin. J Oral Maxillofac Surg 2006; 64(9):1377–80.

54. Robertson D, Smith AJ. The microbiology of the acute dental abscess. J Med Microbiol 2009;58(Pt 2):155–62.

55. Shweta, Prakash SK. Dental abscess: a microbiological review. Dent Res J 2013; 10(5):585–91.

56. Pandey M, Kaur M, Sanwal M, et al. Ludwig's angina in children anesthesiologist's nightmare: Case series and review of literature. J Anaesthesiol Clin Pharmacol 2017;33(3):406–9.

57. Ogle OE. Odontogenic infections. Dent Clin North Am 2017;61(2):235–52.

58. Bodner L, Fliss DM. Parotid and submandibular calculi in children. Int J Pediatr Otorhinolaryngol 1995;31(1):35–42.

59. Francis CL, Larsen CG. Pediatric sialadenitis. Otolaryngol Clin North Am 2014; 47(5):763–78.

60. Hackett AM, Baranano CF, Reed M, et al. Sialoendoscopy for the treatment of pediatric salivary gland disorders. Arch Otolaryngol Head Neck Surg 2012;138(10): 912–5.

61. Ottaviani F, Marchisio P, Arisi E, et al. Extracorporeal shockwave lithotripsy for salivary calculi in pediatric patients. Acta Otolaryngol 2001;121(7):873–6.

62. Krolls SO, Trodahl JN, Boyers RC. Salivary gland lesions in children. A survey of 430 cases. Cancer 1972;30(2):459–69.

63. Lack EE, Upton MP. Histopathologic review of salivary gland tumors in childhood. Arch Otolaryngol Head Neck Surg 1988;114(8):898–906.

64. Ethunandan M, Ethunandan A, Macpherson D, et al. Parotid neoplasms in children: experience of diagnosis and management in a district general hospital. Int J Oral Maxillofac Surg 2003;32(4):373–7.

65. Carlson ER, Ord RA. Benign pediatric salivary gland lesions. Oral Maxillofac Surg Clin North Am 2016;28(1):67–81.

66. Lennon P, Silvera VM, Perez-Atayde A, et al. Disorders and tumors of the salivary glands in children. Otolaryngol Clin North Am 2015;48(1):153–73.

67. Gilowski Ł, Wiench R, Polakiewicz-Gilowska A, et al. Necrotizing sialometaplasia of the palatal mucosa in patient with history of anorexia: review and case report. Am J Otolaryngol 2014;35(3):400–1.

68. Brannon RB, Fowler CB, Hartman KS. Necrotizing sialometaplasia. A clinicopathologic study of sixty-nine cases and review of the literature. Oral Surg Oral Med Oral Pathol 1991;72(3):317–25.

69. Mukaratirwa S, Petterino C, Bradley A. Spontaneous necrotizing sialometaplasia of the submandibular salivary gland in a Beagle dog. J Toxicol Pathol 2015;28(3): 177–80.

70. Swart JG, Lekkas C, Allard RH. Oral manifestations in Cowden's syndrome. Report of four cases. Oral Surg Oral Med Oral Pathol 1985;59(3):264–8.

71. Balachandran K, Kamalanathan S, Gopalakrishnan S, et al. Multiple endocrine neoplasia 2B: delayed presentation, rapid diagnosis. BMJ Case Rep 2013; 2013 [pii:bcr2013009185].

72. Cangiarella J, Jagirdar J, Adelman H, et al. Mucosal neuromas and plexiform neurofibromas: an immunocytochemical study. Pediatr Pathol 1993;13(3):281–8.

73. Giannini PJ, Shetty KV. Diagnosis and management of oral candidiasis. Otolaryngol Clin North Am 2011;44(1):231–40, vii.

74. Islam NM, Bhattacharyya I, Cohen DM. Common oral manifestations of systemic disease. Otolaryngol Clin North Am 2011;44(1):161–82, vi.

75. Newburger JW, Takahashi M, Gerber MA, et al. Diagnosis, treatment, and long-term management of Kawasaki disease: a statement for health professionals from the Committee on Rheumatic Fever, Endocarditis and Kawasaki Disease, Council on Cardiovascular Disease in the Young, American Heart Association. Circulation 2004;110(17):2747–71.

76. Saguil A, Fargo M, Grogan S. Diagnosis and management of kawasaki disease. Am Fam Physician 2015;91(6):365–71.

77. Miller RW, Young JL, Novakovic B. Childhood cancer. Cancer 1995;75(1 Suppl): 395–405.

78. Perez EA, Kassira N, Cheung MC, et al. Rhabdomyosarcoma in children: a SEER population based study. J Surg Res 2011;170(2):e243–51.

79. Turner JH, Richmon JD. Head and neck rhabdomyosarcoma: a critical analysis of population-based incidence and survival data. Otolaryngol Head Neck Surg 2011;145(6):967–73.

80. Brady JS, Chung SY, Marchiano E, et al. Pediatric head and neck bone sarcomas: an analysis of 204 cases. Int J Pediatr Otorhinolaryngol 2017;100:71–6.

81. Qaisi M, Eid I. Pediatric head and neck malignancies. Oral Maxillofac Surg Clin North Am 2016;28(1):11–9.

82. Patel SG, Meyers P, Huvos AG, et al. Improved outcomes in patients with osteogenic sarcoma of the head and neck. Cancer 2002;95(7):1495–503.

83. Huh WW, Holsinger FC, Levy A, et al. Osteosarcoma of the jaw in children and young adults. Head Neck 2012;34(7):981–4.

84. Guadagnolo BA, Zagars GK, Raymond AK, et al. Osteosarcoma of the jaw/craniofacial region: outcomes after multimodality treatment. Cancer 2009; 115(14):3262–70.

Periodontal Diseases and Traumatic Dental Injuries in the Pediatric Population

Belinda Nicolau, DDS, MSc, PhD[a],*, Geneviève Castonguay, BSc, PhD[a],
Sreenath Madathil, BDS, MSc[a], Thien Vuong[a],
Tahyna Duda Deps Almeida, DDS, MSc[a,b]

KEYWORDS

- Children • Quality of life • Periodontal diseases • Traumatic dental injuries
- Oral health

KEY POINTS

- Periodontal diseases and traumatic dental injuries (TDIs) are highly prevalent worldwide.
- Gingivitis and periodontitis are common forms of periodontal diseases in children.
- Behavioral factors (eg, smoking and poor oral hygiene) and environmental factors (eg, low socioeconomic status [SES] and high stress) increase the risk of periodontal diseases.
- Sports are the main causes of TDIs in several populations.
- Both periodontal diseases and TDIs can lead to pain, impairment of function, esthetic problems, and psychosocial effects, with major consequences on quality of life.

INTRODUCTION

How many children leave healthy teeth under their pillow for the tooth fairy?

Unfortunately, not many! Oral health problems, including injuries and chronic inflammation in the soft tissues, specifically periodontal diseases, are a leading cause of health problems in children in all but a few parts of the world. Despite the major improvements seen in both general and oral health in the past century, millions of people around the world have not benefited from the socioeconomic development and scientific advances that have substantially contributed to improved health. Thus, disadvantaged and socially marginalized populations bear the greatest burden of oral diseases.

---

[a] Faculty of Dentistry, McGill University, 2001 McGill College Avenue, Suite 500, Montreal, Quebec H3A 1G1, Canada; [b] Faculty of Dentistry, Federal University of Minas Gerais, Av. Presidente Antônio Carlos, 6627 Pampulha, Belo Horizonte, Minas Gerais, Brazil
* Corresponding author. Division of Oral Health and Society, Faculty of Dentistry, McGill University, 2001 McGill College, Suite 527, Montréal, Quebec H3A 1G1, Canada.
E-mail address: belinda.nicolau@mcgill.ca

Pediatr Clin N Am 65 (2018) 1051–1061
https://doi.org/10.1016/j.pcl.2018.05.010
0031-3955/18/© 2018 Elsevier Inc. All rights reserved.

pediatric.theclinics.com

Due to their high prevalence and incidence in all regions of the world, oral diseases, including periodontal diseases and traumatic dental injuries (TDIs), are major public health problems. Oral disease not only has a major impact on quality of life in terms of pain, suffering, and impairment of function[1] but is also associated with major chronic diseases (eg, diabetes and cardiovascular disease).[2,3]

As with most chronic diseases, infancy, childhood, and adolescence are the most important periods for oral disease development. Moreover, a history of chronic oral disease is an excellent predictor of future disease. Similarly, risk behaviors linked to chronic diseases seem to track from childhood to adulthood. Strong evidence suggests that adult chronic disease, including chronic oral disease, results from interactive exposures throughout an individual's life course.[4] These interactions include intrinsic factors, such as individual social resources (eg, social competence, self-esteem, decision making, problem-solving skills, and coping strategies) and behavior, and extrinsic factors (eg, material circumstances and sociocultural influences).[4] The potential for chronic oral disease is determined by these interactive factors and so is the potential to prevent these diseases.

This article provides an update for health professionals on the current literature concerning periodontal diseases and TDIs in children and teenagers. The epidemiology, prevention, and individual and societal impact of 2 common conditions affecting children's oral health are discussed. When selecting the publications to include in this article, the authors considered features of study design, sample size and representativeness of the sample. Including studies that did not adequately describe the diagnostic criteria used for periodontal diseases or TDIs and those that used nonstandard and nonvalidated methods were avoided. This review starts with an overview of the distribution of TDIs and periodontal diseases in children and their main risk factors, followed by their impact on children's quality of life as well as their economic burden. The article concludes with a discussion on potential prevention strategies and some recommendations for health care professionals based on these strategies.

PERIODONTAL DISEASES

Periodontal diseases are among the most common oral diseases affecting the oral soft tissues and teeth of children. They are infections of structures in the oral area covering the teeth, such as the gingiva, the cementum, the periodontal ligaments, and the alveolar bone. They can take many forms and have many stages, the least severe ones being those affecting the gingiva only.[5] The 2 most prevalent forms of periodontal diseases in children and adolescents (up to 20 years of age) are plaque-associated chronic gingivitis and periodontitis. The former, an inflammatory process of the marginal gingiva, is characterized by clinical signs of inflammation confined to the gingiva without any destruction of the supporting tissue (bone and ligament), whereas periodontitis is deeper.

Plaque-associated chronic gingivitis, hereafter referred to as gingivitis, is a common disease affecting a large proportion of children and adolescents.[5,6] A national survey on the oral health of American children showed that 82% of adolescents have overt gingivitis and signs of gingival bleeding.[7] A high prevalence of gingivitis among children and adolescents is also observed in other studies worldwide.[1]

Periodontitis is characterized by the destruction of the periodontal supporting tissue resulting in an apical loss of epithelial attachment along with bone loss around the tooth. There are 3 main types of periodontitis: chronic periodontitis, which is rare in children and adolescents, and aggressive periodontitis that can be localized (usually affecting the first molars and incisors) or generalized. This early-onset periodontitis happens around the age of puberty and is a rapidly destructive disease. One of the characteristics of the disease is that the amount of destruction does not correspond to the amount of plaque or other local irritants.[8]

Varying case definitions of periodontitis combined with different study designs and clinical examination methodologies are major challenges when attempting to synthesize this body of literature. The prevalence of severe periodontal attachment loss on multiple teeth, however, is low in different populations of children and adolescents.[5] For example, the prevalence of aggressive periodontitis among American adolescents varied from 0.06% among white populations to 2.64% in African American populations.[5] The localized form is 4 times more common compared with the generalized form.[9] Although there is strong evidence showing that adult men are at higher risk of developing chronic periodontitis compared with female adults,[10] there is a lack of agreement on whether gender is a risk factor for early-onset periodontitis.[11] A study using a national survey in the United States, which included a representative sample of 14 to 17 year olds, reported that early-onset periodontitis occurs more often among male African Americans than female African Americans but more often in female whites than male whites. As discussed by Papapanou and Susin,[12] it is important to recognize that the same level of periodontal disease severity in people of different ages has very different impacts; for example, the impact of an attachment loss of 6 mm in adolescence is substantially greater than in old age,[12] given the tendency to progress (and not be reversible).

The etiology of periodontal diseases is complex and dynamic, involving the interplay between bacterial infection and the host response, often modified by behavioral factors.[11,13] The bacteria involved in periodontitis are predominantly gram-negative anaerobic bacilli with some anaerobic cocci and a large quantity of anaerobic spirochetes.[14] These bacteria produce several molecules, including lipopolysaccharides, proteases, and other cytotoxic molecules. Lipopolysaccharides and other virulence factors in the gingival tissues initiate and perpetuate immunoinflammation, resulting in the production of high levels of proinflammatory cytokines, such as tumor necrosis factor (TNF)-α. These cytokines induce the production of prostaglandins and matrix metalloproteinases, which in turn destroy the connective tissues of the gingiva, periodontal ligament, and alveolar bone.[13,14]

Behavioral and environmental factors along the life course are also known to increase the risk of periodontal diseases. Children and adolescents who were born and remain in a low socioeconomic position have a greater risk of disease.[4] It is suggested that exposures to adverse environments along the life course contribute additively to oral health problems, including periodontal diseases.[4] Data from the Dunedin Study, a birth cohort among New Zealanders, show that oral hygiene habits and periodontal diseases at age 26 follow a biological gradient according to childhood socioeconomic status (SES), with adult experience of any of those markers lower among those of higher childhood SES. The adverse influence of low childhood SES persisted after controlling for childhood oral health and current adult SES.[15,16] Similarly, Brazilian children who remained in low SES throughout their childhood and adolescence were more likely to have high levels of periodontal diseases by the time they were 13 years old.[17,18] Psychosocial factors along an individual's life also play a role in the development of the disease; children from non-nuclear families and those experiencing high levels of stress are more likely to develop gingivitis.[17,18] Behavioral factors, such as smoking and poor oral hygiene, also increase the risk of periodontal diseases.[19–24] Likewise, alterations in hormone levels (steroid hormones) during adolescence may modify the host response to dental plaque, increasing gingivitis. Finally, there is strong evidence for the link between periodontal diseases and general health outcomes, such as coronary heart disease, diabetes, and obesity. For example, changes in insulin levels with diabetes could modulate a host's immune and inflammatory system, rendering an individual more susceptible to the effects of microbial dental plaque. Although the nature of these associations is debatable, the evidence supports that at least periodontitis commonly co-occurs with other chronic diseases that have an inflammatory component (eg, diabetes and atherosclerosis).[2,3]

Similarly, children who have a weak immune system, which results in an impaired response to plaque, are more likely to have periodontal bone loss and premature tooth loss.[11,25] Neutrophil dysfunction also increases the likelihood of having gingivitis, periodontitis, premature tooth loss, and oral mucous membrane infection.[26] Moreover, patients with systemic genetic disorders have more periodontal diseases. Individuals with Down syndrome showed a prevalence of periodontal diseases of 58% to 96% at the age of 35 years or younger.[27,28] In Papillon-Lefèvre syndrome[a], there is periodontitis as soon as the first teeth erupt, resulting in rapid damage; there is a dysfunctional and irregular inflammatory response in the soft tissues, which destroys them. Neutropenia also increases the risk of oral infections, due to a lack of neutrophils.[29]

The short-term and long-term effects of periodontal diseases in children go beyond the teeth and oral health status. Changes in body function and structure brought about by these diseases may also impair physical and psychosocial functions. Although major consequences of severe periodontal diseases (eg, tooth loss) may be rare in children and adolescents, the literature supports that this population experiences negative psychosocial effects (eg, halitosis and unesthetic red swollen gums).[30] Moreover, periodontal inflammation in children and adolescents may increase systemic inflammation. For example, obese children and metabolically unhealthy children have higher levels of TNF-α in the gingival crevicular fluid compared with nonobese and metabolically healthy children.[31–33]

In summary, periodontal diseases result from complex interactions between the biological make-up of individuals and exposures along their lives. Periodontal disease is a cumulative chronic condition, and its different forms may reflect the timing, duration, and levels of individual exposures. Investigating these conditions as they develop, starting early in life, may provide information about the mechanisms involved. In addition, this may allow the identification of groups of individuals who are more prone to the condition, using the severity of the disease to make distinctions among them, to target prevention efforts at these groups. Together, the available evidence demonstrates the importance of monitoring and preventing this disease in children and adolescents. Pediatricians could play a significant role in achieving this goal by familiarizing themselves with common oral health conditions among children and referring children with need for care to dentists. **Table 1** provides examples of questions that may help pediatricians to identify these oral health conditions.

TRAUMATIC DENTAL INJURIES

As the doorway to the body, the mouth is constantly challenged by aggressors (eg, bacteria and viruses). Therefore, dental caries and periodontal diseases, which have an infectious component, are the most common oral diseases. Head and face injuries, however, including tooth fracture (also known as TDI), are also prevalent.

---

[a] This rare disorder of autosomal recessive inheritance is characterized by redness, palmar-plantar hyperkeratosis, and early onset of severe destructive periodontitis, leading to premature loss of both primary and permanent dentitions.

Table 1			
Simple questions to assess dental treatment need among children			
1	Have you observed any bleeding from your gums recently?	Yes	No
2	Do any of your teeth seem longer than they used to?	Yes	No
3	Do you have pain in your gums?	Yes	No
4	Do you feel any of your teeth are loose?	Yes	No
5	Do you think any of your front teeth may be broken?	Yes	No

Participants who answer "Yes" to any of the questions should be sent for a dental consultation.

The common belief that injuries occur at random and, therefore, cannot be prevented is questionable. Most injuries and their associated events are predictable and preventable,[34,35] which has led some investigators to argue that there is no scientific basis to separate injury from disease.[36]

A majority of orofacial injuries affect the soft tissues, whereas dental trauma most commonly involves tooth fracture, avulsion (in which the tooth is torn away from the mouth), or subluxation (in which the tooth is loosened and pressed into the gum but not displaced).[37] Overall, nearly all orofacial and dental trauma involves the upper lip, maxilla, and central upper incisors.[37]

TDI occurs in both primary and permanent dentitions, and its prevalence varies according to the age of the sample and location of the study, both within and between countries. As with periodontal diseases, differences in prevalence can also be explained by variations in the disease definition, diagnostic criteria, and sampling techniques used. Approximately 33% of preschool and 25% of schoolchildren worldwide experience TDI in primary teeth and permanent dentition, respectively. In North America, the prevalence of TDIs is 24% and 12% among 11 to 12-year-old Quebec and American children, respectively.[38] In the United Kingdom, the permanent anterior teeth of 9% of schoolchildren are affected by a TDI.[39]

Injuries overall are a real public health problem due to their prevalence, high treatment cost, and occurrence at an early age.[40] Specifically, head injuries and other facial injuries are a leading cause of mortality in childhood.[41] Moreover, these injuries, including TDIs, may severely influence an individual's quality of life.[42] Tooth fractures, unlike bone fractures, do not heal, and, depending on their severity, their prognosis is ambiguous. For example, severe cases of TDI involving large crown fractures, luxations, and avulsions, may lead to pain, loss of function (eg, eating, chewing, and talking) and esthetic problems (reluctance to smile and discolored tooth) with major physical, emotional, and social consequences for children and their families.[42] Furthermore, such injuries and their impact may restrict home and school activities, causing the loss of school hours.[42]

Similar to other disorders, the etiology of head and facial injuries is complex, involving oral factors (eg, overjet), environmental factors (eg, SES and material deprivation), and human behavior (eg, risk taking and hyperactivity), which can be further categorized into intentional and unintentional.[37] While the intentional category alludes to abusive and violent behaviors, the unintentional category refers to sports, falls, unsafe playgrounds or schools, and motor vehicle injuries. TDIs specifically may also be caused by foreign objects in the mouth or present in food.[43]

For preschool and school-aged children, injuries most commonly take place at home and in the neighborhood.[44] Although a significant proportion of TDIs in young children are due to physical leisure activities at home, at playgrounds, and in schools,[45–47] sport activities, traffic accidents, and some forms of violence (eg, fights, assault, and battery) are among the most common reasons for TDIs among teenagers.[48–50]

Among American girls and boys, 69% and 75%, respectively, participate in organized and team sports.[51] Children and adolescents spend significant amounts of time in such recreational and sport activities. For example, Canadian children spend an average of 15 to 18 hours per week in leisure physical activities depending on their age; school-aged children (5–12 years old) spend slightly more time than 13 to 17 year olds.[44] The younger group is most susceptible to sports-related oral injuries.[49,52] Although the reported incidences of sports-related oral injuries in the literature vary widely based on the sport played, the level of competition, and participant age and gender,[53–55] sports activities are considered one of the "principal causes of craniofacial injuries."[56] Approximately one-third of all dental injuries[56–58] and 1 in 6 sports-related injuries occur in the craniofacial area.[59]

Although sports are the main causes of TDIs in several populations, the etiology of TDI is influenced by several factors and, therefore, like prevalence, the proportion of TDIs attributed to a cause varies according to the population (eg, age, culture, environment, and geographic location). For example, violence is a more common cause of TDI than sports in some countries. Baghdady and colleagues[60,61] reported that among Iraqi and Sudanese 6 to 12-year-old children, 36% and 71%, respectively, of TDIs were due to violence, whereas only 3% were caused by sports. Data from Brazil, including the authors' work, showed similar proportions of TDIs due to sports and violence.[62,63] The proportion reported to be from unknown causes in 1 of these studies was high (40%).[63] It is known in the literature that individuals tend to report unknown causes when they do not feel comfortable reporting the true cause. Results of this study also showed that children from non-nuclear families and those who reported high levels of paternal punishment had a higher risk of TDI, suggesting that the hidden causes of TDI included violence and adverse psychosocial environments. This is an important finding to be aware of for those treating children because it may alert them to child abuse.

Attention-deficit/hyperactivity disorder (ADHD) has also been considered a risk factor for TDI. Hyperactive children compared with nonhyperactive children have more TDIs, and the risk lessens after treatment of the ADHD.[64] Similarly, children who engage in risk-taking behavior or who are bullied have a higher risk of TDI compared with other children; prosocial behavior seems to protect against TDI. Obesity also has been reported as a risk factor for TDI.[65] These associations might seem counterintuitive; however, being obese may decrease physical ability, increasing the risk of falls and accidents. Similarly, preschoolers who have a higher height for their age have a higher risk of TDI compared with other children.[66,67] Finally, orofacial characteristics, such as increased overjet and inadequate lip coverage, are important causes of TDIs.[44] These anatomic characteristics seem to be risk factors for children of all age groups, including preschool age children.

The numerous behavioral and environmental causes of TDI explain its high prevalence (discussed previously). This condition not only has a major impact on the quality of life of the children and adolescents who experience TDI but also carries a major economic burden. For example, the average estimated cost to treat a patient with a TDI in the permanent incisor is $858.[68] Similarly, the annual cost of treating TDIs per million inhabitants of Denmark has been estimated to be between $2 and $5 million.[69] In the United States, treatment of the 5 million teeth avulsed annually amounts to approximately $500 million.[70] Over a lifetime, a single avulsed tooth costs $5000 to $20,000 to treat.[71] Considering these data and the important impact TDIs have on children, adolescents, and their families, acknowledging the preventable nature of most accidents and working to prevent them are critical.

DISCUSSION AND SUMMARY

An overview of 2 major oral health conditions affecting children and adolescents is provided. The World Health Organization defines health as "a complete state of physical, mental, and social well-being, and not just the absence of infirmity." Having good oral health is part of overall health not only with regard to the presence or absence of a disease but also because of the impact of oral conditions on individual quality of life. Thus, it must be recognized that oral health is an integral part of general health that needs to be considered in health care delivery systems and public health policies.

The World Health Organization definition also addresses the old question of nature versus nurture, because it considers that both are inseparable and necessary for full health. Human biology becomes imprinted in and by the environment, and the environment interacts with body/cells. This interactive process happens over an individual's life span. The authors' work has shown the importance of a life course perspective to study the etiology of periodontal disease and TDI conditions given the important role of early life events and circumstances. The wider perspectives discussed previously can help better appreciate the impact of periodontal diseases and TDIs and offer avenues to develop specific preventive strategies. For example, it is well established that periodontal diseases in adults co-occur with several chronic conditions (eg, diabetes) and it seems that these links start in childhood.[31,32] Moreover, systemic conditions, periodontal diseases, and TDIs share common risk behaviors, which also start in childhood (eg, smoking habits). Promoting a healthy environment in schools, for example, may put children in health trajectories, which not only benefits their oral health but also lowers their risk of obesity and other inflammatory conditions throughout their lives. Similarly, social and physical environments play a role in the etiology of TDI. Improving these environments to make them safer would not only reduce TDIs but also increase the well-being and overall health of children, their family, and their community. As the famous saying, "the mouth is a mirror of the body" implies, looking at periodontal diseases and TDIs allows us to see into a child's whole body, habits, and environment, from nutritional deficiencies to playgrounds in the child's neighborhood. It may also help target interventions for the benefit of the whole society.

REFERENCES

1. Petersen PE. The World Oral Health Report 2003: continuous improvement of oral health in the 21st century–the approach of the WHO Global Oral Health Programme. Community Dent Oral Epidemiol 2003;31(Suppl 1):3–23.

2. Humphrey LL, Fu R, Buckley DI, et al. Periodontal disease and coronary heart disease incidence: a systematic review and meta-analysis. J Gen Intern Med 2008;23(12):2079–86.

3. Keller A, Rohde JF, Raymond K, et al. Association between periodontal disease and overweight and obesity: a systematic review. J Periodontol 2015;86(6): 766–76.

4. Nicolau B, Thomson WM, Steele JG, et al. Life-course epidemiology: concepts and theoretical models and its relevance to chronic oral conditions. Community Dent Oral Epidemiol 2007;35(4):241–9.

5. Albandar JM, Tinoco EM. Global epidemiology of periodontal diseases in children and young persons. Periodontol 2000 2002;29:153–76.

6. Botero JE, Rosing CK, Duque A, et al. Periodontal disease in children and adolescents of Latin America. Periodontol 2000 2015;67(1):34–57.

7. Albandar JM, Kingman A, Brown LJ, et al. Gingival inflammation and subgingival calculus as determinants of disease progression in early-onset periodontitis. J Clin Periodontol 1998;25(3):231–7.

8. Jenkins WM, Papapanou PN. Epidemiology of periodontal disease in children and adolescents. Periodontol 2000 2001;26:16–32.

9. Loe H, Brown LJ. Early onset periodontitis in the United States of America. J Periodontol 1991;62(10):608–16.

10. Albandar JM. Periodontal diseases in North America. Periodontol 2000 2002;29: 31–69.

11. Albandar JM, Rams TE. Risk factors for periodontitis in children and young persons. Periodontol 2000 2002;29:207–22.

12. Papapanou PN, Susin C. Periodontitis epidemiology: is periodontitis under-recognized, over-diagnosed, or both? Periodontol 2000 2017;75(1):45–51.

13. Page RC. The etiology and pathogenesis of periodontitis. Compend Contin Educ Dent 2002;23(5 Suppl):11–4.

14. Van Dyke TE, Sheilesh D. Risk factors for periodontitis. J Int Acad Periodontol 2005;7(1):3–7.

15. Poulton R, Caspi A, Milne BJ, et al. Association between children's experience of socioeconomic disadvantage and adult health: a life-course study. Lancet 2002; 360(9346):1640–5.

16. Thomson WM, Poulton R, Milne BJ, et al. Socioeconomic inequalities in oral health in childhood and adulthood in a birth cohort. Community Dent Oral Epidemiol 2004;32(5):345–53.

17. Nicolau B, Marcenes W, Hardy R, et al. A life-course approach to assess the relationship between social and psychological circumstances and gingival status in adolescents. J Clin Periodontol 2003;30(12):1038–45.

18. Nicolau B, Netuveli G, Kim JW, et al. A life-course approach to assess psychosocial factors and periodontal disease. J Clin Periodontol 2007;34(10):844–50.

19. Grossi S. Smoking and stress: common denominators for periodontal disease, heart disease, and diabetes mellitus. Compend Contin Educ Dent Suppl 2000;(30):31–9 [quiz: 66].

20. Johnson GK, Slach NA. Impact of tobacco use on periodontal status. J Dent Educ 2001;65(4):313–21.

21. Kinane DF, Chestnutt IG. Smoking and periodontal disease. Crit Rev Oral Biol Med 2000;11(3):356–65.

22. Nunn ME. Understanding the etiology of periodontitis: an overview of periodontal risk factors. Periodontol 2000 2003;32:11–23.

23. Papapanou PN. Epidemiology of periodontal diseases: an update. J Int Acad Periodontol 1999;1(4):110–6.

24. Rivera-Hidalgo F. Smoking and periodontal disease. Periodontol 2000 2003;32: 50–8.

25. Meyle J, Gonzales JR. Influences of systemic diseases on periodontitis in children and adolescents. Periodontol 2000 2001;26:92–112.

26. Van Dyke TE, Hoop GA. Neutrophil function and oral disease. Crit Rev Oral Biol Med 1990;1(2):117–33.

27. Morgan J. Why is periodontal disease more prevalent and more severe in people with Down syndrome? Spec Care Dentist 2007;27(5):196–201.

28. Lopez-Perez R, Borges-Yanez SA, Jimenez-Garcia G, et al. Oral hygiene, gingivitis, and periodontitis in persons with Down syndrome. Spec Care Dentist 2002; 22(6):214–20.
29. Alrayyes S, Hart TC. Periodontal disease in children. Dis Mon 2011;57(4):184–91.
30. Petersen PE, Bourgeois D, Ogawa H, et al. The global burden of oral diseases and risks to oral health. Bull World Health Organ 2005;83(9):661–9.
31. Ka K, Rousseau MC, Lambert M, et al. Metabolic syndrome and gingival inflammation in Caucasian children with a family history of obesity. J Clin Periodontol 2013;40(11):986–93.
32. Kâ K, Rousseau MC, Tran SD, et al. Association between metabolic syndrome and gingival inflammation in obese children. Int J Dent Hyg 2017. [Epub ahead of print].
33. Khosravi R, Tran SD, Lambert M, et al. Adiposity and gingival crevicular fluid tumour necrosis factor-alpha levels in children. J Clin Periodontol 2009;36(4): 301–7.
34. Doege TC. Sounding board. An injury is no accident. N Engl J Med 1978;298(9): 509–10.
35. Loimer H, Guarnieri M. Accidents and acts of God: a history of the terms. Am J Public Health 1996;86(1):101–7.
36. Haddon W Jr, Baker SP. Injury control. In: Clark DW, MacMahon B, editors. Preventive and community medicine. 2nd edition. Boston: Little Brown; 1981. p. 109–40.
37. Glendor U, Marcenes W, Andreasen JO. Classification, epidemiology and etiology. In: Andreasen JO, Andreasen FM, Andersson L, editors. Textbook and color atlas of traumatic injuries to the teeth. 4th edition. Oxford (England): Blackwell Munksgaard; 2007. p. 228.
38. Galarneau C, Boiteau V, Hamel D, et al. Étude clinique sur l'état de santé buccodentaire des élèves québécois du primaire 2012-2013 – (ÉCSBQ) – Rapport national. Montréal (Canada): Institut national de santé publique du Québec; 2018.
39. Blokland A, Watt RG, Tsakos G, et al. Traumatic dental injuries and socioeconomic position - findings from the Children's Dental Health Survey 2013. Community Dent Oral Epidemiol 2016;44(6):586–91.
40. Glendor U. Epidemiology of traumatic dental injuries–a 12 year review of the literature. Dent Traumatol 2008;24(6):603–11.
41. Atabaki SM. Pediatric head injury. Pediatr Rev 2007;28(6):215–24.
42. Zaror C, Martinez-Zapata MJ, Abarca J, et al. Impact of traumatic dental injuries on quality of life in preschoolers and schoolchildren: a systematic review and meta-analysis. Community Dent Oral Epidemiol 2018;46(1):88–101.
43. Hyman FN, Klontz KC, Tollefson L. Eating as a hazard to health: preventing, treating dental injuries caused by foreign objects in food. J Am Dent Assoc 1993; 124(11):65–9.
44. Glendor U. Aetiology and risk factors related to traumatic dental injuries–a review of the literature. Dent Traumatol 2009;25(1):19–31.
45. Blinkhorn FA. The aetiology of dento-alveolar injuries and factors influencing attendance for emergency care of adolescents in the north west of England. Endod Dent Traumatol 2000;16(4):162–5.
46. O'Neil DW, Clark MV, Lowe JW, et al. Oral trauma in children: a hospital survey. Oral Surg Oral Med Oral Pathol 1989;68(6):691–6.
47. Onetto JE, Flores MT, Garbarino ML. Dental trauma in children and adolescents in Valparaiso, Chile. Endod Dent Traumatol 1994;10(5):223–7.

48. Petersson EE, Andersson L, Sorensen S. Traumatic oral vs non-oral injuries. Swed Dent J 1997;21(1–2):55–68.

49. Rodd HD, Chesham DJ. Sports-related oral injury and mouthguard use among Sheffield school children. Community Dent Health 1997;14(1):25–30.

50. Skaare AB, Jacobsen I. Dental injuries in Norwegians aged 7-18 years. Dent Traumatol 2003;19(2):67–71.

51. Nowjack-Raymer RE, Gift HC. Use of mouthguards and headgear in organized sports by school-aged children. Public Health Rep 1996;111(1):82–6.

52. Tesini DA, Soporowski NJ. Epidemiology of orofacial sports-related injuries. Dent Clin North Am 2000;44(1):1–18, v.

53. Bijur PE, Trumble A, Harel Y, et al. Sports and recreation injuries in US children and adolescents. Arch Pediatr Adolesc Med 1995;149(9):1009–16.

54. Echlin PS, Upshur RE, Peck DM, et al. Craniomaxillofacial injury in sport: a review of prevention research. Br J Sports Med 2005;39(5):254–63.

55. Kumamoto DP, Maeda Y. A literature review of sports-related orofacial trauma. Gen Dent 2004;52(3):270–80 [quiz: 281].

56. U.S. Department of Health and Human Services. Oral health in America: a report of the surgeon general. Rockville (MD): National Institutes of Health, National Institute of Dental and Craniofacial Research; 2000.

57. Borssen E, Holm AK. Traumatic dental injuries in a cohort of 16-year-olds in northern Sweden. Endod Dent Traumatol 1997;13(6):276–80.

58. Lephart SM, Fu FH. Emergency treatment of athletic injuries. Dent Clin North Am 1991;35(4):707–17.

59. Center for Disease Control and Prevention (CDC). Nonfatal Sports- and Recreation-Related Injuries Treated in Emergency Departments — United States, July 2000–June 2001. MMWR Morb Mortal Wkly Rep 2002;23(51):736–40.

60. Baghdady VS, Ghose LJ, Alwash R. Traumatized anterior teeth as related to their cause and place. Community Dent Oral Epidemiol 1981;9(2):91–3.

61. Baghdady VS, Ghose LJ, Enke H. Traumatized anterior teeth in Iraqi and Sudanese children–a comparative study. J Dent Res 1981;60(3):677–80.

62. Marcenes W, Alessi ON, Traebert J. Causes and prevalence of traumatic injuries to the permanent incisors of school children aged 12 years in Jaragua do Sul, Brazil. Int Dent J 2000;50(2):87–92.

63. Nicolau B, Marcenes W, Sheiham A. Prevalence, causes and correlates of traumatic dental injuries among 13-year-olds in Brazil. Dent Traumatol 2001;17(5): 213–7.

64. Sabuncuoglu O, Irmak MY. The attention-deficit/hyperactivity disorder model for traumatic dental injuries: a critical review and update of the last 10 years. Dent Traumatol 2017;33(2):71–6.

65. Correa-Faria P, Petti S. Are overweight/obese children at risk of traumatic dental injuries? A meta-analysis of observational studies. Dent Traumatol 2015;31(4): 274–82.

66. Feldens CA, Kramer PF, Feldens EG, et al. Socioeconomic, behavioral, and anthropometric risk factors for traumatic dental injuries in childhood: a cohort study. Int J Paediatr Dent 2014;24(3):234–43.

67. Granville-Garcia AF, de Menezes VA, de Lira PI. Dental trauma and associated factors in Brazilian preschoolers. Dent Traumatol 2006;22(6):318–22.

68. Wong FS, Kolokotsa K. The cost of treating children and adolescents with injuries to their permanent incisors at a dental hospital in the United Kingdom. Dent Traumatol 2004;20(6):327–33.

69. Borum MK, Andreasen JO. Therapeutic and economic implications of traumatic dental injuries in Denmark: an estimate based on 7549 patients treated at a major trauma centre. Int J Paediatr Dent 2001;11(4):249–58.
70. Welch CL, Thomson WM, Kennedy R. ACC claims for sports-related dental trauma from 1999 to 2008: a retrospective analysis. N Z Dent J 2010;106(4): 137–42.
71. Ranalli DN. Prevention of craniofacial injuries in football. Dent Clin North Am 1991; 35(4):627–45.

Preventing Oral Disease
Alternative Providers and Places to Address This Commonplace Condition

Susan A. Fisher-Owens, MD, MPH[a,b,*], Elizabeth Mertz, PhD[c]

KEYWORDS

- Children's oral health • Primary care • Integrated medical home
- Preventive services • Interdisciplinary care

KEY POINTS

- Pediatric primary care providers can and should use their prevention-focused approach to help better prevent the most common chronic condition of childhood.
- Multiple other providers can be used to help decrease oral disease.
- Other settings, keeping in mind patients' family and community contexts, can help expand opportunities to prevent disease.

INTRODUCTION

Since the early middle ages, dentistry has been a field separated from medicine[1]; however, there is no other part of the body for which medicine cedes responsibility of care. As stated multiple times in this edition, dental caries is the most common chronic disease of childhood, and more needs to be done to address it. In the United States, children at greatest risk for oral health problems, based on socioeconomic status, are least likely to receive care. Despite dental professionals' unified goal of children's first visit by age 1,[2–5] almost 10% of children at this age already have dental caries (data from National Survey on Children's Health), but fewer than 2% have seen a dentist.[6] Caries is a progressive disease, especially if left untreated; by age 11, 42% of children have had dental caries in their primary teeth (untreated in roughly half of the children),[7] and by adulthood, 92% of adults age 20 to 64 have had dental caries in their permanent teeth.[8]

Disclosure Statement: The authors have nothing to disclose.
[a] Department of Pediatrics, UCSF School of Medicine, Zuckerberg San Francisco General Hospital, 1001 Potrero Avenue/MS6E37, San Francisco, CA 94110, USA; [b] Department of Preventive and Restorative Dental Sciences, UCSF School of Dentistry, 505 Parnassus Avenue, San Francisco, CA 94143, USA; [c] Faculty, Healthforce Center for Research and Leadership Development, 3333 California Street, Suite 410, San Francisco, CA 94143, USA
* Corresponding author. Department of Pediatrics, UCSF School of Medicine, Zuckerberg San Francisco General Hospital, 1001 Potrero Avenue/MS6E37, San Francisco, CA 94110.
E-mail address: Susan.Fisher-Owens@UCSF.edu

Pediatr Clin N Am 65 (2018) 1063–1072
https://doi.org/10.1016/j.pcl.2018.05.011
0031-3955/18/© 2018 Elsevier Inc. All rights reserved.

Prevention efforts are critical to stemming this "silent epidemic."[9] Research shows that children who are started on preventive care before they develop oral health problems actually cost the health system less money than those who initiate care at an older age.[10] Additional research is emerging about improved outcomes and lower cost of care overall for adult diseases when oral health is improved, including for diabetes,[11–13] stroke,[14] Alzheimer[15–20] and other cognitive loss/dementia,[21,22] and chronic kidney disease and end-stage renal disease.[23,24] Given this great need and the opportunity to have a significant positive impact on oral health, and as a consequence the health care system as a whole, there is a clarion call to engage the broad health care workforce in activities to prevent oral disease. This article describes prevention-focused activities that can be performed by nondentists, the workforce available to deploy in these efforts, and the settings in which they can be done to help prevent this disease and its effects.

CLASSIC PREVENTION IN PRIMARY CARE OFFICES

In the United States, more than 90% of children see a pediatric primary care provider (PCP)[a] in the first year of life. Pediatric PCPs are prevention-oriented: they assess risk (eg, with sleep position and sudden infant death syndrome), counsel with targeted anticipatory guidance (eg, with obesity and food introduction or family history of disease), and provide appropriate preventive interventions (eg, vaccinations). Increasingly, pediatric PCPs are embracing the use of these techniques to prevent dental caries, the most common chronic disease of childhood.

Risk Assessment

Assessing risk for caries can be done by almost any type of professional, and in any care setting. For example, pediatric PCPs already screen for risk factors for obesity, diabetes, and other conditions that also share risk factors for caries. These include consumption of sugar-sweetened beverages (for obesity, but which also increases risk of caries) or medications (which can dry the mouth and thus lessen the effectiveness of saliva to prevent caries). Others are closely related, such as the oral health of a parent and/or sibling when taking the family history. These questions are already part of, or can easily be integrated into, a pediatric PCP's routine.

There are formal Caries Risk Assessment (CRA) tools available to PCPs, including CRAs from the American Academy of Pediatric Dentistry (see http://www.aapd.org/media/Policies_Guidelines/G_CariesRiskAssessment.pdf), the American Academy of Pediatrics (AAP) (see https://www.aap.org/en-us/Documents/oralhealth_Risk AssessmentTool.pdf), and a smart form app format from Smiles for Life (http://www.smilesforlifeoralhealth.org/). All CRAs evaluate the risk factors and preventive habits most likely to influence oral health, and, again, include questions that are normally already being asked in the clinical visit, such as family history and food and beverage habits. Risk assessments easily can be integrated into pediatric medical care[25,26] and help identify, for example, those at high risk who would benefit most from the topical application of fluoride varnish. The effectiveness of CRA use was recently confirmed in a randomized controlled trial performed in a community dental setting,[27] re-creating the positive results from a similar study in a university setting.[28] Both studies demonstrated that proper use of CRA tools resulted in better preventive care, with targeted treatment, decreasing the percentage of children classified as

---

[a] Of note, PCPs may be physicians trained as pediatricians, family practitioners, or others, and may also be nurse practitioners or physician assistants.

high-risk for caries in their communities. Similar results of using a CRA in the medical setting have been presented at a conference.[29]

Anticipatory Guidance

Screening questions provide teachable moments for *anticipatory guidance*. For instance, if a parent reaches for a bottle to silence the baby during a visit, the provider can offer other soothing techniques while talking about not using a bottle for behavior control; this has an additional benefit for obesity prevention. This also segues to the topic of putting only fluoridated tap water in the bottle once a child has weaned from breastmilk or formula.

Some such moments are captured simply by an astute clinician in the office. One of the authors reports regularly seeing parents lick a pacifier that has fallen on the ground, in an effort to "clean" it before popping it back in the child's mouth (See the article "Infant Oral Health" by Charlotte Lewis and Erica Brecher in this issue.); this is a teachable moment to discuss the microbiology of caries transmission, and ways to prevent it. Noting the color of the beverage in a bottle offered to a waiting child is another opportunity to discuss healthy eating and drinking habits, including the role of community water fluoridation.

A recent pilot project from the AAP tested the use of the "Brush, Book, Bed" campaign in the pediatrician's office (materials are free to members). This campaign springboards off of the success of the Reach Out and Read campaign (which encourages child literacy) by systematically adding toothbrushing into the bedtime routine. This approach provides structure to the bedtime routine. An added bonus for parents is that this has shown to result in decreased latency to sleep, greatly appreciated by caregivers.[30]

Preventive Intervention

A brief intervention available for pediatric PCPs is the application of *fluoride varnish* in the office. Ideally, it is given based on risk assessment. It especially benefits high-risk patients and has been shown to safely decrease the risk of early childhood caries (37%–73%, depending on if used once or multiple times)[31,32] For the provider, it can be integrated seamlessly into flow (taking only a few minutes during the visit),[25] and is a billable activity. The US Preventive Services Task Force now recommends fluoride varnish be applied to all children with teeth until their sixth birthday (of note, their recommendation does not require a risk assessment).[33]

There are multiple models of providers working to integrate oral health into their clinical practice. Some providers take this on entirely, talking about the mouth, and diet, while examining the patient; some even apply the varnish while examining the patient. Others have their staff trained to apply the varnish and provide anticipatory guidance.

Nutritionists can be colocated with medical or dental providers, or on their own. So many of the messages that nutritionists address with obesity counseling can be extended to preventing oral disease. Similarly, many of the messages around parenting provided by behavioral health can underscore the importance of setting and maintaining a regimen of limits and of preventive care.

EXTENSION OF PRIMARY CARE PREVENTION BY ADDITION OF ALLIED HEALTH PROFESSIONALS

There are different models for improving access to oral health care. The first generation of collaborative effort usually involves referrals to dental care, as pediatric PCPs do with other diseases; this was only minimally effective at improving rates. The second generation features collocation of medical and dental care. Surprisingly, this results in only approximately 40% of the patients receiving dental care. The third generation improved the system by offering integrated care, when patients are receiving anticipatory guidance and preventive intervention. This can be done with medical staff, as mentioned previously, or by hiring dental staff to provide services mentioned previously (and even more) in the PCP office. A fourth generation involves teledentistry as a consult service.[34] Not surprisingly, patients most prefer the integrated model (Hilton I, personal communication, 2016).

PCPs are familiar with working with many types of allied health professionals. For decades, nurse practitioners and physician assistants have enriched the practices of physicians. Also, most PCPs are comfortable working directly or indirectly with community health workers, individuals who may not have had as much formal training in the health field, but who are culturally competent with their communities, and thus can provide messaging that is positively received. "Promotores de Salud" are one example of community health workers who work in the Latinx/Hispanic community; they can effectively promote oral health messages.[35] Either in the PCP office or in the field, domestically or internationally, community health workers influence health behaviors positively.[36–38]

Similarly, there are multiple types of dental care professionals who can help expand the existing workforce and increase access for patients. Dentists are trained to perform the full range of dental care, but especially restorative and surgical practices, skills that are not always necessary for primary prevention of disease. The pediatric PCP should be familiar with the existence and abilities of other dental professionals who can provide preventive screening and/or oral care in the medical office. Adding these allied dental providers may allow improved patient care, including the administration of additional preventive or restorative treatments, such as sealants, silver diamine fluoride, or interim therapeutic restoration.

In the United States, for example, *dental hygienists* and *dental therapists* have received similar training, just with a greater emphasis on prevention or therapeutics, respectively. They both work under the general (but not necessarily direct) supervision of a dentist. Licensing varies by state, so in some states, these providers can be quite independent.

Although working in dozens of other countries around the world, the first introduction of *dental therapists* in the United States was in the Alaska Native Tribal Health Consortium in 2006, where they serve the Alaska Native Populations. Both Oregon and Washington tribal health systems now employ dental therapists.[39] In Minnesota, the state adopted dental therapy in 2009, with a further category of advanced dental therapist, which is a dual therapist/hygiene model. In each state or setting, the scope of practice ranges based on local regulations, but in general they can do preventive and basic restorative procedures with the same clinical effectiveness as dentists.[40] The dental therapy model is now used in 54 countries.[41,39]

In the United States, a specific subgroup of hygienists who have received additional training and work more independently are *registered dental hygienist in alternative practice*.[42] These professionals are well positioned to support patients in the community health setting who have compromised access, such as nursing homes, prisons, or schools.[43,44] Most data on the effectiveness of *registered dental hygienists in alternative practice* have been derived from studies that involved the elderly and imprisoned populations. Bell and Coplen[45] showed rapidly improved access to oral health care in Oregon through work in schools. In Colorado, hygienists work integrated in medical offices,[34] and in Kansas, in school-based care, all with improvements in oral health.[46,47]

Dental assistants generally work under direct supervision of a dentist and may, but do not have to, be officially trained at an accredited program. In some states, expanded functions have been added to dental assistants' scope of work to increase efficiency of dental practice. If able to practice under the supervision of a dentist instead of direct supervision, this group has been postulated to be able to increase care in retirement communities, where at least half of the patients do not need the higher skills of a dentist.[48] In Kansas, where dental assistants are trained to scale (scrape plaque from teeth, although only supragingival), adults' receipt of care was increased.[49]

Other countries also work with allied professionals. Several countries have a similar professional group known as the *dental nurse*, with related skills. Dental nurses are particularly helpful in settings in which there are insufficient dentists, to help provide prevention messages and staff rural health centers and community hospitals. Thailand has used this model for almost 2 decades. There, a cadre of dental nurses were established to run rural health centers and community hospitals. A central element of this new Thai initiative, faced with a shortage of dentists, was and continues to be promoting toothbrushing with fluoridated toothpaste in primary schools. The results have been encouraging and a decrease in tooth decay has been noted.[50] In the United Kingdom, extended dental nurses can apply fluoride varnish. Dental therapists were first introduced in New Zealand, where they are trained for 2 years before working in underserved areas. Finally, Austria successfully introduced qualified dental health educators, who visit mothers after birth and provide them with a comprehensive set of instructions. This approach significantly decreased caries of children at age 5.[51]

The dental equivalent of a community health worker (CHW) is a community health dental coordinator, who provides education and assistance, as well as limited clinical preventive skills, particularly varnish, coronal polishing, and placement of sealants.[52] Their cultural competency is counted as a key element in their success.[53] Certainly, CHWs can be trained to incorporate oral health education and guidance with their other health messages.

Most of the previously described workforce categories, except the registered dental hygienist in alternative practice, are licensed to be working under the direct supervision of dentists. Several states have altered dental practice acts to allow more limited supervision; this loosening of regulation can afford settings, especially those with vulnerable population, more access to services,[45,47] including allowing these staff to work in medical practices.

Several research programs were funded by the National Institute of Dental and Craniofacial Research in 2015 to investigate different modalities of oral health messaging from nondental sites, be it in person, decentralized to homes, or provided in group settings, or even via text message. It will be informative to see the results from those studies, which have yet to be published.

EXTENSION OF PRIMARY CARE IN ALTERNATIVE SETTINGS

It is clearly possible to extend oral health services beyond the medical or dental home. Most notably, these services can be provided in community settings, where the patients and families are located, such as Women, Infant, and Children (WIC) settings, Head Start/Early Health Start, and schools. WIC, Head Start, and Early Head Start education already includes oral health promotion, but research is ongoing regarding investigating ways to improve the messaging and preventive services. Given this large population of economically at-risk children, this could be an excellent way to expand to other settings for providing preventive care.

Perhaps one of the most ideal settings for preventive, and even for restorative, care, is the school-based health clinic. These clinics allow children and teenagers to be seen in an environment they can access easily, where they are comfortable, and where less time will be missed from school. It also frees the parents from having to miss time from work. School-based health clinics have been shown to improve oral health.[54] The most developed programs involve dental prophylaxis, radiographs, and restoration,[46,55] but simpler models that include only screening or structured fluoride mouth-rinsing programs are also effective.[56] The services of many school-based programs include sealant application, and in the United States have the potential to reach 7 million more low-income children who do not otherwise have access to sealants.[57] Parents do need to consent for care, and information obtained during oral health care is sent back to them.[46,47] In this setting, the school nurse, if there is one, is an essential member of the team.[54,58]

Another manner to access dental care in poorly resourced settings is the use of teledentistry. Teledentistry is an evolving field that allows a dentist to provide services from afar. This provides access in rural communities, as well as inner-city schools.[59–61] Currently this field has focused on supporting ancillary providers working on their own, but could potentially become available to PCPs, especially if other dental professionals are collocated and looking for supervision/confirmation.

Last, the home is another ideal setting to support oral health behaviors. Direct messaging through text messages sent to parents has been shown not only to be effective at influencing heath behaviors,[62] but specifically to improve oral health behaviors in the United States[63] as well as other countries such as Iran.[64] This is a modality that may be able to be disseminated more widely, such as through Text4Baby, for greater impact. Most systems do not offer texting direct to children, because of limited access to cell phones and other issues with consent and messaging to teenagers.

SUMMARY

Pediatric PCPs are inherently prevention-focused. In the primary care office, familiar tactics of assessing risk, providing anticipatory guidance, and using preventive interventions easily can be applied to oral health promotion. There are ways care can and should be extended, with more types of the workforce working together, as well as expanding to more settings. Interprofessional care that engages patients in their domains of the family and community are important for continuing to decrease this pervasive and yet largely preventable disease.

REFERENCES

1. Mertz EA. The dental-medical divide. Health Aff (Millwood) 2016;35(12):2168–75.

2. American Academy of Pediatric Dentistry. Guideline on periodicity of examination, preventive dental services, anticipatory guidance/counseling, and oral treatment for infants, children, and adolescents. Pediatr Dent 2013;37(6):123–30.

3. American Academy of Pediatrics Section on Oral Health. Maintaining and improving the oral health of young children. Pediatrics 2014;134(6):1224–9.

4. American Dental Association, Statement on Early Childhood Caries (Policy). 2000. 454. Available at: https://www.ada.org/en/about-the-ada/ada-positions-policies-and-statements/statement-on-early-childhood-caries. Accessed January 13, 2018.

5. American Academy of Public Healthy Dentistry, First Oral Health Assessment Policy. 2004. Available at: https://www.aaphd.org/oral-health-assessment-policy. Accessed January 13, 2018.
6. American Academy of Pediatrics. Profile of pediatric visits. Elk Grove Village (IL): AAP; 2010. p. 16.
7. NIDCR. Dental Caries in Children (Ages 2-11). 2018. Available at: https://www.nidcr.nih.gov/research/data-statistics/dental-caries/children. Accessed January 13, 2018.
8. NIDCR. Dental Caries (Tooth Decay) in Adults (Age 20 to 64). 2018. Available at: https://www.nidcr.nih.gov/research/data-statistics/dental-caries/adults. Accessed January 13, 2018.
9. US Department of Health and Human Services. Oral health in America: a report of the surgeon general. Rockville (MD): US Department of Health and Human Services; 2000.
10. Savage MF, Lee JY, Kotch JB, et al. Early preventive dental visits: effects on subsequent utilization and costs. Pediatrics 2004;114(4):e418–23.
11. Taylor GW, Nahra TA, Manz MC, et al. Is periodontal treatment associated with lower medical costs in adults with diabetes? Findings in Blue Care Network 2001-2005. 2009.
12. Borgnakke WS, Ylöstalo PV, Taylor GW, et al. Effect of periodontal disease on diabetes: systematic review of epidemiologic observational evidence. J Periodontol 2013;84(4 Suppl):S135–52.
13. Nasseh K, Greenberg B, Vujicic M, et al. The effect of chairside chronic disease screenings by oral health professionals on health care costs. Am J Public Health 2014;104(4):744–50.
14. Tonetti MS, Van Dyke TE, working group 1 of the joint EFP/AAP workshop. Periodontitis and atherosclerotic cardiovascular disease: consensus report of the Joint EFP/AAP Workshop on Periodontitis and Systemic Diseases. J Periodontol 2013;84(4 Suppl):S24–9.
15. Cheng SB, Ferland P, Webster P, et al. Herpes simplex virus dances with amyloid precursor protein while exiting the cell. PLoS One 2011;6(3):e17966.
16. Olsen I, Singhrao SK. Can oral infection be a risk factor for Alzheimer's disease? J Oral Microbiol 2015;7:29143.
17. Singhrao SK, Harding A, Poole S, et al. Porphyromonas gingivalis periodontal infection and its putative links with Alzheimer's disease. Mediators Inflamm 2015;2015:137357.
18. Ide M, Harris M, Stevens A, et al. Periodontitis and cognitive decline in Alzheimer's disease. PLoS One 2016;11(3):e0151081.
19. Olsen I, Taubman MA, Singhrao SK. Porphyromonas gingivalis suppresses adaptive immunity in periodontitis, atherosclerosis, and Alzheimer's disease. J Oral Microbiol 2016;8:33029.
20. Pritchard AB, Crean S, Olsen I, et al. Periodontitis, microbiomes and their role in Alzheimer's disease. Front Aging Neurosci 2017;9:336.
21. Batty GD, Li Q, Huxley R, et al. Oral disease in relation to future risk of dementia and cognitive decline: prospective cohort study based on the Action in Diabetes and Vascular Disease: Preterax and Diamicron Modified-Release Controlled Evaluation (ADVANCE) trial. Eur Psychiatry 2013;28(1):49–52.
22. Li J, Xu H, Pan W, et al. Association between tooth loss and cognitive decline: a 13-year longitudinal study of Chinese older adults. PLoS One 2017;12(2):e0171404.

23. Ruospo M, Palmer SC, Craig JC, et al. Prevalence and severity of oral disease in adults with chronic kidney disease: a systematic review of observational studies. Nephrol Dial Transplant 2014;29(2):364–75.

24. Palmer SC, Ruospo M, Wong G, et al. Dental health and mortality in people with end-stage kidney disease treated with hemodialysis: a multinational cohort study. Am J Kidney Dis 2015;66(4):666–76.

25. Dooley D, Moultrie NM, Heckman B, et al. Oral health prevention and toddler well-child care: routine integration in a safety net system. Pediatrics 2016; 137(1):e1–8.

26. Rozier RG, Sutton BK, Bawden JW, et al. Prevention of early childhood caries in North Carolina medical practices: implications for research and practice. J Dent Educ 2003;67(8):876–85.

27. Rechmann P, Chaffee BW, Rechmann BMT, et al. Changes in caries risk in a practice-based randomized controlled trial. Adv Dent Res 2018;29(1):15–23.

28. Featherstone JD, White JM, Hoover CI, et al. A randomized clinical trial of anti-caries therapies targeted according to risk assessment (caries management by risk assessment). Caries Res 2012;46(2):118–29.

29. Ellsworth TT et al. #T19. An interdisciplinary approach to preventing and managing early childhood caries. Presented at: National Association of Pediatric Nurse Practitioners Annual Conference. Boston, March 11-14, 2014.

30. Barone LF. Brush, book, bed - 3 simple steps to good oral health and improved literacy. Pediatrics 2018;141(1 MeetingAbstract):597.

31. Weintraub JA, Ramos-Gomez F, Jue B, et al. Fluoride varnish efficacy in preventing early childhood caries. J Dent Res 2006;85(2):172–6.

32. Braun PA, Widmer-Racich K, Sevick C, et al. Effectiveness on early childhood caries of an oral health promotion program for medical providers. Am J Public Health 2017;107(S1):S97–103.

33. US Preventive Services Task Force (USPSTF). Final Recommendation Statement: Prevention of Dental Caries in Preschool Children: Recommendations and Rationale. 2014. Available at: https://www.uspreventiveservicestaskforce.org/Page/Document/RecommendationStatementFinal/dental-caries-in-children-from-birth-through-age-5-years-screening. Accessed January 13, 2018.

34. Braun PA, Cusick A. Collaboration between medical providers and dental hygienists in pediatric health care. J Evid Based Dent Pract 2016;16(Suppl):59–67.

35. Hoeft KS, Barker JC, Shiboski S, et al. Effectiveness evaluation of Contra Caries Oral Health Education Program for improving Spanish-speaking parents' preventive oral health knowledge and behaviors for their young children. Community Dent Oral Epidemiol 2016;44(6):564–76.

36. Tiwari T, Albino J, Batliner TS. Challenges faced in engaging American Indian mothers in an early childhood caries preventive trial. Int J Dent 2015;2015:179189.

37. Mathu-Muju KR, Kong X, Brancato C, et al. Utilization of community health workers in Canada's Children's Oral Health Initiative for indigenous communities. Community Dent Oral Epidemiol 2018;46(2):185–93.

38. Mathu-Muju KR, McLeod J, Donnelly L, et al. The perceptions of First Nation participants in a community oral health initiative. Int J Circumpolar Health 2017;76(1):1364960.

39. Nash DA, Friedman JW, Mathu-Muju KR, et al. A review of the global literature on dental therapists. Community Dent Oral Epidemiol 2014;42(1):1–10.

40. Bolin KA. Assessment of treatment provided by dental health aide therapists in Alaska: a pilot study. J Am Dent Assoc 2008;139(11):1530–5 [discussion 1536–9].
41. Nash DA, Mathu-Muju KR, Friedman JW. The dental therapist movement in the United States: a critique of current trends. J Public Health Dent 2018;78(2): 127–33.
42. Mertz E, Glassman P. Alternative practice dental hygiene in California: past, present, and future. J Calif Dent Assoc 2011;39(1):37–46.
43. Langelier M, Continelli T, Moore J, et al. Expanded scopes of practice for dental hygienists associated with improved oral health outcomes for adults. Health Aff (Millwood) 2016;35(12):2207–15.
44. Naughton DK. Expanding oral care opportunities: direct access care provided by dental hygienists in the United States. J Evid Based Dent Pract 2014;14(Suppl): 171–82.e1.
45. Bell KP, Coplen AE. Evaluating the impact of expanded practice dental hygienists in Oregon: an outcomes assessment. J Dent Hyg 2015;89(1):17–25.
46. Simmer-Beck M, Walker M, Gadbury-Amyot C, et al. Effectiveness of an alternative dental workforce model on the oral health of low-income children in a school-based setting. Am J Public Health 2015;105(9):1763–9.
47. Simmer-Beck M, Wellever A, Kelly P. Using registered dental hygienists to promote a school-based approach to dental public health. Am J Public Health 2017;107(S1):S56–60.
48. Monaghan NP, Morgan MZ. What proportion of dental care in care homes could be met by direct access to dental therapists or dental hygienists? Br Dent J 2015; 219(11):531–4 [discussion: 534].
49. Mitchell TV, Peters R, Gadbury-Amyot CC, et al. Access to care and the allied oral health care workforce in Kansas: perceptions of Kansas dental hygienists and scaling dental assistants. J Dent Educ 2006;70(3):263–78.
50. Treerutkuarkul A, Gruber K. Prevention is better than treatment. Bull World Health Organ 2015;93:594–5.
51. Wagner Y, Greiner S, Heinrich-Weltzien R. Evaluation of an oral health promotion program at the time of birth on dental caries in 5-year-old children in Vorarlberg, Austria. Community Dent Oral Epidemiol 2014;42(2):160–9.
52. American Dental Association. Breaking down barriers to oral health for all Americans: the community dental health coordinator. 2012. p. 12. Available at: https://www.ada.org/en/~/media/ADA/Publications/ADA%20News/Files/ADA_Breaking_Down_Barriers. Accessed January 13, 2018.
53. Braun PA, Quissell DO, Henderson WG, et al. A cluster-randomized, community-based, tribally delivered oral health promotion trial in Navajo Head Start children. J Dent Res 2016;95(11):1237–44.
54. Carpino R, Walker MP, Liu Y, et al. Assessing the effectiveness of a school-based dental clinic on the oral health of children who lack access to dental care. J Sch Nurs 2017;33(3):181–8.
55. Caring for Kids: School-based Dental Care. Available at: http://www.healthinschools.org/issue-areas/school-based-dental-health/#sthash.WDWRgPKv.dpbs. Accessed January 13, 2018.
56. Divaris K, Rozier RG, King RS. Effectiveness of a school-based fluoride mouthrinse program. J Dental Res 2012;91(3):282–7.
57. CDC. Dental Sealants Prevent Cavities. 2016. Available at: https://www.cdc.gov/vitalsigns/dental-sealants/index.html. Accessed January 13, 2018.

58. Peterson J, Niessen L, Lopez GMN. Texas public school nurses' assessment of children's oral health status. J Sch Health 1999;69(2):69–72.

59. Glassman P. Virtual dental home. J Calif Dent Assoc 2012;40(7):564–6.

60. Glassman P, Harrington M, Namakian M, et al. The virtual dental home: bringing oral health to vulnerable and underserved populations. J Calif Dent Assoc 2012; 40(7):569–77.

61. Kopycka-Kedzierawski DT, Billings RJ. Teledentistry in inner-city child-care centres. J Telemed Telecare 2006;12(4):176–81.

62. U.S. Department of Health and Human Services. Promoting Maternal and Child Health Through Health Text Messaging: An Evaluation of the Text4baby Program - Final Report, U.S.D.o.H.a.H. Services, Editor. 2015. Available at: file:///C:/Users/FisherOwens/Downloads/text4babysummary.pdf. Accessed January 13, 2018.

63. Hashemian TS, Kritz-Silverstein D, Baker R. Text2Floss: the feasibility and acceptability of a text messaging intervention to improve oral health behavior and knowledge. J Public Health Dent 2015;75(1):34–41.

64. Makvandi Z, Karimi-Shahanjarini A, Faradmal J, et al. Evaluation of an oral health intervention among mothers of young children: a clustered randomized trial. J Res Health Sci 2015;15(2):88–93.

Oral–Health–Related Quality of Life in Children and Adolescents

William Murray Thomson, PhD[a],*, Hillary L. Broder, PhD[b]

KEYWORDS

• Children • Quality of life • Self-report • Dental care • Health services research

KEY POINTS

• Child oral–health–related quality of life (OHRQOL) measures enable determination of the impact of a child's oral condition on the child's life.

• Several scales are available for use, and all have acceptable psychometric properties.

• Child OHRQOL measures can be used to gauge the effect of clinical interventions, such as dental treatment under general anesthesia, orthodontic treatment, and treatment of orofacial clefting.

Health is a subjective state, and oral health is no exception.[1] Locker defined oral health as "a standard of the oral tissues which contributes to overall physical, psychological and social well-being by enabling individuals to eat, communicate and socialise without discomfort, embarrassment or distress and which enables them to fully participate in their chosen social roles."[2] His introduction of the concept of oral–health–related quality of life (OHRQOL) and adaptation of the World Health Organization model of the International Classification of Impairments, Disabilities and Handicaps to oral health[3] spurred a great deal of research effort over the following 2 decades. This focused largely on the development and validation of what are commonly known as "OHRQOL measures" but which, in fact, represent the impact of oral conditions on people's lives. Those impacting conditions might be disease-related (such as dental caries) or anatomic (such as malocclusion or orofacial clefting). Initially, the developmental work focused on adults, with measures developed for use among older people but subsequently validated for use with younger adults, with much attention to their testing and validation in different cultures and settings.

Disclosure Statement: The authors declare no conflicts of interest in relation to this article.
[a] Faculty of Dentistry, The University of Otago, PO Box 56, Dunedin 9054, New Zealand;
[b] Cariology and Comprehensive Care, NYU College of Dentistry, New York University, 345 East 24th Street, New York, NY 10010, USA
* Corresponding author.
E-mail address: murray.thomson@otago.ac.nz

Pediatr Clin N Am 65 (2018) 1073–1084
https://doi.org/10.1016/j.pcl.2018.05.015   pediatric.theclinics.com
0031-3955/18/© 2018 Elsevier Inc. All rights reserved.

By the turn of the last century, attention had somewhat inevitably shifted to the issue of OHRQOL measurement in children. It was not that it had been avoided, rather that children's self-reporting on their oral health posed more challenges. Very young children tend to be unreliable informants, while their ongoing social and cognitive development meant that it was likely that different measures would be needed for different ages. Moreover, the development and rollout of adult OHR-QOL measures was seen as having been laborious and inefficient, with the typical pattern being to develop a measure in one age group and culture and then to validate and test it in other cultures, age groups, and settings. Such work was onerous and repetitive, and there was always the chance that any version tested and developed in another culture would end up markedly different from the original measure, with cross-cultural comparability sacrificed for intracultural validity. A prime example of this phenomenon was the development of the Malay version of the Oral Health Impact Profile,[4] which resulted in a measure with markedly different item content from the original one.

Accordingly, Broder, Reisine, and Locker obtained US National Institutes of Health funding and convened an international group of dental health services researchers in 2000 with the aim of developing a child OHRQOL measure simultaneously in a wide range of cultures and settings. It was hoped that coordinating this work would make the testing and validation stages considerably more efficient. Consideration also had to be given to the readability and formatting of the child questionnaires to safeguard that the language was age-appropriate and they were designed and constructed to be easily and reliably completed (such as through using appropriate font sizes and alternate line colors). That work resulted eventually in 2 measures (known as the Child Perceptions Questionnaire [CPQ] and the Child Oral Health Impact Profile [COHIP]), and these have been the most widely used in recent years. They are not the only scales that have been developed for use with children, however. **Table 1** presents an overview of the available child OHRQOL measures. Five are used directly with children, and 3 require proxy informants—typically caregivers or parents—because they are intended for use with much younger children.

Gilchrist and coworkers[14] systematically appraised the 3 most commonly used child-report measures (CPQ, Child-OIDP, and COHIP). They found that, although the CPQ had been the most frequently used measure, there was sound evidence for the validity and reliability of each. Most of the 199 articles reporting fieldwork had been from cross-sectional studies. With only 3 longitudinal studies published, there was a need for more data on the responsiveness and evaluative properties of those scales. Considerably more longitudinal work with the 2 scales, which use proxy informants (the Early Childhood Oral Health Impact Scale [ECOHIS] and the Parent[P]-CPQ), has provided good evidence for their responsiveness.[15,16] Satisfactory demonstration of test-retest reliability, however, remains an issue with the latter. To date, only 1 study has examined it, finding it acceptable in a Saudi Arabian clinical sample.[17] The relative lack of test-retest data is largely because the longitudinal work has been confined to clinical samples of children undergoing dental treatment under general anesthesia. Researchers (and ethics committees) are understandably wary of increasing respondent burden unnecessarily, requiring already stressed parents to complete another questionnaire would have been onerous for them and likely to have affected the studies' follow-up rates.[16] Studies such as these underline the challenges encountered in developing, testing, and using OHRQOL measures with children and their families: the work can be exacting and unpredictable, and there is no such thing as the perfect study; all have had to make compromises in some way.[18]

Measure	Year First Published	No of Items	Short Form Available?	Age Range	Any Positive Items?	Usage to Date
Child as informant						
CPQ[5]	2002[a]	37	Yes (8 items and 16 items)	8–14[b]	No	Considerable
Child Oral Impacts on Daily Performances[7]	2004[c]	8	No	11–12	No	Moderate
COHIP[8]	2007[d]	34	Yes (19)	7–16	Yes	Moderate
Pediatric Oral-Health-related Quality of Life[9]	2011[e]	10	No	<16	No	Low
Scale of Oral Health Outcomes[10]	2012[f]	5	Not needed	5	No	Moderate
Proxy as informant						
Parent-CPQ[11]	2003[g]	33	Yes (8 items and 16 items)	<8	No	Considerable
ECOHIS [12]	2007[h]	9	Not needed	<8	No	Considerable
COHIP-Preschool[13]	2017[i]	9	No	<2–6	Yes	Low

Table 1
Overview of child oral–health–related quality of life measures

[a] Jokovic and Locker, 2002.
[b] This has separate (but similar) versions for 11-year-olds to 14-year-olds and 8-year-olds to 10-year-olds, but recent work (Foster Page and colleagues,[6] 2013) has shown that the former works just as well for the latter.
[c] Gherunpong and colleagues, 2004.
[d] Broder and colleagues, 2007.
[e] Huntington and colleagues, 2011.
[f] Tsakos and colleagues, 2012.
[g] Jokovic and colleagues, 2003—this also has a family impact component, not included here.
[h] Pahel and colleagues, 2007—this also has a family impact component, not included here.
[i] Ruff and colleagues, 2017.

HOW CHILD ORAL-HEALTH–RELATED QUALITY OF LIFE MEASURES WORK

It has been argued that child OHRQOL measures are a way of placing sufferers (whether children or their families) accurately on what would effectively be a continuum of misery and then observing their treatment-associated movement toward the less severe end of such a continuum.[16] With the exception of the COHIP,[8] the higher the scale score, the more severe the impact that poor oral health (or orofacial aesthetics or function) has on a child. Despite the movement toward including positive health items in health-related quality-of-life measures, most of the available OHRQOL measures that have been validated clinically and epidemiologically use negatively worded items, with only the COHIP differing; 4 of the 34 items in the COHIP have positive items; for the short-form COHIP, 2 of the 19 items are positively worded. At the analysis stage, those items are reverse-coded for consistency with the remainder. The inclusion of positive items is considered useful, because it enables the capture of information about the beneficial aspects of a child's condition on the child's life, and completing the questionnaire does not become an exercise in rating a catalog of unrelentingly negative aspects of life. Given that contemporary definitions of health emphasize both positive and negative aspects, it is appropriate to include the former in measures that aim to reflect people's health-related quality of life.[19] Moreover, it may be that the absence of a negative condition does not fully reflect treatment outcome in longitudinal clinical research. In short, treatment can serve to enhance the well-being of an individual, thereby underscoring the principle that outcome measures can be more robust when tapping into both positive and negative oral health perceptions.

USES OF CHILD ORAL-HEALTH–RELATED QUALITY OF LIFE MEASURES

OHRQOL measures have several applications.[20] They can be used to identify children with poor oral health, whether in clinical or epidemiologic contexts. They can identify the oral conditions with the greatest impact on children's day-to-day lives and functioning. They are useful in epidemiologic surveys, not only to complement the more traditional clinical indices but also as oral health measures in their own right. They can be used as outcome measures in health services research or in clinical trials.[21] Health economists can use them in cost-utility analysis. At the political level, the information gleaned from such measures can be used in advocating for the allocation of scarce resources toward orofacial care and research,[22] or the retention (or rationing) of services which may be threatened.[16] If it can be shown that poor oral health has a substantially impact on quality of life, well-being, and productivity, policy-makers and planners are more likely to regard child oral disease as an important public health issue and to allocate resources toward treating and preventing oral ill health. OHRQOL measures can also be used in clinical practice to monitor an individual patient's condition or to facilitate the decision-making process for a patient who is faced with choosing among various treatment options. In other words, evidence-based care can and should incorporate patient-reported outcomes. Thus, there is much that OHRQOL measures can contribute to knowledge and practice in pediatric dentistry.

OUTCOME EXAMPLES

Some examples of the longitudinal use of child OHRQOL measures in assessing the outcomes of interventions are discussed. The first involves a brief overview of the work done internationally on improvements in child OHRQOL, which are associated with dental treatment under general anesthesia. The second illustrates the measurement of improvements in adolescent OHRQOL as a result of orthodontic treatment. The third describes changes in child/adolescent OHRQOL as a result of surgical treatment for orofacial clefts among school-aged youth.

Child Oral-Health–Related Quality of Life and Dental Treatment Under General Anesthesia

Child OHRQOL scales enable researchers to place children accurately on the continuum of misery, discussed previously, and then observe their treatment-associated movement toward the less severe end of that continuum. Studies to date have usually been a preintervention/postintervention one, with the same children assessed before treatment and again sometime after it. To date, 13 such studies have been published,[23–34] with patient numbers at baseline ranging from 31 to 311. Effect sizes observed in those studies were large (**Table 2**), with marked improvements in OHRQOL observed. Several of those studies also investigated the wider effects on the children's families, with similar effect sizes.

   An important practical issue is how sustainable those effects are. In other words, how long does the improvement in child OHRQOL last after treatment? Is it generalizable across locations and/or across oral conditions? A Lithuanian study examined the sustainability after 6 months of the changes observed in OHRQOL in the same group

Table 2
Treatment-associated effect sizes detected in before-after studies of children undergoing treatment of early childhood caries under general anesthesia, by scale

	Scale Which Was Used	
Authors and Year	Parent-Child Perceptions Questionnaire	Early Childhood Oral Health Impact Scale
Malden et al,[23] 2008	0.9	—
Klaasen et al,[24] 2009	—	0.9
Lee et al,[25] 2011	—	0.6
Gaynor et al,[26] 2012	0.9	—
Baghdadi,[17] 2014	1.6	—
Jankauskiene et al,[28] 2014	—	1.6
Cantekin et al,[29] 2014	—	0.9
Almaz,[27] 2014	—	1.0
Ridell et al,[30] 2015	0.7	—
Abanto et al,[31] 2016	—	2.2
Yawary et al,[32] 2016	—	1.1
De Souza et al,[33] 2017	1.0	—
Mean effect size detected	1.0	1.2

for which ECOHIS score changes had been documented after 1 month[30] and found that the effect sizes (over baseline) remained large. Using the P-CPQ, Baghadi[34] observed large effect sizes persisting after 6 months, and another study observed large effect sizes (with a modified CPQ_{11-14}) after 1 year in a clinical sample of special needs children who had been rehabilitated dentally under general anesthesia.[35] These data suggest that the improvements are maintained in the medium term (ie, months), but further work is required to determine their longer-term sustainability. Challenges to be overcome in this respect include both response shift (respondents recalibrating/adjusting to their child's new health state) and the effects of ongoing early childhood caries (that is, new lesions producing new impacts).

Improvements in Adolescents' Oral-Health–Related Quality of Life After Orthodontic Treatment

Although the stated aims of orthodontic treatment are to improve appearance, correct the function of the dentition, and correct occlusion that could have a negative impact on long-term oral health,[36] most treatment is undertaken for psychosocial reasons.[37] Moreover, the cost of orthodontic treatment is substantial. Accordingly, it is important to determine its impact on adolescents OHRQOL, yet reports from longitudinal studies of such improvements are surprisingly scarce.[38,39] Prior to 2016, any such studies had been conducted with patients in dental school orthodontic clinics,[39–43] and in none of those adolescent studies were the medium-term treatment-associated changes in OHRQOL determined. Real-world observations of treatment-associated changes in malocclusion and OHRQOL data were needed, using data from patients treated outside dental schools, given that most orthodontic treatment is undertaken outside that particular sector.

Such a study was recently conducted in New Zealand, with the investigators recruiting 174 adolescent patients who were undergoing 2-arch, fixed-appliance treatment in 19 private-sector orthodontic practices from throughout the country and observing them in a 4-year prospective study.[44] Participants were assessed before treatment, at debond (the removal of the braces, when 87.4% of the baseline sample were reassessed, with mean treatment time 26 months) and a mean 21 months post-debond (when 59.4% of the baseline sample were reassessed). OHRQOL was measured using CPQ_{11-14}.

Among the 104 individuals who took part in all 3 assessments, little change in OHR-QOL overall was detected by the end of their orthodontic treatment (a phase referred to as the debond stage), despite a considerable improvement being noted in their malocclusion. The mean CPQ_{11-14} was slightly greater at debond, and this was most notable with its functional limitations subscale. By the end of the study, the decreases in CPQ_{11-14} overall and subscale scores were all substantial, especially in the emotional well-being and social well-being subscales (**Fig. 1**). Effect sizes were moderate to large. The lag time in CPQ_{11-14} score reduction (indicating improved OHR-QOL) may reflect the participants having had time in which to adjust to their improved occlusions and occlusal settling and to reflect on the aesthetic, social, and emotional outcomes of their treatment and on the absence of their appliances. Thus, a temporary increase in symptomatic impacts observed at the debond stage seems to ameliorate with time, with the OHRQOL benefits of orthodontic treatment manifesting themselves some months later.

Improvements in Child Oral-Health–Related Quality of Life with Treatment of Orofacial Clefts

Clefting is the most common facial birth defect worldwide.[45] Cleft care in developed countries is delivered by a multidisciplinary team due to the special needs associated with cleft, including speech/language challenges, facial differences, atypical dental development, malocclusion, learning disabilities, chronic ear infections, and associated psychosocial sequelae. Cleft specialists (including plastic surgeons, dentists, psychologists, social workers, speech/language therapists, and so forth) provide ongoing evaluations and interventions from infancy to late adolescence or young adulthood. In addition to dental and adjunct therapies prior to treatment completion, cleft habilitation can include up to 20 surgical procedures through late adolescence.

An overview of cleft care quality-of-life outcomes for school-aged youth was recently published.[46] As with many other OHRQOL studies, the studies represented

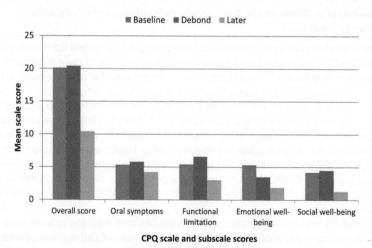

Fig. 1. Changes in OHRQOL among adolescents undergoing orthodontic treatment.

cross-sectional evaluations. Cleft professionals generally assume that sequential surgical procedures and adjunct therapies improve patient well-being, although scant empirical longitudinal evidence is available to support that contention. Because the majority of cleft patients are children, a longitudinal multicenter study was undertaken by 6 large multidisciplinary teams in the United States, including an ethnically diverse sample of 1200 7-year-old to 18-year-old youth and their caregivers, using the COHIP.

Appearance and speech ratings by the plastic surgeons, speech pathologists, and participants (as well as participants' OHRQOL) improved over time among the 43% of the participants who underwent lip/nose revision, orthognathic surgery, secondary palatal revisions, and/or alveolar bone grafting. Multilevel modeling was used to examine the data more thoroughly, revealing that female youth participants had lower (worse) self-rated emotional well-being and overall COHIP scores than their male counterparts.[47] Youth 12 years of age and older had lower emotional well-being, school, and overall COHIP scores than those who were younger. Those with nonprivate insurance had lower scores on oral symptoms, functional and emotional well-being, school, and overall COHIP scores than those with private insurance. Youth with cleft palate only had higher scores on oral symptoms, emotional well-being, and the overall COHIP than participants with cleft lip and palate. Relative to those with a visible surgical recommendation (such as lip/nose revisions), youth with invisible surgical recommendations (such as fistula repairs) scored higher on functional and emotional well-being, school, and overall COHIP. A novel finding was a negative association between the number of prior surgical procedures and scores on oral symptoms, functional well-being, school, and overall COHIP. Further analysis indicated that a higher number of previous surgical procedures was associated with poorer self-rated and caregiver-rated OHRQOL.[47] By early adolescence (12 years of age), there were differences in the average number of procedures by cleft type, but these were not fully explained by the extent of facial difference. This finding may indicate that those with a greater number of previous procedures (11–20) had had more severe cleft-related defects and/or unrealistic expectations associated with surgery treatment and/or familial conflict in decision-making.[48] An alternative explanation could be that surgery may reach a point of diminishing returns. Although the timing of surgery and number of procedures may be important to individuals OHRQOL, these findings suggest that adjunct psychological counseling could provide support to patients and their families undergoing the stress and expectations associated with surgery.[49,50] The effects of other influences on well-being (such as gender, age, family function, depression, anxiety, and/or resilience) remains to be elucidated. In summary, unlike treating caries or malocclusion, cleft habilitation is complex and its evaluation requires a large sample to fully examine potential impacts on OHRQOL scores.

Because cleft lip and palate is a more severe and visible condition, it is important to identify risk and protective factors for OHRQOL and psychosocial well-being. With the cultural emphasis on appearance, exploring ways to foster resilience in this patient population is vital.[51,52] Moreover, the type of payer may be a cultural factor in the United States[52–54] that may not be relevant in countries with socialized health care systems that ensure that families have access to revisional care.

These findings underscore that patient-reported outcome measures—in this case, the COHIP—have evaluative properties that are responsive to change and clearly capture a different perspective than surgeons' ratings of their patients' facial appearances and/or functional status. Despite the costs of care and associated expenses in time and effort, the findings suggest a positive impact of surgical interventions on OHRQOL regardless of age group, ethnicity, or family payer status.

Table 3
Child Oral Health Impact Profile and Child Oral Health Impact Profile–Short Form scores by visit

	Baseline		First Follow-up[a]		Second Follow-up	
	Mean	SD	Mean	SD	Mean	SD
Child						
COHIP	96.9	18.7	100.3	18.4	102.4	17.2
COHIP-SF	53.3	11.3	56.1	10.9	57.9	10.2
Pearson correlation	0.96	—	0.96	—	0.96	—
Caregiver						
COHIP	93.8	19.7	95.6	19.9	97.1	18.7
COHIP-SF	51.6	11.6	53.5	11.8	54.5	11.2
Pearson correlation	0.97	—	0.97	—	0.97	—

[a] Follow-up was at approximately 1 year and 2 years after the baseline assessment; note that an increase in COHIP score reflects an improvement in OHRQOL.

Despite the thrust to develop short OHRQOL forms for practicality purposes, there is little evidence comparing the short and long forms of OHRQOL measures. Recent analyses reveal that the short form (COHIP-SF) corresponds well to the original COHIP. **Table 3** presents a comparison of the long and short forms for the child and caregiver scores, respectively; these data were derived from Broder's longitudinal study of school-aged children with cleft.[18] As with the original measure, the child COHIP-SF scores improve over time. The correlation between the short and long forms was uniformly high, exceeding 0.96 at each data collection time point. Computing the effect sizes[a] for the child scores in **Table 3** relative to baseline is informative: for the first and second follow-ups, they are 0.2 and 0.3, respectively, for the long form; for the short form, they are 0.2 and 0.6, respectively. Thus, treatment affords a small effect using the long form, but with the short form, the effect seems to get greater with time; this may reflect less background noise in the short-form version of the COHIP. Similarly, **Table 4** presents the COHIP and COHIP-SF scores for surgical and nonsurgical participants along with their caregiver proxy ratings. Children who had cleft-related surgery had poorer self-rated and caregiver-rated OHRQOL over time (represented by their lower scale scores) than children who did not have surgery.[46]

WHERE TO FROM HERE?

Although the past 2 decades' work on child OHRQOL instruments has resulted in several measures that are used effectively to bolster the knowledge base underpinning the practice of pediatric dentistry, further work remains to be done. Future child OHRQOL research includes determining the minimally important difference, which has been underutilized in children's quality-of-life assessments and would be useful in distinguishing children/adolescents with clinically meaningful improvements in score from those with only minor changes. Additionally, mixed-methods approaches—which use qualitative and quantitative assessments—can be particularly useful for

[a] The effect size is determined by dividing the mean change score by the standard deviation of the pretreatment scores to give a dimensionless measure of effect. Effect size statistics of less than 0.2 indicate a small clinically meaningful magnitude of change, 0.2 to 0.7 a moderate change, and greater than 0.7 a large change.

Table 4
Mean Child Oral Health Impact Profile and Child Oral Health Impact Profile–Short Form scores by surgery and visit

	First Follow-up (SD)[a]		Second Follow-up (SD)		Third Follow-up (SD)	
	Surgery	No Surgery	Surgery	No Surgery	Surgery	No Surgery
Child						
COHIP	97.6 (19.2)	99.3 (18.3)	102.2 (17.1)	103.2 (17.7)	102.9 (18.4)	111.5 (10.8)
COHIP-SF	51.7 (11.3)	55.1 (11.1)	53.8 (10.8)	58.3 (10.7)	56.0 (11.4)	64.2 (6.1)
Caregiver						
COHIP	94.8 (26.2)	95.9 (19.9)	97.1 (20.2)	98.2 (19.3)	99.1 (19.8)	106.5 (7.0)
COHIP-SF	49.2 (11.2)	52.1 (11.9)	50.6 (11.8)	53.9 (11.6)	52.2 (11.2)	61.3 (94.8)

[a] Follow-up was at approximately 1 year and 2 years after the baseline assessment; note that an increase in COHIP score reflects an improvement in OHRQOL.

research on new patient populations and understudied OHRQOL issues (such as satisfaction with care and family functioning). They can contribute to designing and evaluating interventions to improve not only OHRQOL but also psychosocial functioning in patients and their caregivers. Personality is known to influence people's self-reported oral health, with those scoring higher on negative affectivity (or neuroticism) likely to report more negative impacts, other factors being equal,[55] yet there have been no investigations yet on how parental personality influences proxy reports for child OHRQOL. Finally, it seems that child OHRQOL measures are here to stay, with their value having been repeatedly demonstrated, and the next few years should see their routine use in clinical and public health practice.

REFERENCES

1. Cohen LK, Jago JD. Toward the formulation of sociodental indicators. Int J Health Serv 1976;6:681–98.
2. Locker D. Does dental care improve the oral health of older adults? Community Dent Health 2001;18:7–15.
3. Locker D. Measuring oral health: a conceptual framework. Community Dent Health 1988;5:3–18.
4. Saub R, Locker D, Allison P. Derivation and validation of the short version of the Malaysian Oral Health Impact Profile. Community Dent Oral Epidemiol 2005;33: 378–83.
5. Jokovic A, Locker D, Stephens M, et al. Validity and reliability of a questionnaire for measuring child oral-health-related quality of life. J Dent Res 2002;81:459–63.
6. Foster Page LA, Thomson WM, Ukra A, et al. Factors influencing adolescents' oral health-related quality of life (OHRQoL). Int J Paediatr Dent 2013;23:415–23.
7. Gherunpong S, Tsakos G, Sheiham A. Developing and evaluating an oral health-related quality of life index for children; the CHILD-OIDP. Community Dent Health 2004;21:161–9.
8. Broder HL, McGrath C, Cisneros G. Questionnaire development: face validity and item impact testing of the child oral health impact profile. Community Dent Oral Epidemiol 2007;35(Suppl 1):8–19.
9. Huntington NL, Spetter D, Jones JA, et al. Development and validation of a measure of pediatric oral health-related quality of life: the POQL. J Public Health Dent 2011;71:185–93.

10. Tsakos G, Blair YI, Yusuf H, et al. Developing a new self-reported scale of oral health outcomes for 5-year-old children (SOHO-5). Health Qual Life Outcomes 2012;10:62.
11. Jokovic A, Locker D, Stephens M, et al. Measuring parental perceptions of child oral health-related quality of life. J Public Health Dent 2003;63(2):67–72.
12. Pahel BT, Rozier RG, Slade GD. Parental perceptions of children's oral health: the Early Childhood Oral Health Impact Scale (ECOHIS). Health Qual Life Outcomes 2007;5:6.
13. Ruff RR, Sischo L, Chinn CH, et al. Development and psychometric validation of the Child Oral Health Impact Profile – Preschool version (COHIP-PS). Community Dent Health 2017;34:176–82.
14. Gilchrist F, Rodd H, Deery C, et al. Assessment of the quality of measures of child oral health-related quality of life. BMC Oral Health 2014;4:40.
15. Jankauskiene B, Narbutaite J. Changes in oral health-related quality of life among children following dental treatment under general anaesthesia. A systematic review. Stomatologija 2010;12:60–4.
16. Thomson WM. Public health aspects of paediatric dental treatment under general anaesthetic. Dent J 2016;4:20.
17. Baghdadi ZD. Effects of dental rehabilitation under general anesthesia on children's oral health-related quality of life using proxy short versions of OHRQoL instruments. ScientificWorldJournal 2014;2014:308439.
18. Broder HL, Crerand CE, Ruff RR, et al. Challenges in conducting multicentre, multidisciplinary, longitudinal studies in children with chronic conditions. Community Dent Oral Epidemiol 2017;45:317–22.
19. Lin X-J, Lin I-M, Fan S-Y. Methodological issues in measuring health-related quality of life. Tzu Chi Med J 2013;25:8–12.
20. Shearer DM, MacLeod RJ, Thomson WM. Oral-health-related quality of life: an overview for the general dental practitioner. N Z Dent J 2007;103:82–7.
21. Sischo L, Broder HL. Oral health-related quality of life: what, why, how, and future implications. J Dent Res 2011;90:1264–70.
22. Robinson PG. Choosing a measure of health related quality of life. Community Dent Health 2016;33:107–15.
23. Malden PE, Thomson WM, Jokovic A, et al. Changes in parent-assessed oral-health-related quality of life among young children following dental treatment under general anaesthetic. Community Dent Oral Epidemiol 2008;36:108–17.
24. Klaassen MA, Veerkamp JS, Hoogstraten J. Young children's Oral Health-Related Quality of Life and dental fear after treatment under general anaesthesia: a randomized controlled trial. Eur J Oral Sci 2009;117:273–8.
25. Lee GH, McGrath C, Yiu CK, et al. Sensitivity and responsiveness of the Chinese ECOHIS to dental treatment under general anaesthesia. Community Dent Oral Epidemiol 2011;39:372–7.
26. Gaynor WN, Thomson WM. Changes in young children's OHRQoL after dental treatment under general anaesthesia. Int J Paediatr Dent 2012;22:258–64.
27. Almaz EM, Sonmez S, Oba AA, et al. Assessing changes in oral health-related quality of life following dental rehabilitation under general anesthesia. J Clin Pediatr Dent 2014;8:263–7.
28. Jankauskiene B, Virtanen JI, Kubilius R, et al. Oral health-related quality of life after dental general anaesthesia treatment among children: a follow-up study. BMC Oral Health 2014;14:81.

29. Cantekin K, Yildirim MD, Cantekin I. Assessing change in quality of life and dental anxiety in young children following dental rehabilitation under general anesthesia. Pediatr Dent 2014;36:12E–7E.

30. Ridell K, Borgstrom M, Lager E, et al. Oral health-related quality-of-life in Swedish children before and after dental treatment under general anaesthesia. Acta Odontol Scand 2015;73:1–7.

31. Abanto J, Paiva SM, Sheiham A, et al. Changes in preschool children's OHRQoL after treatment of dental caries: responsiveness of the B-ECOHIS. Int J Paediatr Dent 2016;26:259–65.

32. Yawary R, Anthonappa RP, Ekambaram M, et al. Changes in the oral health-related quality of life in children following comprehensive oral rehabilitation under general anaesthesia. Int J Paediatr Dent 2016;26:322–9.

33. De Souza MC, Harrison M, Marshman Z. Oral health-related quality of life following dental treatment under general anaesthesia for early childhood caries – a UK-based study. Int J Paediatr Dent 2017;27:30–6.

34. Baghdadi ZD. Children's oral health-related quality of life and associated factors: mid-term changes after dental treatment under general anesthesia. J Clin Exp Dent 2015;7:e106–13.

35. El-Meligy O, Maashi M, Al-Mushayt A, et al. The effect of full-mouth rehabilitation on oral health-related quality of life for children with special health care needs. J Clin Pediatr Dent 2016;40:53–61.

36. Roberts-Harry D, Sandy J. Orthodontics. Part 1: who needs orthodontics? Br Dent J 2003;195:433–7.

37. Plunkett DJ. The provision of orthodontic treatment: some ethical considerations. N Z Dent J 1997;93:17–20.

38. Zhou Y, Wang Y, Wang X, et al. The impact of orthodontic treatment on the quality of life a systematic review. BMC Oral Health 2014;14:66.

39. Javidi H, Vettore M, Benson PE. Does orthodontic treatment before the age of 18 years improve oral health-related quality of life? A systematic review and meta-analysis. Am J Orthod Dentofacial Orthop 2017;151:644–55.

40. Agou S, Locker D, Muirhead V, et al. Does psychological well-being influence oral-health-related quality of life reports in children receiving orthodontic treatment? Am J Orthod Dentofacial Orthop 2011;139:369–77.

41. Chen M, Wang DW, Wu LP. Fixed orthodontic appliance therapy and its impact on oral health-related quality of life in Chinese patients. Angle Orthod 2010;80:49–53.

42. Feu D, Miguel JA, Celeste RK, et al. Effect of orthodontic treatment on oral health-related quality of life. Angle Orthod 2013;83:892–8.

43. Palomares NB, Celeste RK, Oliveira BH, et al. How does orthodontic treatment affect young adults' oral health-related quality of life? Am J Orthod Dentofacial Orthop 2012;141:751–8.

44. Healey DL, Gauld RDC, Thomson WM. Treatment-associated changes in malocclusion and OHRQoL: a four-year cohort study. Am J Orthod Dentofacial Orthop 2016;150:811–7.

45. Mossey PA, Little J, Munger RG, et al. Cleft lip and palate. Lancet 2009;374:1773–85.

46. Sischo L, Wilson-Genderson M, Broder HL. Quality-of-life in children with orofacial clefts and caregiver well-being. J Dent Res 2017;96(13):1474–81.

47. Broder HL, Wilson-Genderson M, Sischo L. Oral health-related quality of life in youth receiving cleft-related surgery: self-report and proxy ratings. Qual Life Res 2016;26:859–67.

48. Ruff RR, Sischo L, Broder HL. Minimally important difference of the Child Oral Health Impact Profile for children with orofacial anomalies. Health Qual Life Outcomes 2016;14:140.

49. Feragen KB, Borge A, Rumsey N. Social experience in 10-year-old children born with a cleft: exploring psychosocial resilience. Cleft Palate Craniofac J 2009;46: 65–74.

50. Strauss RP. "Only skin deep": health, resilience, and craniofacial care. Cleft Palate Craniofac J 2001;38:226–30.

51. Sischo L, Broder HL, Phillips C. Coping with cleft: a conceptual framework of caregiver responses to nasoalveolar molding. Cleft Palate Craniofac J 2015;52: 651–9.

52. Seid M. Barriers to care and primary care for vulnerable children with asthma. Pediatrics 2008;122:994–1002.

53. US Department of Health and Human Services. Oral health in America: a report of the surgeon general. Rockville (MD): National Institute of Dental and Craniofacial Research; 2000.

54. Rumsey N, Stock NM. Living with a cleft: psychological challenges, support and intervention. In: Berkowitz S, editor. Cleft lip and palate: diagnosis and management. 3rd edition. New York: Springer; 2013. p. 907–16.

55. Thomson WM, Caspi A, Poulton R, et al. Personality and oral health. Eur J Oral Sci 2011;119:366–72.

Pediatric Oral Health Policy

Its Genesis, Domains, and Impacts

Burton L. Edelstein, DDS, MPH[a,b,*]

KEYWORDS

- Oral health policy • Insurance coverage • Health workforce • Prevention
- Health safety net • Health surveillance

KEY POINTS

- Public policymaking – a complex iterative process amenable to influence by child advocates – has increasingly addressed pediatric oral health and dental care over time.
- Policy domains of particular import to children's health, including their oral health, are insurance coverage, workforce, safety net, prevention, and surveillance.
- The Affordable Care Act's nearly 2 dozen dental provisions provide a framework for comprehensive improvements in children's oral health and dental care.
- Policymaking has improved pediatric access, utilization, and outcomes, yet inequitable children's oral health remains a significant policy concern.
- Change drivers in US health care delivery and financing are promoting increasing integration of medical and dental care for children and greater accountability to health outcomes.

In 1997, the American Academy of Pediatrics (AAP) Washington office supported the creation of the Children's Dental Health Project (CDHP) and thereby formalized efforts to include pediatric oral health as a bona fide pediatric health policy issue. With active support from the AAP and the American Academy of Pediatric Dentistry, the CDHP networked widely to press Congress for inclusion of pediatric oral health in federal legislation, oversight hearings, and congressional studies. The need for this effort was evident in Congress' decision earlier that year to establish dental benefits as optional rather than mandatory coverage in the State Children's Health Insurance Program (S-CHIP) that insured approximately 7 million children of working-poor families. Partnering with children's advocates, dental groups, and a variety of national associations of state officials, governors, health directors, Medicaid directors, dental

Disclosure: The author reports no financial conflicts of interest.
[a] Population Oral Health, Columbia University College of Dental Medicine, Columbia University Medical Center, 622 West 168th Street, PH7-311, Box 20, New York, NY 10032, USA;
[b] Children's Dental Health Project, 1020 19th Street NW, Suite 400, Washington, DC 20036
* Corresponding author. Population Oral Health, Columbia University College of Dental Medicine, Columbia University Medical Center, 622 West 168th Street, PH7-311, Box 20, New York, NY 10032.
E-mail address: ble22@columbia.edu

directors, and public health officials, advocates for children encouraged each state to elect the dental option. Once universally achieved, this tactic prepared Congress to mandate dental services when S-CHIP was reauthorized 10 years later as CHIP. Success securing the dental benefit in CHIP was followed shortly thereafter by the congressional mandate that pediatric dental coverage be required under the Affordable Care Act (ACA).

These coverage accomplishments illustrate that proven strategies to influence Congressional policymaking, including grooming legislative champions, assembling and activating the necessary coalitions, levering the press, and persistently promoting well-crafted policies, can result in meaningful action that benefits children. The story, however, does not end with these significant decade-old achievements. In 2018, Congress delayed the required reauthorization of CHIP and undermined key provisions of the ACA thereby demonstrating a fundamental characteristic of policymaking: it is a process that is never over. For this reason, the pediatric health community is obliged to actively engage in policymaking (or support those who do) to ensure that children's health and welfare are given a consistent and strenuous voice.

This contribution explores how and why pediatric oral health evolved from an afterthought in both pediatric medicine and public policymaking to a featured policy issue; how policymakers have integrated oral health into pediatric medical policy's domains of coverage, workforce, safety-net, prevention, and surveillance; and how policymaking has positively impacted children's oral health and dental care. This contribution looks forward in time to examine medical-dental integration in ways that may stimulate truly seamless pediatric health promoting systems. It briefly explores other advanced country's forays into pediatric oral health policy to consider how those endeavors may inform future US policy.

POLICY, POLICYMAKERS, AND POLICYMAKING

Policy delineates how things are done. It sets the rules, specifies the procedures, and describes the processes to accomplish defined ends. "It establishes priorities, promotes the common good, and maximizes use of available resources. Expressed as legislation, regulation, rules, and procedures, policy … creates options, sets limits, and dictates processes and outcomes. It determines who is authorized to take actions under specified circumstances, including where, when, and how those actions are permissible."[1] Policy is authoritative and, once established, tends to be resistant to change until circumstances call it into question and create demand for updated or totally new policies.

Policymakers operate in multiple institutions, including government, academia, professional associations, businesses, nonprofits, and even families. They achieve the authority to establish and enforce policies and resultant programs through status, appointment, precedent, or election. Power, politics, and influence are closely affiliated with the process of making policy. Importantly, those who actively and persistently influence policymakers are as influential as those who actually make policy. That is why lobbyists, advocates, academics, journalists, constituents, analysts, and community-based professionals are all critical to the process.

Problems are then prioritized for policy action according to agendas established by those with political power. These agendas are influenced by a wide range of inputs, including current events, political and personal interests, advocates and lobbyists, the press, and other branches of government. The congressional policymaking process—a complex competitive interplay of priorities, politics, power, and processes that typically run in parallel between the US Senate and US House of

Representatives—results in authorizing legislation that, once finalized and then confirmed by the president, establishes policies and programs. Congress must then plan for and determine dollars to implement its policies and programs through budget and appropriations legislation. In addition to authorizing and providing dollars for policies and programs, Congress' third role is to conduct oversight strategies (hearings, investigations, and reports) to evaluate outcomes and ensure that the policies and programs are executed as intended. This review process typically identifies new problems, due to unintended consequences of prior action[2] and environmental changes, including changes in the political makeup of Congress. Newly identified problems then initiate the cycle anew.

PEDIATRIC ORAL HEALTH: FROM AFTERTHOUGHT TO MAINSTREAM

In practice, pediatric oral health policy is a subset of pediatric health policy that is a subset of health policy, itself a subset of domestic policy. This niche placement suggests that oral health must be mainstreamed as a core element of pediatric general health if it is to be addressed as a serious policy issue. However, the observation that issues related to children's oral health and dental care are estranged from policies and programs affecting children's general health is a reflection of the historical separation of the medical and dental professions. Dentistry's relation to mainstream medicine has been variously characterized as "divorced and severe[d],"[3] "separated and divided,"[4] "siloed,"[5] and "ignored."[6] Physicians have been both credited for professionalizing dentistry[3] and blamed for its separation in education and training, credentialing and licensing, staffing, practice, and insurance.[7] Since the time of the ancient Egyptians, Assyrians, and Greeks, oral infection and inflammation have been recognized as threats to systemic health. In the early twentieth century, this awareness resulted in inappropriate wholesale dental extractions based on the outmoded focal theory of infection. Today this oral-systemic awareness is again evident in the multiple studies detailing the roles of dental infections and periodontal inflammation in a wide range of chronic systemic diseases.[6]

Interests in whole-child health, health equity, and person- and family centered care are now coupled with environmental drivers for accountability and value in health care purchasing to drive medical-dental integration across coverage, workforce, safety net, prevention, and surveillance policies. Policies to integrate medical and dental insurance design and affordability are being advanced through embedding, bundling, and administrative strategies (eg, states that require applicants to purchase both pediatric medical and dental coverage before being allowed to exit their exchange [ie, ACA Marketplaces] Web site).[8] Workforce policies to engage primary care providers in oral health screening, risk assessment, anticipatory guidance, fluoride management, and referral (as described in Susan A. Fisher-Owens and Elizabeth Mertz's article, "Preventing Oral Disease: Alternative Providers and Places to Address this Commonplace Condition," in this issue) are now long-standing and substantial.[9] Policies and programs promoting education of primary care medical providers have been advanced by the federal government's Integration of Oral Health and Primary Care Practice initiative,[10] multiple health care professional associations' endorsement of "Smiles for Life" national oral health curriculum,[11] and multiple states' requirement for physician education as a prerequisite for Medicaid paying physicians for oral health services.[12] National and state health foundations have advanced policies and strategies for engaging physicians in systems of care that incorporate oral health for children[13,14] as have academic and professional leaders[15,16] and safety net providers.[17] Crediting the US Surgeon General's 2000 Report Oral Health in America with raising public awareness about the poor state of children's oral health in the United States, Douglass and colleagues[9] detailed the education, training, and practice opportunities for pediatricians and family physicians to join with dentists to "ensure improvement of the oral health of America's children."[9] Others have focused on the potential for electronic health records to integrate, align, and enhance oral health[18] despite few private dentists qualifying for meaningful use incentives and requirements under the HITECH (Health Information Technology for Economic and Clinical Health) Act of 2009. In contrast, federally qualified health centers that colocate medical and dental care are leading efforts to integrate electronic health records (EHRs) for both pediatric and adult populations.[19,20]

As childhood caries is reconceptualized as a chronic condition amenable to behavioral and pharmacologic interventions rather than as only an acute surgical problem,[21] pediatric dentistry's clinical caries management policies[22] increasingly reflect medical approaches to addressing asthma, diabetes, and obesity in young children.[23] AAP's Bright Futures program[24] also provides clinical policies for medical providers on the prevention and management of caries in children. Consistent with these policies, the US Preventive Services Task Force has found supportive evidence for medical providers prescribing fluoride tablets and/or applying fluoride varnish while calling for additional evidence of effectiveness for physician counseling on oral health.

Federal agency policies and requirements reflect the importance of children's oral health within the larger contexts of population health surveillance and program performance. Annually reportable oral health measures are included in Head Start's Program Information Reports; Maternal and Child Health Block Grants' National Performance Measures; Healthy People 2020's Objective updates; and Medicaid's Early and Periodic Screening, Diagnostic, and Treatment (EPSDT) 416 Reports. The last uniquely requires reporting of oral health services delivered by "a non-dentist-provider"[25] defined as "any qualified health care practitioner who is neither a dentist nor providing services under the supervision of a dentist."[25]

National surveys that pediatric medicine relies on for input to policymaking also include measures of both oral health and dental care. Findings from national surveillance studies (National Health and Nutrition Examination Survey, National Health Interview Survey, and National Children's Health Survey) risk studies (Behavioral Risk Factor Surveillance System), and health care expenditures studies (Medical Panel Expenditure Survey) assist in evaluating the impact of policies and programs and in identifying problems needing policy action. Members of Congress also rely on evaluation studies that they commission from the Government Accountability Office (GAO) when assessing the performance of policies and program. Since Congress first considered CHIP in 1996, there have been 31 major GAO reports pertinent to pediatric oral health surveillance, workforce, coverage, and access, as well as the impact of governmental programs to address these domains.[26]

UNITED STATES CONGRESSIONAL ACTION ON PEDIATRIC ORAL HEALTH AND DENTAL CARE

Three enactments by Congress highlight the explicit inclusion and progression of pediatric oral health in federal legislation: the addition of pediatric dentistry to the Title VII Section 747 Training in Primary Care Medicine and Dentistry Program in 1998, the CHIP reauthorization in 2010, and the ACA in 2010. Each sequentially expanded consideration of pediatric dentistry and oral health by first addressing workforce (Title VII), then coverage (CHIP reauthorization), and ultimately the full range of public policies impacting children's oral health (ACA).

The Health Professions Education Partnerships Act

Modifications to the then 35-year-old health professions training law in 1998 addressed pediatric dentistry workforce for the first time. The Training in Primary Care Medicine and Dentistry Program had begun as a medical school construction program in 1963, expanded to support hospital-based physician and general dentist postgraduate training in 1971, next established financing for hospital-based postdoctoral general dentistry residency programs in 1976, then included university-based general dentistry education in 1985, and promoted medical and dental innovation in 1992 before finally expanding to include funding of pediatric dentistry training in 1998.[27] The ACA in 2010 also addressed this Title VII program by creating a separate administrative cluster for dental programs and broadening the use of funds for pediatric dentistry faculty development, predoctoral training in pediatric dentistry, and faculty loan repayment.[28]

The Children's Health Insurance Program

Unlike Medicaid that provides comprehensive dental care for children through a back door, CHIP's 2010 reauthorization addressed comprehensive dental care for children directly. Medicaid's back-door access to dental coverage is its 1967 pediatric EPSDT benefit that requires that any medically necessary care needed by a beneficiary younger than 21 years must be covered. Because dental care is noted to be medically necessary, it has become a defined benefit by default. In sharp contrast, the CHIP dental authorization was the first in US history to explicitly authorize dental care for socially vulnerable children.

The inclusion of the defined dental benefit in CHIP reflects well on the policymaking process, as Congress was influenced by the full range of outside and inside interests. These interests included states' elective adoption of the earlier optional S-CHIP dental benefit; an active coalition of dental, medical, social welfare, and business groups that persistently advocated for children's oral health; policy shops that provided Congress with analyses demonstrating the need for and value of dental care; the press that featured the death of a 12-year-old Maryland Medicaid beneficiary who died of sequelae of a dental abscess; legislative champions in both the House and Senate; a US Surgeon General's Report, Oral Health in America, that characterized childhood caries as a silent epidemic; and federal agency actions.[29] Activating Congressional interest were formal hearings and informal briefings, supportive Dear Colleague Letters that circulated among members of Congress, professional lobbying by a variety of groups, Congressional Research Service and GAO reports, issue briefs by a variety of advocacy groups, and press attention.

CHIP expanded health coverage to children who were ineligible for Medicaid because their families' incomes exceeded Medicaid eligibility levels but who were uninsured because their working-parents could not access or afford dependent coverage through their employer or the private individual insurance market. Some members of Congress, primarily liberal Democrats, argued for a straightforward Medicaid expansion to be secured by raising the income threshold for eligibility. Others, primarily conservative Republicans, argued for creating a totally different insurance program for these children of the working poor. The fundamental difference between these two approaches was whether the child or the state would be entitled to the federal dollars that pay for coverage. Medicaid expansion proponents sought an expansion of the individual entitlement such that all eligible children would be assured of coverage. New program proponents called for a state entitlement of federal funds such that states could close their programs to further enrollment if their federal dollar allocation became depleted. Compromise was reasonably simple: each state was allowed to choose whether it would use federal dollars to expand Medicaid, establish a separate CHIP program, or institute a combination of both approaches. Nine states expanded Medicaid, 13 created a new CHIP program, and 29 elected a combination of both approaches.[30]

States that expanded Medicaid did so with the understanding that EPSDT's comprehensive dental coverage would extend to the newly covered children and adolescents. States that created a new CHIP program were required to provide somewhat less comprehensive but still significant dental benefits. Those benefits, defined in legislation, called for dental care that is "necessary to prevent disease and promote oral health, restore oral structures to health and function, and treat emergency conditions." States elected a variety of benchmarks (commercial or government-employee plans) and implementation approaches[31] resulting in substantial but less uniformity across states in CHIP dental coverage than in Medicaid dental coverage.

The Children's Health Insurance Program Reauthorization Act (CHIPRA) in 2010 also established the Medicaid and CHIP Payment and Access Commission as "a non-partisan legislative branch agency that provides policy and data analysis and makes recommendations to Congress, the Secretary of the U.S. Department of Health and Human Services, and the states on a wide array of issues affecting Medicaid and the S-CHIP."[32] The legislation specified that the 17 commissioners contribute expertise in a variety of health policy disciplines, including pediatric medicine along with experts in safety net, health care finance, health plans, integrated delivery systems, consumers, and others (Public Law 111–3.Sec 506[2] [A]). The law's specification that a dentist must be appointed as one of the commissioners further evinced that oral health had continued to emerge as a bona fide public policy issue requiring ongoing attention.

The Affordable Care Act

The ACA provides a veritable menu of pediatric oral health provisions addressing coverage, workforce, safety net, prevention, and surveillance. Although many of the provisions have not been implemented for lack of appropriations and the law may be further modified or repealed over time, its pediatric oral health provisions can be readily recycled in future legislation. For that purpose, CDHP has developed 3 guides for legislators and advocates: a catalog of ACA dental provisions that includes intent, citation, and legislative language for each of more than 20 provisions[33] and 2 implementation roadmaps, one on oral health[34] and one on dental care provisions.[35]

Highlights of these provisions include

- Coverage provisions: Coverage was addressed by establishing dental care as an essential health benefit within the larger category of pediatric services. Dental coverage must meet standards of coverage in a state-selected benchmark plan and, unlike typical dental coverage, cannot impose annual or lifetime limits.[36]
- Workforce provisions: Workforce was addressed extensively through authorizations to expand federal primary care medical and dental training grants; prioritize integration among public health, medical, and dental training; establish a 15-state workforce innovation program to incentivize development of dental therapists and other new midlevel dental providers; and create a dental faculty loan repayment program that prioritizes interdisciplinary care of underserved populations.

- Safety-net provisions: The ACA reinforced an existing policy priority supporting school-based health systems by expanding funding for school-based dental care.
- Prevention provisions: Prevention of childhood dental disease was addressed in authorizations of a national public education campaign on childhood caries; promotion of chronic disease management approaches to pediatric caries; and an expanded grant program to support school-based dental sealant programs.
- Oral health surveillance provisions: Surveillance was significantly enhanced by the ACA that included a mandate for prenatal oral health assessment in the Pregnancy Risk Assessment Monitoring System; strengthening dental measures in Medical Expenditure Panel Survey by adopting the same look-back validation procedures required of medical measures; mandated participation by all states in the Centers for Disease Control and Prevention's (CDC) National Oral Health Surveillance System; and charging the CDC's Center for Health Statistics with maintaining detailed dental disease monitoring in the National Health and Nutrition Examination Survey.

IMPACT OF FEDERAL POLICYMAKING ON PEDIATRIC ORAL HEALTH AND DENTAL CARE

Federal policymaking to address children's oral health and dental care has resulted in substantive improvements over time. CHIP and ACA dental coverage combined with Medicaid and employer-sponsored insurance have ensured that most US children have financial access to dental care.

The number of children with public dental coverage through Medicaid and CHIP has increased by 1.7 times between 1997, a time before CHIPRA and the ACA, and 2017, after CHIPRA and the ACA, from 28.8% to 48.4% of children having public coverage—an increase from 20.4 million children with Medicaid in 1997[37] to 35.7 million with Medicaid or CHIP in 2017.[38] An additional 1 million children have gained private individual-market coverage through the ACA marketplaces (ie, exchanges),[39] most with federal subsidies to offset premium and out-of-pocket expenses.

Paralleling this coverage expansion has been an increase in dental utilization. By 2013, dental utilization by children in Medicaid had increased to a national average of 48.3% (range across states: 27.9% to 64.3%), whereas utilization by children with private coverage increased to a national average of 64% (range across states: 47.7% to 75.9%). Over time, there has been a significant narrowing of the gap in dental care utilization between Medicaid-enrolled children and children with private dental benefits with a 53% decrease in this gap between 2005 and 2013 nationally (range across states: 8.8% to 192.6%).[40]

But oral health disparities remain. Because children from poor and low-income families experience higher rates of dental caries and other dental problems, this remarkable increase in equitable utilization has not resulted in equitable oral health outcomes. An analysis of the 2011 to 2012 National Children's Health Survey revealed that "parents of publicly insured children were less likely to report that the condition of their child's teeth was excellent or very good and more likely to report that the child had had a dental problem in the past 12 months" despite equivalent use of dental services. This finding suggests that "Medicaid is meeting its mandate to ensure that dental care is as available for children in the program as it is for privately insured children, but refinements in Medicaid policy are needed to improve poor children's oral health"[41] outcomes.

Federal policies that have increased support for pediatric dental training since 1998 have similarly demonstrated a strong positive impact. A 10-year assessment showed that this program has succeeded in "building general and pediatric dental training capacity, diversifying the dental workforce, providing outreach and service to underserved and vulnerable populations, stimulating innovations in dental education, and engaging collaborative and interdisciplinary training with medicine."[27] Since that time, the sponsoring agency, the Health Resources and Services Administration (HRSA), has dramatically expanded its medical-dental integration efforts through funding and resource development.[42]

Federal policy action has additionally stimulated a positive impact on the dental safety-net's facility, EHR, and workforce dental capacity. HRSA reports that in 2016, 5.7 million people received dental services at 1367 centers by 6699 dentists, dental hygienists, and dental therapists and that half of all eligible children treated received recommended dental sealants.[43] These figures represent dramatic increases in access and utilization from 2000 when 1.3 million people received dental services from 1258 dental professionals,[44] stimulated in part by a federal $100 million dental program expansion grant program. School-based dental clinics have similarly experienced rapid growth with a 20% increase between 2011 and 2014 alone.[45]

Nonetheless, reflecting the historical separation of medicine and dentistry, some federal policies that benefit pediatric medicine have not been extended to pediatric dentistry. For example, the ACA authorized the so-called 'primary care fee bump' designed to encourage primary care providers to increase care of Medicaid beneficiaries and the HITECH incentives failed to address pediatric dental providers.

LOOKING TO THE FUTURE

As pediatric oral health has become increasingly recognized as a core component of whole-child health and child-centered care, efforts to better coordinate and integrate primary dental and medical care have evolved to include colocation of services; formalized referral networks; Bright Futures, health home, and professional guidelines; inclusion of dental benefits in health insurance plans; training and incentivizing primary care medical providers in oral health counseling, screening, and fluoride varnish application; and early integration of dental services within accountable care organizations and patient-centered medical homes. Because pediatricians see children at earlier ages than do dentists, pediatricians hold a unique opportunity to address children's oral health, including their risks for early childhood caries, potentially managing this chronic disease directly through strategies to arrest caries progression that involve substantive counseling in nutrition, appropriate use of fluoridated toothpaste, and direct application of topical fluorides or by delegating to medical assistants and referring to nutritionists, health educators, or social workers. Shifts in US health care delivery and financing that increasingly reward outcomes over procedures and value over volume, though alternative payment mechanisms that support value-based care can be expected to further drive medical-dental integration.

INTERNATIONAL PERSPECTIVES ON PEDIATRIC DENTAL CARE

The long-standing separation of pediatric medicine and dentistry is reflected in the variety of approaches that countries have adopted in determining how to integrate pediatric oral health services into their national health plans and delivery systems. Decisions involve whether and how extensively to provide coverage for dental services, the types of dental delivery systems to support, and how to pay providers for dental services and finance dental care. These decisions are substantially grounded in the political philosophy of any given country. For example, Germany provides a substantial pediatric dental benefit through a mostly independent dental delivery system supported by mostly private financing under a conservative political philosophy. In sharp contrast, Denmark's substantial dental benefit is supported by a mixed public and private delivery system with mostly public payment and all government financing predicated on a socialist political philosophy. Sitting between these two examples is the United Kingdom's approach to covering pediatric dental services through a mostly private delivery system funded by the government and grounded in a liberal political philosophy (Lowell-Shlansky E. Cross-national dental care models. Unpublished student research at Columbia University College of Dental Medicine, 2013). Unlike these advanced peer countries, the US approach to providing dental care for children is a hodge-podge of disparate public and private delivery, payment, and financing mechanisms that generally provide reasonably comprehensive dental benefits for children but not for adults.

Dental training and dental personnel also vary across developed countries with US and Canadian dentist training requiring postbaccalaureate education, whereas most other developed countries train dentists at the baccalaureate level. Similarly, most other countries train and deploy midlevel dental therapists, particularly for care of children in safety net programs, whereas dental therapy remains nascent in the United States.

Leading-edge thinkers around the globe are increasingly reconceptualizing pediatric dental caries as a chronic disease amenable to behavioral and pharmacologic management rather than as an acute surgical problem. Through their professional interactions, they share proposals to support this shift in care and can be expected to drive change in childhood caries management through a variety of demonstrations that will inform the future of US dental care for children.

SUMMARY

Judging by legislation, public and private programs, insurance coverage, and increasing dental utilization and associated improvements in oral health, it is clear that pediatric oral health policy has become institutionalized, increasingly attended to, and beneficial to the health and welfare of children. Nonetheless, public and private policies continue to change and evolve requiring that pediatric health advocates and practitioners remain engaged in consistently advocating for children who depend on adults to voice their needs.

REFERENCES

1. Edelstein BL. Policy and personalized oral health care. In: Polverini PJ, editor. Personalized oral health care: from concept design to clinical practice. Springer; 2015. p. 134. Available at: http://www.springer.com/us/book/9783319232966.
2. Institute of Medicine. Unintended consequences of health policy programs and policies: workshop summary. Washington, DC: National Academy Press; 2001. Available at: https://www.nap.edu/read/10192/chapter/2.
3. Simon L. Overcoming historical separation between oral and general health care: interprofessional collaboration for promoting health equity. AMA J Ethics 2016; 18(9):941–9.
4. Beck J. Why dentistry is separate from medicine: the divide sometimes has devastating consequences. The Atlantic 2017. Available at: https://www.theatlantic.com/

health/archive/2017/03/why-dentistry-is-separated-from-medicine/518979/. Accessed December 29, 2017.

5. Glurich I, Schwel KM, Lindberg S, et al. Integrating medical-dental care for diabetic patients: qualitative assessment of provider perspectives. Health Promot Pract 2017;19(4):531–41.
6. Vieira CL, Caramelli B. The history of dentistry and medicine relationship: could the mouth finally return to the body? Oral Dis 2009;15(8):538–46.
7. Otto M. Teeth: the story of beauty, inequality, and the struggle for oral health in America. New York: The New Press; 2017. p. 304.
8. Snyder A, Kanchinadam K, Hess C, et al. Improving integration of dental health benefits in health insurance marketplaces. Washington, DC: National Academy for State Health Policy; 2014.
9. Douglass AB, Douglass JM, Krol DM. Educating pediatricians and family physicians in children's oral health. Acad Pediatr 2009;9(6):452–6.
10. Health Resources and Services Administration. Integration of oral health and primary care practice. Rockville (MD): U.S. Department of Health and Human Services; 2014. Available at: https://www.hrsa.gov/sites/default/files/oralhealth/integrationoforalhealth.pdf.
11. Society of Teachers of Family Medicine. Smiles for Life: a national oral health curriculum. 3rd edition. Available at: https://www.smilesforlifeoralhealth.org/buildcontent.aspx?pagekey=62947&lastpagekey=64336&userkey=13563525&sessionkey=3886221&tut=555&customerkey=84&custsitegroupkey=0.
12. Sams LD, Rozier RG, Quinonez RB. Training requirements and curriculum content for primary care providers delivering preventive oral health services to children enrolled in Medicaid. Fam Med 2016;48(7):556–60.
13. Grantmakers in Health. Returning the mouth to the body: integrating oral health & primary care. 2012. Issue Brief No.40. Washington, DC. Available at: http://www.gih.org/files/FileDownloads/Returning_the_Mouth_to_the_Body_no40_September_2012.pdf.
14. Edelstein BL, Rubin MS, Douglass JM. Improving children's oral health by crossing the medical-dental divide. Hartford (CT): Connecticut Health Foundation; 2015. Available at: https://www.cthealth.org/publication/improving-childrens-oral-health-medical-dental-divide/.
15. Harvard School of Dental Medicine. Integrating oral health and medicine initiative. Available at: https://oralhealth.hsdm.harvard.edu/.
16. Jones JA, Snyder JJ, Gesko DS, et al. Integrated medical-dental delivery systems: modesl in a changing environment and their implications for dental education. J Dent Educ 2017;81(9):eS21–9.
17. Hilton IV. Creating medical-dental integration: helpful hints and promising practices. Denver (CO): National Network for Oral Heatlh Access; 2014. Available at: http://www.nnoha.org/nnoha-content/uploads/2014/06/Creating-Medical-Dental-Integration_2014-06-23.pdf.
18. Acharya A, Shimpi N, Mahnke A, et al. Medical care providers' perspectives on dental information needs in electronic health records. J Am Dent Assoc 2017;148(5):328–37.
19. Tinanoff N, Bernstein J, Vargas C, et al. Integration of oral health and pediatric medical primary care in community health centers. Boston (MA): Boston University Center to Reduce and Eliminate Dental Disparities; 2015. Available at: http://www.bu.edu/creedd/files/2016/05/Final-report-NIDCR-Protocol-11-013.pdf.
20. National Network for Oral Health Access. Electronic medical and dental record integration options. 2012 Presentation to the National Association of Community

Health Centers. Available at: http://www.nnoha.org/nnoha-content/uploads/2013/08/Electronic-Medical-and-Dental-Record-integration-options-slides.pdf.

21. Ng MW, Ramos-Gomez F, Lieberman M, et al. Disease management of early childhood caries: ECC Collaborative Project. Int J Dent 2014;2014:327801.

22. American Academy of Pediatric Dentistry Council on Clinical Affairs. Policy on early childhood caries (ECC): unique challenges and treatment options. Reference manual 2017-18. Pediatr Dent 2017;39(6):62–3.

23. Edelstein BL, Ng MW. Chronic disease management strategies of early childhood caries: support from the medical and dental literature. Pediatr Dent 2015;37(3):28107.

24. Casamassimo P, Holt K, editors. Bright futures: oral health—pocket guide. 3rd edition. Washington, DC: National Maternal and Child Oral Health Resource Center; 2016.

25. Center for Medicare and Medicaid Services. Instructions for completing form CMS-416: annual early and periodic screening, diagnostic, and treatment (EPSDT) participation report. Available at: https://www.medicaid.gov/medicaid/benefits/downloads/cms-416-instructions.pdf. Accessed January 13, 2018.

26. Huang T, Edelstein BL. Analaysis of Government Accountability Office (GAO) Reports on Children's Oral Health 1990-2016, in press.

27. Ng MW, Glassman P, Crall J. The impact of Title VII on general and pediatric dental education and training. Acad Med 2008;83(11):1039–48.

28. American Academy of Pediatric Dentistry. 2017 legislative fact sheet, HRSA Title VII pediatric dentistry appropriations. Undated. Available at: http://www.aapd.org/assets/1/7/2017_HRSA_Title_VII_Fact_Sheet.pdf. Accessed January 15, 2018.

29. Edelstein BL. Putting teeth in CHIP: 1997-2009 retrospective of congressional action on children's oral health. Acad Pediatr 2009;9(6):467–75.

30. Henry J. Kaiser Family Foundation. State Health Facts: CHIP Program Name and Type. Available at: https://www.kff.org/other/state-indicator/chip-program-name-and-type/?currentTimeframe=0&sortModel=%7B%22colId%22:%22Location%22,%22sort%22:%22asc%22%7D. Accessed January 13, 2018.

31. National Maternal and Child Oral Health Policy Center. CHIP dental coverage: an examination of state oral health benefit changes as a result of CHIPRA. 2011. Available at: file:///C:/Users/ble22/Downloads/CHIP%20Dental%20Coverage_%20An%20Examination%20of%20State%20Benefit%20Changes%20as%20a%20Result%20of%20CHIPRA.pdf. Accessed January 13, 2018.

32. Medicaid and CHIP payment and access commission. About MACPAC. Available at: https://www.macpac.gov/about-macpac/. Accessed January 13, 2018.

33. Children's Dental Health Project. Summary or oral health provisions in the ACA. 2010. Available at: file:///C:/Users/ble22/Downloads/Guide%20for%20Advocates%20&%20Policymakers%20(2010)%20(6).pdf. Accessed January 13, 2018.

34. Children's Dental Health Project. A roadmap for implementation, part i: oral health provisions in health reform. Washington DC: 2011. Available at: file:///C:/Users/ble22/Downloads/A%20Roadmap%20for%20Implementation%20-%20Part%20I_%20Oral%20Health%20Provisions%20in%20Health%20Reform%20(1).pdf. Accessed January 15, 2018.

35. Children's Dental Health Project. A roadmap for implementation, part ii: dental care provisions in health reform. Washington DC: 2011. Available at: https://www.cdhp.org/resources/195-a-roadmap-for-implementation-part-ii-dental-care-provisions-in-health-reform. Accessed January 15, 2018.

36. Booth M, Reusch C, Touschner J. Pediatric dental benefits under the ACA: Issues for state advocates to consider. Washington, DC: Georgetown University Center for Children and Families and the Children's Dental Health Project; 2012. Available at: file:/// C:/Users/ble22/Downloads/Pediatric%20dental%20benefits%20under%20the%20AC A_%20Issues%20for%20state%20advocates%20to%20consider.pdf. Accessed January 13, 2018.

37. Provost C, Hughes P. Medicaid: 35 years of service. Health Care Financ Rev 2000;22(1):141–74.

38. Source: KFF.org Available at: https://www.kff.org/medicaid/state-indicator/total-medicaid-and-chip-child-enrollment/?currentTimeframe=0&sortModel=%7B%22 colId%22:%22Location%22,%22sort%22:%22asc%22%7D. Note: US child population source for both 1997 and 2017 is Census Bureau Available at: https:// www.childstats.gov/americaschildren/tables/pop1.asp.

39. Whitener K, Volk J, Miskell S, et al. Children in the marketplace. Washington, DC: Georgetown University Health Policy Institute Center for Children and Families; 2016. Available at: https://ccf.georgetown.edu/wp-content/uploads/2016/06/ Kids-in-Marketplace-final-6-02.pdf. Accessed January 13, 2018.

40. Vujicic M, Nasseh K. Gap in dental care utilization between medicaid and privately insured children narrows, remains large for adults. Chicago (IL): American Dental Association Health Policy Institute; 2016. Available at: http://www.ada.org/ ~/media/ADA/Science%20and%20Research/HPI/Files/HPIBrief_0915_1.pdf? la=en. Accessed January 13, 2018.

41. Shariff J, Edelstein BL. Medicaid meets its equal access requirement for dental care, but oral health disparities remain. Health Aff (Millwood) 2016;35(12): 2259–67.

42. Oral Health and Primary Care Integration. Health Resources and Services Administration. Available at: https://bphc.hrsa.gov/qualityimprovement/clinicalquality/ oralhealth. Accessed January 15, 2018.

43. Health Resources and Services Adminstartion, Bureau of primary care. 2016 Health Center Data, National Data. Available at: https://bphc.hrsa.gov/uds/data-center.aspx?q=tall&year=2016&state=. Accessed January 19, 2018.

44. National Association of Community Health Centers. NACHC's policy update presentation to the national network for oral health access in dallas Texas, 2008 by Craig A. Kennedy MPH. Available at: slideplayer.com/slide/12989251/.

45. School-Based Health Alliance. National School-Based Health Care Census. Available at: http://www.sbh4all.org/school-health-care/national-census-of-school-based-health-centers/. Accessed January 19, 2018.

UNITED STATES POSTAL SERVICE ®

Statement of Ownership, Management, and Circulation
(All Periodicals Publications Except Requester Publications)

1. Publication Title	2. Publication Number	3. Filing Date
PEDIATRIC CLINICS OF NORTH AMERICA	424 – 66	9/18/2018

4. Issue Frequency	5. Number of Issues Published Annually	6. Annual Subscription Price
FEB, APR, JUN, AUG, OCT, DEC	6	$216.00

7. Complete Mailing Address of Known Office of Publication *(Not printer)* *(Street, city, county, state, and ZIP+4®)*

ELSEVIER INC.
230 Park Avenue, Suite 800
New York, NY 10169

Contact Person
STEPHEN R. BUSHING

Telephone *(Include area code)*
215-239-3688

8. Complete Mailing Address of Headquarters or General Business Office of Publisher *(Not printer)*

ELSEVIER INC.
230 Park Avenue, Suite 800
New York, NY 10169

9. Full Names and Complete Mailing Addresses of Publisher, Editor, and Managing Editor *(Do not leave blank)*

Publisher *(Name and complete mailing address)*

TAYLOR E BALL, ELSEVIER INC.
1600 JOHN F KENNEDY BLVD. SUITE 1800
PHILADELPHIA, PA 19103-2899

Editor *(Name and complete mailing address)*

KERRY HOLLAND, ELSEVIER INC.
1600 JOHN F KENNEDY BLVD. SUITE 1800
PHILADELPHIA, PA 19103-2899

Managing Editor *(Name and complete mailing address)*

PATRICK MANLEY, ELSEVIER INC.
1600 JOHN F KENNEDY BLVD. SUITE 1800
PHILADELPHIA, PA 19103-2899

10. Owner *(Do not leave blank. If the publication is owned by a corporation, give the name and address of the corporation immediately followed by the names and addresses of all stockholders owning or holding 1 percent or more of the total amount of stock. If not owned by a corporation, give the names and addresses of the individual owners. If owned by a partnership or other unincorporated firm, give its name and address as well as those of each individual owner. If the publication is published by a nonprofit organization, give its name and address.)*

Full Name	Complete Mailing Address
WHOLLY OWNED SUBSIDIARY OF REED/ELSEVIER, US HOLDINGS	1600 JOHN F KENNEDY BLVD. SUITE 1800 PHILADELPHIA, PA 19103-2899

11. Known Bondholders, Mortgagees, and Other Security Holders Owning or Holding 1 Percent or More of Total Amount of Bonds, Mortgages, or Other Securities. If none, check box   ▶ ☐ None

Full Name	Complete Mailing Address
N/A	

12. Tax Status *(For completion by nonprofit organizations authorized to mail at nonprofit rates)* *(Check one)*
The purpose, function, and nonprofit status of this organization and the exempt status for federal income tax purposes:

☒ Has Not Changed During Preceding 12 Months
☐ Has Changed During Preceding 12 Months *(Publisher must submit explanation of change with this statement)*

PS Form **3526**, July 2014 *(Page 1 of 4 (see instructions page 4))* PSN: 7530-01-000-9931   PRIVACY NOTICE: See our privacy policy on www.usps.com.

---

13. Publication Title			14. Issue Date for Circulation Data Below
PEDIATRIC CLINICS OF NORTH AMERICA			JUNE 2018

15. Extent and Nature of Circulation			Average No. Copies Each Issue During Preceding 12 Months	No. Copies of Single Issue Published Nearest to Filing Date
a. Total Number of Copies *(Net press run)*			549	789
b. Paid Circulation *(By Mail and Outside the Mail)*	(1)	Mailed Outside-County Paid Subscriptions Stated on PS Form 3541 (Include paid distribution above nominal rate, advertiser's proof copies, and exchange copies)	286	370
	(2)	Mailed In-County Paid Subscriptions Stated on PS Form 3541 (Include paid distribution above nominal rate, advertiser's proof copies, and exchange copies)	0	0
	(3)	Paid Distribution Outside the Mails Including Sales Through Dealers and Carriers, Street Vendors, Counter Sales, and Other Paid Distribution Outside USPS®	191	287
	(4)	Paid Distribution by Other Classes of Mail Through the USPS (e.g., First-Class Mail®)	0	0
c. Total Paid Distribution *(Sum of 15b (1), (2), (3), and (4))*		▶	477	657
d. Free or Nominal Rate Distribution *(By Mail and Outside the Mail)*	(1)	Free or Nominal Rate Outside-County Copies included on PS Form 3541	60	114
	(2)	Free or Nominal Rate In-County Copies Included on PS Form 3541	0	0
	(3)	Free or Nominal Rate Copies Mailed at Other Classes Through the USPS (e.g., First-Class Mail)	0	0
	(4)	Free or Nominal Rate Distribution Outside the Mail (Carriers or other means)	0	0
e. Total Free or Nominal Rate Distribution *(Sum of 15d (1), (2), (3) and (4))*		▶	60	114
f. Total Distribution *(Sum of 15c and 15e)*		▶	537	771
g. Copies not Distributed *(See Instructions to Publishers #4 (page #3))*		▶	12	18
h. Total *(Sum of 15f and g)*		▶	549	789
i. Percent Paid *(15c divided by 15f times 100)*		▶	88.83%	85.21%

* If you are claiming electronic copies, go to line 16 on page 3. If you are not claiming electronic copies, skip to line 17 on page 3.

16. Electronic Copy Circulation		Average No. Copies Each Issue During Preceding 12 Months	No. Copies of Single Issue Published Nearest to Filing Date
a. Paid Electronic Copies	▶	0	0
b. Total Paid Print Copies (Line 15c) + Paid Electronic Copies (Line 16a)	▶	477	657
c. Total Print Distribution (Line 15f) + Paid Electronic Copies (Line 16a)	▶	537	771
d. Percent Paid (Both Print & Electronic Copies) (16b divided by 16c × 100)	▶	88.83%	85.21%

☒ I certify that 50% of all my distributed copies (electronic and print) are paid above a nominal price.

17. Publication of Statement of Ownership

☒ If the publication is a general publication, publication of this statement is required. Will be printed   ☐ Publication not required.

in the   OCTOBER 2018   issue of this publication.

18. Signature and Title of Editor, Publisher, Business Manager, or Owner

STEPHEN R. BUSHING - INVENTORY DISTRIBUTION CONTROL MANAGER

(signature)   Date   9/18/2018

I certify that all information furnished on this form is true and complete. I understand that anyone who furnishes false or misleading information on this form or who omits material or information requested on the form may be subject to criminal sanctions (including fines and imprisonment) and/or civil sanctions (including civil penalties).

PS Form **3526**, July 2014 *(Page 3 of 4)*   PRIVACY NOTICE: See our privacy policy on www.usps.com.

Moving?

Make sure your subscription moves with you!

To notify us of your new address, find your **Clinics Account Number** (located on your mailing label above your name), and contact customer service at:

Email: **journalscustomerservice-usa@elsevier.com**

800-654-2452 (subscribers in the U.S. & Canada)
314-447-8871 (subscribers outside of the U.S. & Canada)

Fax number: **314-447-8029**

Elsevier Health Sciences Division
Subscription Customer Service
3251 Riverport Lane
Maryland Heights, MO 63043

*To ensure uninterrupted delivery of your subscription, please notify us at least 4 weeks in advance of move.